PSYCHOLOGY OF SPORTS, EXERCISE, AND FITNESS

PSYCHOLOGY OF SPORTS, EXERCISE, AND FITNESS
Social and Personal Issues

Edited by
Louis Diamant
University of North Carolina at Charlotte

⬤HEMISPHERE PUBLISHING CORPORATION
A member of the Taylor & Francis Group
New York   Philadelphia   Washington   London

PSYCHOLOGY OF SPORTS, EXERCISE, AND FITNESS: Social and Personal Issues

Copyright © 1991 by Hemisphere Publishing Corporation. All rights reserved. Printed in the United States of America. Except as permitted under the United States Copyright Act of 1976, no part of this publication may be reproduced or distributed in any form or by any means, or stored in a database or retrieval system, without the prior written permission of the publisher.

1 2 3 4 5 6 7 8 9 0   E B E B   9 8 7 6 5 4 3 2 1

Photographs courtesy of Wade Bruton.

This book was set in Times Roman by Hemisphere Publishing Corporation. The editors were Andrew N. Bartlett and Debbie Klenotic; the production supervisor was Peggy M. Rote; and the typesetters were Cynthia B. Mynhier and Lori Knoernschild. Cover design by Debra Eubanks Riffe. Printing and binding by Edwards Brothers, Inc.

A CIP catalog record for this book is available from the British Library.

Library of Congress Cataloging-in-Publication Data

Psychology of sports, exercise, and fitness: social and personal issues / edited by Louis Diamant.
   p. cm.
   Includes bibliographical references and index.

   1. Sports—Psychological aspects. 2. Exercise—Psychological aspects. 3. Physical fitness—Psychological aspects. 4. Sports—Social aspects. I. Diamant, Louis.
GV706.4.P695   1991
796.01—dc20
           90-19467
           CIP

ISBN 1-56032-170-9

Contents

Contributors

STEPHEN H. BOUTCHER, Department of Human Movement Sciences, University of Wollongong, New South Wales 2500, Australia.

LES BRINSON, Department of Psychology, North Carolina Central University, Durham, North Carolina 27707.

ARNIE CANN, Department of Psychology, University of North Carolina at Charlotte, Charlotte, North Carolina 28223.

LOUIS DIAMANT, Department of Psychology, University of North Carolina at Charlotte, Charlotte, North Carolina 28223.

BRAD D. HATFIELD, Department of Physical Education, University of Maryland, College Park, Maryland 20742.

PAMELA S. IMM, Medical University of South Carolina, Charleston, South Carolina 29401.

RUTH V. KAPPIUS, Department of Psychology, University of North Carolina at Charlotte, Charlotte, North Carolina 28223.

JO ANN LEE, Department of Psychology, University of North Carolina at Charlotte, Charlotte, North Carolina 28223.

GARY THOMAS LONG, Department of Psychology, University of North Carolina at Charlotte, Charlotte, North Carolina 28223.

ALBERT A. MAISTO, Department of Psychology, University of North Carolina at Charlotte, Charlotte, North Carolina 28223.

MICHAEL L. MASTERSON, Department of Psychology, University of North Carolina at Charlotte, Charlotte, North Carolina 28223.

JEFFREY F. MEYER, Department of Religious Studies, University of North Carolina at Charlotte, Charlotte, North Carolina 28223.

JULIE A. PRUITT, Department of Psychology, University of North Carolina at Charlotte, Charlotte, North Carolina 28223.

ELWOOD L. ROBINSON, Department of Psychology, North Carolina Central University, Durham, North Carolina 27707.

MICHAEL L. SACHS, Department of Physical Education, Temple University, Philadelphia, Pennsylvania 19122.

RONALD B. SIMONO, Department of Psychology, University of North Carolina at Charlotte, Charlotte, North Carolina 28223.

JANET R. STEPHENS, Department of Psychology, University of North Carolina at Charlotte, Charlotte, North Carolina 28223.

LINDA L.WEINHOLD, Behavior Pharmacology Unit, D-5 West Francis Scott Key, Baltimore, Maryland 21224.

Preface

In the preface to another book that could be thought of as a companion-piece for this volume, I supported the need for its publication with a passionate but true picture of the current fervor for sports, exercise, and fitness (SEF). Nothing changes here, although I have avoided repeating words used to depict the universality of involvement with SEF. The same zest for psychological research that brings to bear theoretical acumen and its application to empirical investigation may be seen in *Psychology of Sports, Exercise, and Fitness: Social and Personal Issues*.

The social psychology of sports and the problems of personal adjustment and mental health are herein encountered with the same regard for the innovative approach, the same respect for the theoretical framework, and the same value for and emphasis on research. The ensuing chapters will explore relationships between the most important areas in SEF and the human psychological condition.

Contributing authors are from a number of psychological specialties: sports psychopharmacology, clinical, industrial, social, developmental, sports medicine, exercise, physiology, physical education, and philosophy. The variety of areas and disciplines provides an eclectic balance of professional, academic, and theoretical backgrounds. The book will be an invaluable source of information and reference for readers whose academic and professional interests include sports psychology, physical education, the social psychology or sociology of sports, exercise, and fitness, developmental psychology, health and fitness education, and sports medicine. The material presented in *Psychology of*

Sports, Exercise, and Fitness: Social and Personal Issues is suitable for advanced undergraduate and graduate students, the professional who likes to keep up with things, and the general reader who is serious about this topic.

The book is divided into three sections, but still is holistic in concept. The section to which a chapter has been assigned does not imply a discrete division from another but rather designates the emphasis given it by the material's editor and author.

Part I, *Introduction,* familiarizes the reader with some of the theoretical bases for doing SEF position papers and empirical research. It provides the reader with ways in which theory and research may be used in the attempt to relate SEF activities to mental states, moods, emotions, and behaviors and, from a social psychological view, how societal variables relate to SEF.

The chapters in Part II examine the elaborate on the intricate interactions of sports, exercise, and fitness with mental health and adjustive processes. A variety of subjects bear the scrutiny of the authors. The relationships of sports, exercise, and fitness to moods, anxiety, physical illness, and eating disorders are among the topics covered. Part III, *Society and the Individual Performer,* basically considers the ways that social variables affect individuals where sports perspective, exercise, and fitness are involved. The range of topics includes the physical recreation problems of the mentally retarded, the value of sports programs in industrial organizations, running as a psychosocial phenomenon, and psychological perspectives on the Afro-American athlete.

I wish, at this point, to express gratitude to those who have been helpful, kind, tolerant, understanding, and generous during my labors on this project. I thank the friends and colleagues I have met while putting this project together. Their grasp of the psychological aspects of sports, exercise, and fitness has been a source of professional enrichment. I am grateful, also, to many others whom I have never met—both historical and contemporary figures—whose names and works enhance these pages. I extend my appreciation to my colleague and friend, Professor Kim Buch, for astute observations. I am immeasurably indebted to the Department of Athletics at the University of North Carolina at Charlotte, especially to Mark Colone, Coach Jeff Mullins, and Director Judy Rose for creating an ideal atmosphere for me to approach a variety of sports and performers and for sharing a holistic view of athletic performance. Also, my thanks to Winifred Swinson for contributing her great organizational skills in behalf of this book, and to Kathy for her willingness to carry out the many details that seemed too much, and to our children, in whom the epigenesis of mind, body, and maturity through sports, exercise, and fitness provides me with constant affirmation.

Louis Diamant

I

INTRODUCTION

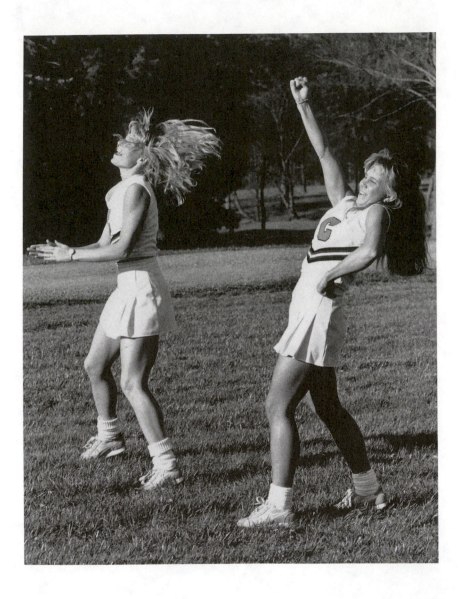

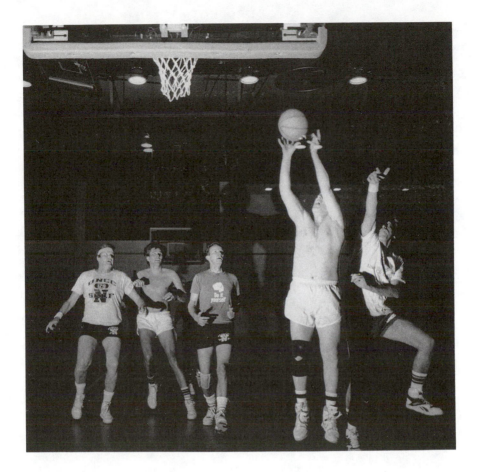

1

THEORY AND RESEARCH IN SPORTS, EXERCISE, AND FITNESS PSYCHOLOGY

Louis Diamant

University of North Carolina at Charlotte

I hope that the reader can tolerate a personal approach, but sitting here, pushed against a printer's deadline, fidgeting and missing my workout, I live the dilemma that psychology, it is hoped, can explain. To wit: within myself an adjustment process apparently inextricably woven to my need to perform aerobically and athletically, as well as to assess my role in this youthful enterprise, while eschewing the more doctrinaire role (at least for my generation) of the constant age-appropriate professional achiever. At once the major themes of this book come into focus—the oddness of myself as an older athletic performer struggling with barbells and demanding to win at squash, and the mental health and mood stability that I have related to my exercise. One might say that these are matters of mind, body, and maturity, a theme continued from the companion volume (Diamant) and herein looked at specifically as the relation between sports, exercise, and fitness as they relate to mental health and adjustment and as social variables affecting the participants at varying levels of performance.

Psychologists employ the tools of science to attempt to explain and understand how societal and adjustive variables affect individual and group behavior and mental states. Sports writers and various wise journalists, including athletes turned writers and exercise–fitness proponents of various stripes and dimensions, including film stars, models, and television personalities, frequently write insightfully, knowledgeably, and interestingly on the topics germane to this book. I have found many of their conjectures helpful and well presented—not to be dismissed. But—and the conjunction is important—ordinarily those writings lack the balance supplied by the rigors of psychological theory and research and the particular intellectual ambience it provides. In making this statement I ask your indulgence again, because I believe that psychological contributions are also made by creative contributors who do not employ the rigorous methods of research psychology, although, by and large, our profession demands, for existence, the scrutiny of human behavior, thoughts, and emotions with acceptable research methods and theoretical frameworks.

Among the nonpsychologists who do not rely on tight scientific discipline but who, in my opinion, have viewpoints that are faithful to psychological thought, George Sheehan comes instantly to mind. At 70 years of age, he is a runner, physician, writer, and, by his own definition, with which I do not disagree, an athlete. His attitude toward sports—particularly his sport of running—has psychological theoretical validity.

Sheehan (1978) espouses a holistic–humanistic view of sports, that, although playing a negligible part in sports, exercise, and fitness (SEF) psychology, nevertheless is represented in the therapeutic work of a considerable number of psychologists. Humanistic psychology deals with personal growth, as an intrinsic addition to conventional psychiatry's "return to functional normality." It is often associated with existential psychology, which elaborates on freedom, personal control, and self-responsibility in whom we become.

Another, Kostrubala (1976), a psychiatrist, bases treatment programs on running, which he supports theoretically by a humanistic position largely enhanced by Jungian psychology in which he sees running as a means of accessing the layers of conscious, unconscious, and collective unconscious to the behavior pattern of our animal and prehuman archetypal inhabitant as postulated by Jung (1953).

In Chapter 8, a philosopher, Jeffrey Meyer, employs an oriental psychology that relates to the physical expression of "oriental fixity, harmony, at-oneness with the body and locality, being at home with the world." Although hardly a set of postulates from which to design an experiment in Western psychology of sports, it nevertheless provides an interesting theoretical framework from which to view a physical approach to mental health, in contrast to the current Western tradition of pushing muscular and aerobic limits.

Even though existential and humanistic postulates appear, by the direction of current SEF research design, to play a small role in the empirical and quantifiable "hard" research that these areas still can provide a theoretical framework for this type of design. For example, the issue of control is deeply embedded in existential thought—namely, that human beings control their own behavior (in variance) with certain psychoanalytic and behavioral postulates that may be seen as explaining human behavior or unconscious drives or environmental manipulations. A measurement of an individual's perception of this control has been developed by the psychologist Jules Rotter (1966) and deals with the concept of "locus of control," the individual differences in expectancies and outcomes. "Internals" believe that their own behavior controls consequences;

"externals" feel that external events, rather than their own behavior, decide what happens to them. The connection, then, between locus of control and the existential position can be seen in acceptance of an internal locus of control. From an SEF framework, having a stronger internal locus of control has been associated with (a) greater knowledge of one's health, (b) positive attitudes about physical exercise, and (c) lower levels of smoking (McAdams, 1990).

One of the small number of studies dealing with psychoanalytic theory and sports and exercise is an empirical study with weight lifters as the experimental subjects. Using a psychosexual framework, Harlow (1951) hypothesized that male weight lifters develop strength to compensate for unconscious femininity and homosexuality. Harlow compared two groups of athletes, with those in the experimental group discriminated by their expressed enthusiastic interest in weight training. Because sexual identity is a major theme in psychoanalytic theory, personality tests that are responsive to these themes were used. The results were based on a comparison of scores between the control and experimental groups. Harlow concluded that those men who were enthusiastic about weight lifting were characterized by abnormally acute feelings of masculine inadequacy, exposure from early in life to a depriving and frustrating environment, failure to have adequate male object identification, and extreme narcissism and dependence. Is anyone blushing? No need to. That was 40 years ago, before there was a fitness center with free weights on every corner and before virtually every athlete in every sport was pushed to weight training by their coaches.

However, I must say with some chagrin that Peterson (1988), writing more recently on psychodynamic personality, captioned a photograph of male body-builders thus: "Fixation at the phallic stage may result in exaggerated masculinity" (p. 165). No empirical evidence supported his comment. Writing in *New York Magazine,* Pooley (1990) described a convicted criminal and suspected murderer who was also a bodybuilder as "a muscle-bound, coke-and-steroid freak" (p. 28)—obviously a stereotypical label. The study of stereotyping and labeling plays an important role in social psychology (e.g., Bodenhausen & Wyer, 1985; Long & Sultan, 1987) and in SEF (Chapter 12). Chapter 11 empirically examines the perceptions of muscular bodies as a social psychological phenomenon rather than a theoretical interpretation of bodybuilders' personalities.

By and large, SEF psychology has been more attuned to examining observations from more succinct postulates than those involving psychodynamic theories (a whole range of Freudian and neo-Freudian concepts) and existential–humanistic framework (encompassing ideas of the self as postulated by theorists like Carl Rogers [1961] and Abraham Maslow [1987]), although the motivational views of Maslow are often mentioned by psychologically oriented sports psychologists.

Maslow shared Rogers's belief that human beings are propelled by a striving for self-actualization. The notion that self-enhancement and personal growth may be related to athletes and physical behavior laces the SEF literature. However "at the same time the relatively general notions espoused by Freud, his followers and others including Maslow are being discarded in favor of ideas that can be more precisely evaluated and measured" (Cratty, 1989, p. 41).

In the preceding paragraphs I introduced the psychological theories that play a role in the analysis of observations of events but do not provide the basis for a lot of the hard, or quantified, research that has become, in most respects, the bedrock of contemporary psychology. As you will see in the ensuing chapters, all that is psychology cannot exist without these evaluative and measurement processes. The articles and research studies on SEF, which could be practically counted on the fingers just a couple of decades ago, now number in the thousands and are held together by the glue of theories, hypotheses, data collections, and statistical inference. In the main, theoretical distribution lies within the psychodynamic (including psychoanalytic), radical behavioral, cognitive behavioral, humanist–existential, psychobiological, and tract domains. Some, more than others, as Cratty (1989) has implied, lend themselves to research that deals with the social psychological and adjustive aspects of SEF.

Many contemporary position papers in social and adjustive psychology have a basis in empirical investigation. For example, in Chapter 15 Maisto and Stephens write on the need for the handicapped (specifically the mentally retarded) individual to have access to physical recreation. Historically, quantifiable data support the positive psychological benefits of such programs. In one of the scarce early studies, Oliver (1958) reported on the physical conditioning and exercise effects on subnormal intellectual adolescents, average IQ 70. He indicated gains in mental and athletic ability. More recently, Tomporowski and Jameson (1985) implied that a motivational characteristic of exercise can lead to skill acquisition in severely mentally retarded adults. And Gleser (1986), following a host of studies on disability since Oliver's research, confirmed the ego-strengthening effects of physical conditioning by reporting that visually handicapped children, many with neurological and psychiatric disorders, found a greater sense of well-being, self-esteem, and social identity through modified judo practice and a motivational framework.

The concept of fitness and exercise or conditioning as behavior that will enhance occupational motivation has worked its way onto the corporate as well as the educational and clinical agenda, with an estimated 50,000 U.S. business firms promoting physical activity. A recent report by the National Chamber Foundation—the research branch of the U.S. Chamber of Commerce—found that family income and physical conditioning were the only reliable factors in predicting employee absenteeism (National Chamber Foundation, 1989). Falkenberg (1987) reviewed a considerable number of the studies examining relations between sports, exercise, and physical fitness and personal and occupational mental states. The studies were mainly concerned with the reduction of mental stress and improvement of employee production. Although Falkenberg's review indicated some division of findings regarding the benefit to employers by the programs in terms of increased production, it was pointed out that long-term participation in physical exercise resulted in individuals showing improved emotional stability, increased personal security, and reduced levels of anxiety and depression. Most important have been her suggestions for relating fitness to psychology, with recommendations for more effective experimentation and research. Because sports participation and spectator involvement are important areas for psychological research, and corporate behavior attempts to control or influence workers' attitudes (e.g., loyalty and job satisfaction) and thus improve performance, an important area of investigation appears to be the value of sports programs in the corporate society. Unfortunately, one finds even less research in this area, and thus I applaud Lee's incursion (Chapter 9) into the organizational use of sports and teams and the psychological concomitants of this use of sports.

An important pursuit for sports psychologists is that of helping athletes anticipate and deal with impeding emotional and mood states created by highly competitive situations, whereas clinical personnel have depended on the tools of sports and exercise to deal with emotional and mood states that originate off the field of competition. In the study of such processes and the application of remedial measures, researchers and practitioners have relied heavily on the scientific delineation of personality traits and the concomitant development of scales to make the necessary individual measurements. Trait theory (Allport, 1961; Cattell, 1970) has been a bedrock upon which such endeavors are built, and psychological measurements (e.g., Cattell, Eber, & Tatsuoka, 1970; McNair, Lorr, & Droppleman, 1971; Martens, 1977; Spielberger, Gorsuch, & Lushene, 1971) are the instruments of construction. Aided also by the precision of exercise physiology, researchers are able to postulate on the promotive (and sometimes deleterious) effects of aerobic exercise behavior, and examine relations to the psychology of emotions, anxiety, and moods. These may serve as examples of the psychobiological (biomedical) or theoretical approach to SEF with a value supported by the fecundity of research.

It is not the intent of this chapter to review the content of the book. The chapters must be read, and their coverage of the social and adjustive processes in SEF will be accessible by their own construction. At the risk of redundancy, this chapter has provided an introduction, a brief guide into the arena where the psychologists do their thing, garnering from myriad observations those consistencies that create hypotheses that support (or undermine) theoretical notions and, further, putting these data to the test that will provide the informational wherewithal to predict behavior and change behavior when it is productive to do so. At the time I was concluding this chapter, I serendipitously thumbed to an article by the neurologist Bruce Dobkin in the *New York Times Magazine*

(Dobkin, 1989) in the regularly featured "Mind and Body." He was writing on the newly classified medical disorder "chronic fatigue syndrome." People with this disorder often have symptoms much like those in clinical depression, and because of its relation to our concerns in this book I noted with some appreciation his concluding sentences. "It's worth," said Dobkin about the etiologically elusive chronic fatigue syndrome, "leaping past the notions of cause and playing the card of physical reconditioning" (p. 37). He opined that the answer for many may involve a closely supervised program of gradually progressive exercise. "Where every thought and movement comes to mean one more possible hurdle [Dobkin was a collegiate hurdler] perhaps the deconditioned victim will finish the race only if heart, will and legs get back in shape" (p. 39). Read on, and you will find chapters that elucidate the relation between psychological methods and SEF and positions such as Dobkin's.

REFERENCES

Allport, G. (1961). *Pattern and growth in personality.* New York: Holt.

Bodenhausen, G. V., & Wyer, R. S. (1985). Effects of stereotypes of decision making and information processing strategies. *Journal of Personality and Social Psychology, 42,* 1042–1050.

Cattell, R. B. (1970). *The scientific analysis of personality.* Baltimore: Penguin.

Cattell, R. B., Eber, H. W., & Tatsuoka, M. M. (1970). *Handbook for the Sixteen Personality Factor Questionnaire (16 PF).* Champaign, IL: Institute for Personality Testing and Ability Testing.

Cratty, J. B. (1989). *Psychology in contemporary sport.* Englewood Cliffs, NJ: Prentice Hall.

Dobkin, B. (1989, July 16). ILL, or just the blahs? *New York Times Magazine,* pp. 36–37.

Falkenberg, L. E. (1987). Employee fitness programs: Their impact on the employee and the organization. *Academy of Management Review, 13*(3), 611–622.

Gleser, J. M. (1986). Modified judo for visually handicapped people. *Journal of Visual Impairment and Blindness, 80*(3), 749–750.

Harlow, R. G. (1951). Masculine inadequacy and compensatory development of physique. *Journal of Personality, 19,* 312–323.

Jung, C. G. (1953). *Two essays on analytical psychology.* New York: Pantheon.

Kostrubala, T. (1976). *The joy of running.* Philadelphia: Lippincott.

Long, G. T., & Sultan, F. E. (1987). Contribution from social psychology. In L. Diamant (Ed.), *Male and female homosexuality: Psychological approaches* (pp. 221–236). Washington, DC: Hemisphere.

Martens, R. (1977). *Sport Competition Anxiety Test.* Champaign, IL: Human Kinetics.

Maslow, A. (1987). *Motivation and personality* (3rd ed.). New York: Harper & Row.

McAdams, D. B. (1990). *The person: An introduction to personality psychology.* New York: Harcourt, Brace, Jovanovich.

McNair, D. M., Lorr, H., & Droppleman, L. F. (1971). *Profile of Mood States manual.* San Diego: Educational and Industrial Testing Service.

National Chamber Foundation. (1989). Determinants of employee absenteeism. Washington, DC: U.S. Chamber of Commerce.

Oliver, J. M. (1958). The effect of physical conditioning activity on the mental characteristics of sub-normal boys. *Journal of Educational Psychology, 28,* 155–168.

Petersen, C. (1988). *Personality.* New York: Harcourt Brace Javanovich.

Pooley, E. (1990, January 29). Death of a hood. *New York Magazine,* pp. 26–33.

Rogers, C. R. (1961). *On becoming a person: A therapist's view of psychotherapy.* Boston: Houghton Mifflin.

Rotter, J. B. (1966). Generalized expectancies for internal versus external control of reinforcement. *Psychological Monographs, 80*(1, Whole No. 609).

Sheehan, G. (1978). *Running and being: The total experience.* New York: Simon and Schuster.

Spielberger, C. D., Gorsuch, R. L., & Lishene, R. F. (1971). *Manual for the State–Trait Anxiety Inventory.* Palo Alto, CA: Consulting Psychologists Press.

Tomporowski, P. D., & Jameson, L. D. (1985). Effects of a physical fitness training program on the exercise behavior of institutionalized mentally retarded adults. *Adapted Physical Fitness Training Quarterly, 2*(3), 197–205.

II

MENTAL HEALTH AND ADJUSTMENT

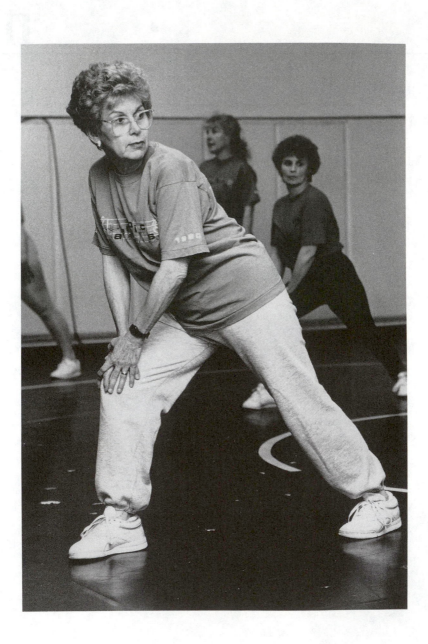

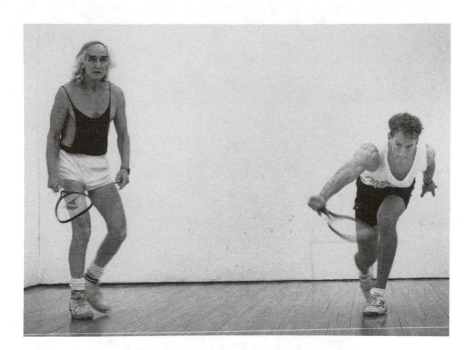

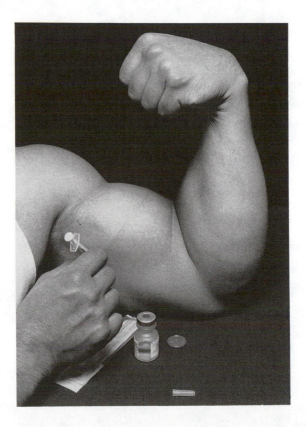

2

EXERCISE AND MENTAL HEALTH: THE MECHANISMS OF EXERCISE-INDUCED PSYCHOLOGICAL STATES

Brad D. Hatfield

University of Maryland, College Park

Anxiety and depression are significant health concerns that affect the lives of a significant number of Americans. In fact, some time ago, Morgan (1979b) indicated that approximately 10 million Americans' daily lives suffer from the effects of stress and that as many as 30–70% of the patients examined by medical practitioners are significantly affected by affective disorders. Of course a number of psychotherapeutic techniques exist to help alleviate stress, anxiety, and depressive disorders, but many individuals have found that physical exercise makes a real contribution to their psychological well-being, helps them to "clear their heads" of cognitive overload, and increases their sense of self-esteem. In fact, some individuals develop exercise habits as an integral part of their life-style because of the psychological reinforcement. Importantly, significant health benefits accrue from participation, too, such as a more desirable body composition, posture, cardiovascular health, and overall physical appearance. As such, there are a number of reasons why some individuals continue exercising for a significant portion of their lives, but the post-exercise affective state or "feel better" phenomenon appears to be a primary one.

The purpose of this chapter is to attempt to explain this "feel better" phenomenon by proposing a number of speculative mechanisms that are neurophysiological, endocrinological, and psychological in nature. As such, I envi-

I wish to express appreciation to Ms. Barbara Foster and Mrs. Lynne Tinsman for their technical assistance in preparing this review. This work was partially supported by research grants of the Department of Health and Human Resources (USA).

sion a number of simultaneously acting phenomena that contribute to a Gestalt or total sense of psychological state. It is naive to assume that any one mechanism (e.g., the popular endorphin hypothesis) could account for these experiential states. The body and mind, with all of their diverse metabolic and physiological functions, are affected by an exercise stimulus. This results in a changes state (i.e., a departure from homeostasis) and a continuous input to the central nervous system (CNS). In addition, and most important, the human brain is characterized by a very malleable phenomenon termed perception or interpretation of the environment and its actions. As such, it continuously evaluates the meaning of its (i.e., the individual's) actions. This is why engagement in the same level of intensity and duration of exercise may result in a variant psychological state and an invariant physiological state characterized by a predictable lactate accumulation, ventilatory effort, heart rate, and so forth. In fact, it seems quite remarkable to me that in spite of the plasticity of the human brain we see such a universal consensus on a subscription to the "feel better" phenomenon. Perhaps, too, it is not that exercise participation is the atypical lifestyle that rewards its "abnormal" participants with great health benefits for their labors. Rather, it may be that the millions of sedentary Americans (i.e., the majority of the population) are living an abnormal life in light of our evolutionary history (i.e., one that has been characterized by movement) and perhaps what we consider normal health profiles in our population are actually substandard compared with the level at which we would be if our culture was less sedentary.

At any rate, I do not propose that exercise is a panacea for our ills. Exercise is a stressor, an ergogenic stress that results in psychological and physiological responses (i.e., acute effects) and adaptations (i.e., chronic effects) that may provide health benefits. This stimulus is characterized by modality (e.g., running, cycling, and rowing) intensity and duration. In terms of modality we could broadly conceive of different activities falling into an aerobic versus resistive (i.e., weight training) domain. The health benefits received from engagement in exercise are largely dependent on the individual and his or her genetic makeup and level of training. In other words, one person's medicine may be another's poison.

Exercise has the capability to promote problems as well as benefits if the stress goes beyond the adaptive capacity of the body. For example, we see such problems as chondromalacia patellae or a softening and shedding of the cartilage on the articular aspect of the kneecap. This is a painful condition that may manifest itself as a difficulty with walking. Arthritis may occur in some joints. If serious congenital heart conditions are present, exercise participation can conceivably result in death (e.g., the case of Jim Fixx).

If consumed in appropriate and individually determined doses, we know that exercise can promote very beneficial effects. In terms of the positive psychological effects, however, it is interesting that the impetus for much of the research involving the psychological effects of acute exercise stemmed from the early reports of Pitts and McClure (1967), who advanced the notion that anxiety states in neurotic and normal subjects could arise from increased blood lactate levels. This hypothesis, which became institutionalized in some medical circles (Morgan, 1979b), held serious implications for the mental health aspects of exercise in light of the significant levels of lactate production resulting from moderate to heavy levels of intensity. Although an early report (Morgan, Roberts, & Feinerman, 1971) did not support a rise in anxiety following exercise, the results were based on relatively mild exercise stressors. Up to this point very little work had been conducted on the psychological effects of acute exercise involvement. Most reports dealt with the personalities of athletes; exercise psychology was undeveloped as an area of study and no firm refutation existed for the Pitts–McClure notion. Could it be that exercise promoted a stressed, nonrelaxed state? A more definitive test of the Pitts–McClure hypothesis required measurement of state anxiety in subjects high in trait anxiety as a consequence of high-intensity, lactate-producing exercise stimuli. Morgan (1973) provided such a test with a series of programmatic efforts that consistently refuted the Pitts–McClure hypothesis and in so doing helped to develop this area of research.

In one study (Gillett, Morgan, & Balke, 1972, as cited in Morgan, 1973) 40 males completed the State–Trait Anxiety Inventory (STAI-1) before, immediately after, and 20–30 min after a vigorous 45-min treadmill run. Anxiety showed a slight elevation immediately after the run, compared with baseline, but a significant reduction was noted 20 min later. This pattern of decline was similarly experienced by the high- and low-trait-anxiety subjects, and the latter point holds particular importance in light of the Pitts–McClure hypothesis.

In another of these investigations Morgan and Nagle (1972) (cited in Morgan, 1973) compared terminal lactate levels and STAI-1 responses in 6 anxiety neurotic males and an equal number of normal subjects assigned to a graded maximal exercise test. Although terminal lactate levels increased in the high- and low-anxiety subjects from rest (12 mg/100 ml) to maximal exertion (95–100 mg/100 ml), this increase was not associated with any reported anxiety attacks. Finally, using a different psychometric scale, Morgan and Balke (1972) (cited in Morgan, 1973) administered the Profile of Mood States (POMS) to 16 adult males before and after an exercise stress test and again a significant decline in tension was observed. Although Morgan's (1973) summary of the work contained consistent evidence and arguments to support the tension reduction effect of exercise, the evidence provided was severely limited by the lack of any control groups to eliminate response bias from demand characteristics and testing reactivity.

However, in addition to the empirical evidence, Morgan (1973) summarized an earlier report (Grosz & Farmer, 1969) that elucidated the lack of ecological validity for the Pitts–McClure hypothesis. The original experiments by Pitts

and McClure (1967) employed injections of buffered sodium lactate to experimentally induce anxiety attacks. But, unlike the endogenous metabolic acidosis
that arises from active muscular exertion, exogenous injections elicit an entirely
different response. Grosz and Farmer found the introduction of sodium lactate
to evoke a state of metabolic alkalosis, and consequent adaptive hypoventila-
tion, which appeared to be engaged to achieve a state of compensatory respiratory acidosis. Apparently, this ventilatory maneuver, and the resultant discomfort from the metabolic disturbance, can result in a negative affective state. This
mechanistic evidence further weakened the role of exercise-induced lactate levels in the etiology of high anxiety states beyond the simple outcome findings
provided by Morgan and his colleagues.

Morgan's (1973) articulation of psychological underpinnings and their relation to psychological states represents an important development. I believe we
must attempt to understand why these cognitive/affective states occur in order
to fully appreciate and predict the phenomenon. Attention to processes rather
than outcomes only will result in greater relief of our ignorance. In essence,
what are the dynamics behind the "feel better" phenomenon?

It is speculative at this time to propose such mechanisms, but a number of
hypothetical models do exist that are grounded in empirical scientific investigations. Some of the building blocks (i.e., scientific reports and theories) used to
construct these models are not directly related to exercise science, but a creative
perspective can appreicate their relevance. The present chapter cannot exhaust
all of the possible mediating mechanisms of exercise-induced psychological
states. Such a thesis would require volumes. In addition, although the present
work is biased toward neurophysiological and physiological mechanisms of
affect, I am in no way insensitive to the paramount role that perception and
cognition play in producing the final outcome.

Finally, this speculative model-building approach provides a conceptual,
methodological, and technological challenge for the research community, but
only by testing such hypotheses in an a priori manner can we advance our
understanding. Even the rejection of testable hypotheses (when well conceived)
is informative!

MECHANISMS OF CHANGE UNDERLYING
THE ACUTE RESPONSE TO EXERCISE

The outcomes associated with acute exercise involvement have been attributed
to a number of mechanisms. For example, Greist et al. (1978, 1979) have
advanced the notion of mastery feelings or the sense of accomplishment that
comes with the successful completion of an exercise workload. Such an explanation rests on a cognitive basis. Others have discussed neurophysiological
models of affective change (deVries, 1968). But, again, reliance on any singu-

lar mechanism to explain the observed consequences appears limited. Such outcomes are probably determined by a number of factors acting and interacting concurrently, temporally overlapping, and acting in series. As such, the resultant mood states may be explained by a number of simultaneous causal agents.

The Hyperthermic Model

One explanation of affective change is a neurophysiological model developed from an early report by Von Euler and Soderberg (1957) that shall be referred to as the hyperthermic model. In essence, this model incorporates the view of the somatopsychic perspective (i.e., the body affects the brain) as well as that of the psychosomatic (i.e., that the brain affects the body), but the dominant influence is the former. The primary stimulus promoting affective change is the elevation in body temperature from the exercise and this alteration in physiological state is manifested in a number of responses that are orchestrated by the hypothalamus. The hypothalamus is a brainstem structure located caudal to the thalamus at the highest level of the brainstem. We know that it assumes a number of homeostatic regulatory roles such as the control of thirst, hunger, and temperature. Typically, exercise scientists focus on the alterations in core temperature and shifts in blood flow to the periphery of the vasculature in order to promote cooling. However, Von Euler and Soderberg (1957) conducted an interesting study involving the passive heating of laboratory rabbits that focused on the CNS's response to hyperthermia; their work holds some very interesting implications for exercise psychology.

In essence, the hyperthermic state is sensed by the hypothalamus, which promotes a number of physical responses that result in temperature control (e.g., peripheral vasodilation), but importantly, there is also an effect on the *brain*. This effect is mediated by the hypothalamic influence on the thalamus, which is believed to serve as the pacemaker for electrocortical activity or the electroencephalographic (EEG) activity of the forebrain cortex. The thalamic generator, when in this hyperthermic state, promotes synchronous firing of the neurons, which results in a predominant slow-wave, high-amplitude EEG profile termed alpha (8–12 Hz) activity. Typically alpha activity is the frequency band of the EEG spectrum that is indicative of a relaxed but alert mental state. Interestingly, this "relaxed" state then affects the peripheral musculature by reducing the volley of neural stimulation from the motor cortex of the brain to the muscles by way of the corticospinal tracts. This reduced "traffic" to the musculature is manifested as a reduction in (a) alpha motoneuron stimulation to the extrafusal fibers or cells of the skeletal muscles and (b) gamma motoneurons, which innervate the intrafusal fibers of the muscle spindles. This latter effect would result in a depression of the tension-producing myotatic stretch reflex. This all adds up to a more relaxed peripheral musculature or sense of physical calm.

In both animals and humans this state would also result in a reduction of sensory or afferent stimuli back to the brainstem reticular formation as well as the somatosensory area of the cortex. The reduction in muscle tension and the associated afferent "traffic" may further promote the feeling of arousal reduction or psychological relaxation. Such a notion is consistent with the practice of other techniques such as progressive muscle relaxation (Jacobson, 1938).

During exercise, the physical demands placed on the muscles would seem to negate the reduction in peripheral afference (although more will be mentioned about the indirect psychological effect of the contracting muscles later), but if our focus remains on the postexercise state then it is important to note that the hyperthermic state or temperature elevation (i.e., the initiating stimulus) remains for some time beyond the termination of the exercise stimulus (depending on the intensity and duration of the workload) when the body is usually in a passive, rested state.

Our bodies are not very efficient work-producing machines: The efficiency of the ratio of energy to force production by the muscles lies in the area of 15–20%. The majority of metabolic processes result in a heat load on the body, but it is this very inefficient state that may well provide one of several paths leading to a state of positive affect.

DeVries (1968) reasoned that exercise-induced hyperthermia could promote the same effect in humans that Von Euler and Soderberg (1957) had observed with passively heated rabbits in the laboratory 20 years earlier and that the perception of change in peripheral tension would contribute to a reduced state of psychological/emotional arousal along the lines of Jacobsonian (1938) principles.

Peripheral Evidence for the Hyperthermic Model

Accordingly, deVries recorded integrated electromyographic (EMG) activity from bipolar placements on the right biceps brachii and quadriceps femoris before and after rest and exercise (i.e., 5 min of bench stepping at a cadence of 30 steps/min). The surface EMG measure used by deVries (1968) represents a rather direct attempt to test the hyperthermic model because EMG activity is a measure of neural input to the muscle tissue and therefore would capture changes in both alpha and gamma motoneuron input. College students (17 males and 12 females ages 19–39) served as their own controls in a repeated-measures design. Pretreatment values of $1.09 + 2.05 \ \mu V$ and $0.64 + 0.87 \ \mu V$ were obtained from the biceps before the exercise and resting control condition, respectively. Compared with pretreatment values, acute exercise promoted a 58% decline in biceps EMG whereas supine rest was associated with a nonsignificant decrease of 1.5%. The quadriceps muscle group showed a similar response but failed to attain statistical significance. DeVries emphasized that the reduced tension was not merely reflective of physical tiredness because EMG increases, rather than decreases, are associated with muscular fatigue. In addition, these findings represented a rather conservative estimate of exercise-induced effects, because the EMG recordings were obtained 1 hr after exercise to minimize electrocardiographic (ECG) artifact, and the young subjects evidenced minimal pretreatment levels of EMG activity at the outset. In other words, little room for improvement would be expected and any significant reductions would have been achieved only with some degree of difficulty. DeVries interpreted the results as supportive of a "tranquilizer" effect.

Unfortunately, no attempt was made to monitor core temperature alteration or the intensity of the exercise. As such, the subjects were probably working at variable levels of effort depending on their aerobic and anaerobic capacities. This lack of control over workloads obviated examination of the intensity/response relation. Nevertheless, the data did reveal evidence for a greater EMG reduction following exercise than rest.[1]

However, as is the case in several other reports, no concurrent psychometric data were obtained along with the psychophysiological measures. Therefore assumptions were made that the EMG was associated with psychological change.

DeVries and Adams (1972) extended this work by contrasting the anxiolytic effects of mild to moderate exercise stress (15 min of steady treadmill walking at heart rate intensities of 100 and 120 bpm) to those of a pharmacological agent (400 mg of meprobamate). Because of the negative side effects associated with such tranquilizing drugs, deVries and Adams believed that a drug-free tranquilizer like exercise would be of considerable benefit to older individuals. Accordingly, 10 elderly subjects (ages 52–70), who evidenced a number of symptoms of chronic anxiety, experienced each of the following conditions: (a) exercise at an intensity of 100 and 120 bpm, (b) meprobamate, (c) a placebo control condition to determine any psychological effects of drug therapy, and (d) a 15-min reading or "standard" control period. Left biceps EMG was compared before and after each treatment. Posttreatment EMG measures were obtained at 30 min, 1 hr, and 1.5 hr after each condition. Subjects were randomly assigned to treatments after baseline assessments in an attempt to control any anticipatory increases in arousal.

Because of small differences noted in baseline EMG prior to the treatments, which were examined on separate days, deVries and Adams employed analysis

[1]Preexercise EMG was somewhat elevated in deVries's (1968) prior study, and therefore the earlier results may have been biased unfairly toward an apparent exercise-induced effect. In that study the subjects knew which treatment they would experience after baseline and it is plausible that they were somewhat keyed up prior to the exercise condition. Such an elevation of tension could have provided more room for change and the resultant decline of EMG could have been caused, alternatively, simply by habituation to the "threatening" testing environment.

of covariance (ANCOVA) "to rule out the effect of even the small non-significant pre-score differences" (1972, p. 135).

Significant reductions in EMG (i.e., 20%, 23%, and 20%), were noted for all three measurement periods after walking at an intensity of 100 bpm. These declines were significantly lower than the values measured after the standard control condition. Notable reductions were also observed after exercise at 120 bpm, but they were not significant. Importantly, the levels of EMG alteration subsequent to drug intervention and placebo control were not differentiated from the standard reading control. Thus physical exercise seemed to promote a superior anxiolytic effect, and again the hyperthermic model was partially supported by the EMG changes, which were indicative of a decrement in motoneuron excitability.

Although one of the major contributions of this study to the literature was its methodological rigor and the comparison of exercise to alterative "tranquilizing" conditions, concurrent measures of self-reported mood again were not obtained from the subjects.[2]

Although the initial studies by deVries (1968) and deVries and Adams (1972) were consistent with the hyperthermic position, there was some concern regarding the muscle site chosen for EMG assessment. A number of studies in the biofeedback literature typically employed the frontalis as the area most sensitive to generalized tension. However, deVries (1968) discussed prior evidence to support the employment of the biceps brachii and argued against the use of the frontalis. This concern was also supported by conflicting results from several studies. For example, some investigations revealed no effect on the frontalis subsequent to graded (Balog, 1983) and steady-state (Farmer et al., 1978) submaximal cycle ergometry, whereas others (Russell, Epstein, & Erickson, 1983; Sime, 1977) reported a decline following mild-intensity walking and running. The explanation for this discrepancy was not apparent from the reports.

Therefore, the EMG evidence to support the hyperthermic model was inconclusive. Perhaps this kind of contradictory evidence is not surprising when one considers the use of single muscle sites and the different signal-processing strategies (i.e., wave form analysis) employed in the different studies. Perhaps future studies would be more definitive if multiple sites were employed. To date, only deVries (1968) has incorporated such a strategy and that attempt was limited to only two such locations.

According to the key muscle hypothesis, forehead measures do not provide any unique information about the state of the general bodily musculature. Rather, forehead EMG measures are primarily responsive to alteration in the activity of the head and neck muscles (Graham et al., 1986).

---

[2]The use of the resting control condition strengthened this conclusion because it provided an attempt to assess the level of activity change that could occur simply with the passage of time or by gaining familiarity with the experimental environment.

To overcome this concern, deVries, Wiswell, Bulbulian, and Moritani (1981) employed an alternate measure of spinal motor neuron excitability, the H/M ratio, derived from evocation of the Hoffmann reflex, as a more general index of anterior motor horn activation. The method of Angel and Hofmann was used, which quantifies muscle action potentials (MAPs) of the calf muscles in response to a single shock to the human tibial nerve. The first spike is that of the stimulus artifact (voltage) and the first MAP is referred to as the M-wave, which results from direct stimulation of motor nerve fibers. The second MAP, the H-wave, is the result of a monosynaptic reflex, which is propagated in afferents from the muscle and back again through efferents to the same muscle. The relative size of the second MAP provided a measure of motoneuron excitability. Accordingly, deVries et al. used a mild exercise stress consisting of 20 min of cycle ergometry at an intensity of 40% heart rate range. Subjects served as their own controls and underwent three separate exercise sessions. Such repeated testing attempted to address the degree of psychophysiological change that can occur simply as a function of situational habituation (Levi, 1972). Equivalent nonexercise control periods consisted of three 20-min sessions during which the subjects simply sat and read. Across all exercise sessions the subjects consistently reduced the magnitude of the ratio by an average of 18.2% from baseline while a slight elevation (i.e., 1.2%) was noted after control. Additional support was thus generated for the hyperthermic model because this finding provided further support for the reduction of generalized alpha motoneuronal excitability, an important component of Von Euler and Soderberg's (1957) model.

A subsequent report (deVries, Simard, Wiswell, Heckathorne, & Carabetta, 1982) also noted a reduction in spinal reflex activation, but failed to demonstrate any inhibition of the gamma motor system. As such, the empirical evidence from this work provides only partial support for the reduction in motor system excitability.

DeVries's studies would have provided a more convincing test of the hyperthermic model if concurrent measures of brain and core temperature had been obtained. However, it is safe to assume that some degree of hyperthermia was present.

Central Evidence for the Hyperthermic Model

None of deVries's programmatic efforts addressed the cortical activation aspects of the hyperthermic model. The first report to examine the central response to acute exercise appeared in 1961 (Pineda & Adkisson, 1961); the results revealed a significant alteration of EEG activation in 16 healthy males (ages 22–36) as a function of exhaustive treadmill running. Exercise consisted of a 3.5-mph walk at increasing grade. The individually determined exercise durations ranged from 35 to 70 min. Physiological assessment of cardiopulmonary activity corroborated that a severe workload was negotiated. EEG alpha

(8–13 Hz) was quantified from left and right frontal and occipital bipolar electrode arrangements using a method called the alpha index (Engel, Romano, Ferris, Webb, & Stevens, 1944). Overall elevations from baseline were of the magnitude of 20%, with the greatest changes occurring in the frontal and right hemispheric locations. These alterations, which were sustained for 30–40 minutes postexercise, prompted Pineda and Adkisson to speculate that the increase was due to a reduction of input from the ascending reticular formation to the cerebral cortex. Although not directly assessed, such a reduction may have been due to a decrease of muscular afference to the reticulum. Furthermore, this electrophysiological response was associated behaviorally with a reduction of attention to the environment and a "median state of consciousness [i.e., mental relaxation]" (Pineda & Adkisson, 1961, p. 340).

Unfortunately, there were a number of problems with this preexperimental study, including (a) failure to employ concurrent psychometric measures, (b) no statistical analysis of the data, and (c) no control group. These problems threaten the internal validity of the study so that any causal effect of exercise on the EEG cannot be inferred. However, the use of a psychophysiological assessment both in this study and by deVries is less confounded by measurement reactivity and is less susceptible to demand characteristics than are self-report measures. Therefore, all that can be concluded from this study is that changes in the CNS were *associated* with aerobic exercise of an intense nature and that such change is associated with affective alterations. The conceptual basis offered for this change, and the modest hemispheric effect noted, is consistent with another of the psychophysiological theories to be presented later.

More recent EEG work (Reeves, Justesen, Levinson, Riffle, & Wike, 1985) has directly assessed exercise-induced changes in central or brain temperature while simultaneously examining alterations in arousal and processing efficiency. Accordingly, 10 athletic subjects were contrasted to 10 resting controls in terms of the flash-evoked N1 component, the pattern reversal P100, and event-related P300 of averaged evoked potentials (AEPs) to simple visual stimuli after 20 min of a standardized series of calisthenic exercises that "produced sweating." Tympanically assessed temperature, an index of cortical thermic state, rose 1.2 °C in the experimentals while core temperature rose 3.0 °C. In addition, mean latencies for the appearance of the AEP indices were reduced 3–9%. Simple reaction time was also reduced compared with control values. It would appear from these results that the CNS was able to process simple visual stimuli faster and more efficiently as a result of the modest bout of exercise-induced hyperthermia. The observed rise in core temperature also compares favorably with moderately intense exercise values observed "in the field," thus enhancing the external validity of the study. Although the enhanced processing efficiency of the CNS would seem to imply activation, as opposed to a relaxed cortical tone, theoretical speculation by Surwillo (1975) indicates that enhanced attentional states are associated with increased EEG alpha activity.

An earlier study by Gliner, Matsen-Twisdale, Horvath, and Maron (1979) also examined changes in the AEPs of male runners performing a signal detection task prior to and following a competitive marathon. Although it failed to demonstrate significant change in the neurophysiological index, improved behavioral performance on the signal detection task was shown after the run. Specifically, a reduction of false-positive identifications was observed. The contradictory findings of the two studies may be resolved in light of the prolonged and variable durations regarding the postexercise testing intervals in the Gliner et al. study. Moreover, the relevance of such a competitive exercise stimulus to the kinds of intensities engaged in for psychological stress reduction seems somewhat limited.

The Cardiac Influence Model—
Visceral Afferent Feedback

An additional conceptual basis for changes in central activation (i.e., obtained from EEG spectral analysis and AEPs) is provided by the cardiac cortical influence model (Lacey & Lacey, 1978). In fact, the effects of the cardiovascular system and somatic afferents acting on the CNS (i.e., arising from the muscular and autonomic activity during exercise) seem to complement those of central hyperthermia.

The cardiovascular–CNS interaction espoused by the Laceys (1978) offers a gross model for explaining these changes in psychological state. These theorists advanced the notion of a fractional arousal construct and attempted to explain the afferent effect of the cardiovascular system on the brain during attentionally demanding situations. Accordingly, when subjects directed their attention to the intake of environmental stimuli, an associated bradycardia response was noted. Conversely, tachycardia was observed when attending to internal cognitive elaboration, accompanied by the rejection of distracting environmental stimuli. These cardiovascular concomitants of attention became known as the intake–rejection hypothesis. In opposition to traditional activation theory, which views autonomic activation as a simple effector response (Duffy, 1962), the intake–rejection model implicates the effect of visceral activity on the CNS. The Laceys explained this phenomenon by resorting to basic neurophysiological principles. They advanced the notion that tachycardia response observed during an internally focused environmental rejection task was accompanied by a pressor response that held adaptive significance. The pressor response resulted in baroreceptor activation within the aortic arch and carotid sinus. This baroreceptor activation, by way of the 9th and 10th cranial nerves, then activated the nucleus tractus solitarius in the brainstem (i.e., medullary area), which in turn promoted a homeostatic reduction in cardiovascular activity by way of vagal efference. As long as the individual was engaged in the attentionally demanding task, the pressor response continued while the body simultaneously and reflexively attempted to inhibit it. This was labeled the visceral afferent feedback hypothesis. The Laceys theorized that the central inhibitory effects were not confined to the psychological consequences, but were also manifested throughout the CNS (particularly the cerebral cortex). Although this arousal model was limited to levels of cardiovascular activity observed during resting attentional states, it may hold relevance for the psychological consequences of acute exercise. Accordingly, concomitant increases in blood pressure and cardiovascular activity associated with such workloads may also promote a relaxation or, at least, an alteration of cortical arousal. (Perhaps this explains why some individuals employ some forms of exercise as a means of "clearing their minds.")

Neurophysiological Mechanisms of Visceral Afferent Feedback

Additional neurophysiological evidence provides further elaboration of this model. According to Bonvallet and Bloch's (1961) work with animal preparations, afferent impulses transmitted from the working muscles are eventually received by a number of brainstem collateral neurons, resulting in increased stimulation of the ascending reticular activating system. Contemporary investigators have also discussed the input of muscle afferents to many areas within the brainstem reticular formation (Iwamoto & Kaufman, 1987). During the initiation of exercise this effect may promote mild stimulation, as opposed to a relaxation effect, by way of the cortical excitation from the reticular formation. However, the achieved level of cortical excitation may eventually reach a point at which activation of an inhibitory mechanism occurs in the bulbar region of the brainstem. This inhibitory site may promote an arresting influence on the reticular formation so that the transmission of somatic afferents to the cortex is reduced. As such, cortical excitation may be decreased. This dampening effect lasts substantially beyond the initiating stimulus (e.g., exercise) such that the impact of the excitation promotes a prolonged poststimulus effect (Bonvallet & Bloch, 1961).

Bonvallet and Bloch (1961) also reported that activation of the bulbar mechanism was enhanced upon presentation of rhythmical repetitive stimuli to the brainstem area. Although speculative, it is tempting to note that most of the studies cited earlier employed rhythmical movements such as walking, cycling, or steady-state treadmill running. In fact, common observation supports the notion that stress reduction workouts are usually repetitive and rhythmical in nature. Byrd (1963) provided earlier support for such a view, noting that health professionals endorsed the role of physical activities for stress reduction—particularly rhythmical movements such as walking, swimming, bowling, and so forth. Interestingly, Morgan (1979b) noted that graded exercise that departs from steady rhythmicity was often associated with anxiety increases. Similarly, Balog (1983) failed to attain a relaxation effect on frontalis EMG subsequent to grade cycle ergometry. Although competing explanations may account for such nonanxiolytic effects, it may be that rhythmical and steady-state work is an important dimension of the exercise stimulus.

Rather direct support for such a somatic influence model using EEG measures as the dependent variable was first provided by the studies of Pineda and Adkisson (1961), Kamp and Troost (1978), and Farmer et al. (1978).[3] Farmer et al. examined EEG alpha before and after 6 min of submaximal cycle ergometry and a 6-min test of maximal work capacity. Two groups of trait-anxious subjects (i.e., Types A and B) were contrasted for postexercise EEG alpha. Electrocortical activation was quantified by the number of seconds above a criterion voltage during a 10-min observation period. For both exercise conditions Type A subjects showed a substantial increase in posttreatment EEG alpha, while Type B subjects evidenced higher alpha at rest, but showed a substantially smaller increase upon completion of exercise.

Although Farmer et al. (1978) did provide evidence consistent with the visceral feedback model, the report was limited by (a) its omission of statistical analysis of EEG differences, (b) a failure to obtain any concurrent assessment of self-reported mood, and (c) failure to report the relative intensity of the submaximal exercise load. This finding was also supported by Hatfield, Vaccaro, Brown, Moore, and Ostrove (1984), who showed that subjects both high and low in cognitive anxiety derived significant EEG alpha change following both moderate (i.e., 60% maximal work capacity) and maximal exercise stimuli.

Finally, a number of investigators have provided evidence that high-trait-anxiety subjects seem to derive even greater anxiolytic effects (Bahrke & Morgan, 1978; deVries & Adams, 1972; Farmer et al., 1978; Hatfield et al., 1984; Morgan et al., 1971; Sime, 1977; Wood, 1977). Although this empirical observation is not readily explained by an agreed on mechanism, it seems plausible to offer some speculation at this stage of development of the exercise and mental health issue. Accordingly, the threshold for stimulation of the bulbar inhibitory mechanism advanced by Bonvallet and Bloch (1961) may be attained more readily by those already high in central arousal (i.e., high-trait-anxiety subjects). In fact, the CNS of the highly anxious subject may exhibit a chronic elevation of EEG activation (Tucker, Cole, & Friedman, 1986). In this manner, the impact of the exercise stimulus may be more profound and prolonged for such individuals.

---

[3]As a separate issue the failure to examine stress reduction effects beyond 1.5 hr did not address the clinical significance of exercise compared with larger or "clinical" dosages of meprobamate.

Lateralization of Visceral Feedback:
The Right-Hemispheric Effect

The effect of the afferent autonomic activation on the brain and, more specifically, the cerebral hemispheres may be lateralized. Evidence of the association
between autonomic nervous system (ANS) activity (specifically heart rate and
blood pressure) and right hemispheric electrocortical activation has been provided by Walker and Sandman (1979, 1982). This lateralized "sensitivity" has
also been noted with skilled marksmen (Hatfield, Landers, & Ray, 1987). Additional evidence has been provided using behavioral measures (Davidson, Horowitz, Schwartz, & Goodman, 1981). However, these relations between the
ANS and CNS have not been directly examined in exercise environments, although Jones and Hollandsworth (1981) did note increased heart rate discrimination or detectability after exercise-induced cardiac activity.[4]

It may be that the substantially increased cardiovascular arousal noted during physical workloads promotes a stronger or preferential effect of alpha activation on the right hemisphere. This model might also explain the lateralized
EEG outcomes observed by Pineda and Adkisson (1961). In addition, Wiese,
Singh, and Yeudall (1983) conducted an experiment in which male and female
college-age subjects were randomly assigned to 40 min of cycle ergometry or
simply rest. The graded exercise stress consisted of 25 min of cycling at 40% of
maximal oxygen uptake (VO_2 max), and 15 min at 60% VO_2 max. The psychophysiological measure consisted of bilateral occipital and parietal EEG alpha
activity generated from eight 30-s sampling periods before and after exercise.
Spectral analysis revealed that the exercised subjects showed greater alpha
power than the controls and the ratios of bilateral activation "showed a change
toward unity" (Wiese et al., 1983, p. 50).

Unfortunately, although the authors noted that statistically significant differences did occur, they failed to provide any values for mean change. However,
the results prompted them to conclude that "since a correlation has been shown
between the dominant brain wave states and their associated subjective feelings,
the increased alpha power after exercise could contribute to an altered state of
consciousness and could help explain the psychological benefits, including reductions in anxiety and depression, that have been reported with regular exercise" (Wiese et al., 1983, p. 50). In addition, the "right-to-left [hemispheric]
changes suggest a decrease in hemispherization in the cortex during exercise
which could further facilitate an atmosphere for psychological change" (p. 50).
However, it is difficult to assess whether the subjects become more right hemi-

---

[4]The EEG changes discussed herein are consistent with a number of hypothetical models, not
just visceral and muscular influence or afference models; for example, such changes are consistent
with the hyperthermic model, too. Thus both models are supported and it is somewhat arbitrary
which model we associated with a given study. What is important to bear in mind is that none of
these studies refute the various models.

sphere oriented or vice versa from this report. The earlier study by Pineda and Adkisson (1961) did show that exhausting physical exercise resulted in somewhat greater change in the right cerebrum.

It is interesting that all of the EEG studies discussed in this section reported increased alpha activation subsequent to spectral analysis. In terms of traditional activation theory, this finding would suggest relative deactivation of the right hemisphere, which Sackeim and Weber (1982) have discussed as the mediator of negative affect.

Such a model is also congruent with the primary process model of cognition that was previously described as characteristic of the postexercise state (Ewing & Scott, 1984). Accordingly, the primary process mode refers to a fantasy-oriented cognitive state involving vivid images or mental pictures. Such a state could be simplistically described as "right hemispheric" and may be partially facilitated or driven by exercise-induced autonomic activity as outlined by the present discussion.

Opponent-Process Model of Affective Change

Another conceptual explanation for exercise-induced affect is the opponent-process theory (Solomon & Corbit, 1973). Although this model is primarily a psychological explanation of outcome, two psychophysiological mechanisms may proceed from it. These are discussed shortly. Basically, this theoretical position holds that engagement in any stressful activity is followed by an opposing, or pleasant, affective state upon cessation of the stressor. On the basis of neurophysiological evidence, this explanation posits a sort of rebound effect of the CNS to a given stress. With long-term adaptation to the stressor, the negative experience (e.g., the perception of fatigue to a given exercise stimulus) becomes reduced, while the opponent experience becomes increasingly positive. In essence, this developmental occurrence represents a shift in the respective amplitudes and durations of the two processes.

Boutcher and Landers (1986) recently tested this model in terms of the mental health effects of acute exercise. The postexercise anxiety (i.e., STAI-1) reports of trained runners were compared with those of an untrained sample after undergoing 20 min of treadmill running at an intensity of 80–85% maximal heart rate. In accord with the hypothesis, trained subjects experienced a significant decline in self-reported anxiety after exercise when contrasted with a comparable baseline period. No such change was observed for the untrained subjects. Such an experimental approach tested an interactional effect between a subject characteristic (i.e., trained and untrained) and the exercise stress. Although the precise mechanism of mood alteration remains unknown, the strength of the study lies in its theoretical and predictive basis for such change. These results show that individuals do not uniformly respond to exercise and that fitness status (and other variables) may significantly mediate such effects.

Possible Mechanisms Mediating the "Rebound Effect" or Opponent Process

Although a number of mechanisms may explain the opponent process, the focus here is on only two of them: (a) the possible role of β-endorphin (β-EP) and other members of the endorphin superfamily and (b) the involvement of the ANS and sympathoadrenal activity.

Beta-endorphins. The endorphin-related literature has focused primarily on the humoral response to exercise, but some studies have examined concomitant psychological and plasma responses as a consequence of exercise (Farrell, Gates, Maksud, & Morgan, 1982; Farrell, Gates, Morgan, & Pert, 1983; Farrell et al., 1986; Grossman et al., 1984; Haier, Quaid, & Mills, 1981; Janal, Colt, Clark, & Glusman, 1984; Markoff, Ryan, & Young, 1982). Only those studies that have directly examined psychological states are discussed here, because the assumption of opioid-induced psychological effects, without direct psychometric assessment, is somewhat tenuous (Morgan, 1985a). Parallel alterations in measured psychological states may not occur even if the levels of endogenous opioids are significantly elevated (Farrell et al., 1982; Goldfarb, Hatfield, Sforzo, & Flynn, 1987; Grossman et al., 1984; Hatfield, Goldfarb, Sforzo, & Flynn, 1987). Conversely, significant elevations in mood state have been noted in the absence of hormonal change (Farrell et al., 1983). Thus the effect of β-EP on mood state bears further consideration beyond that of the popularized notion of a simple direct relation to a "runner's high."

To examine this relation, some investigators have subscribed to a correlation approach, that is, an examination of β-EP level before and after exercise. Accordingly, Farrell et al. (1982) assessed β-EP levels following 30 min of treadmill running at 60%, 80%, and approximately 75% of VO$_2$ max in 6 trained individuals. β-EP levels were significantly elevated only after the 60% condition and the psychological response (as measured by the POMS) was unaltered after each session.[5]

Although the study seemed to provide little evidence of any psychological consequences of exercise in relation to β-EP levels, a number of points need to be raised. First, the ability to detect significant change in the other two exercise conditions (i.e., 75% and 80% of VO$_2$ max) was hampered by the high degree of individual psychoendocrine response variation. Such interindividual variability would be problematic for detecting significant differences with small sample sizes. Second, this variability may not be spurious, as has often been reported by others (Colt, Wardlaw, & Frantz, 1981), and may represent an important

---

[5]The interested reader may also wish to consult Hantas, Katkin, and Reed (1984) and Montgomery and Jones (1984).

individual difference variable that could be examined as a factor in future investigations of the relation between exercise and β-EP. At this time, no studies have examined the β-EP response of individuals to repeated testing and it is difficult to know if there are consistently high and low β-EP responders. Therefore, because the Farrell et al. (1982) study, as all others have, lumped subjects together, an important individual difference variable may have been overlooked. Third, the small subject sample would make the identification of significant self-report effects particularly problematic.[6] Farrell et al. reported that mood was elevated 50% in two of the workloads but a high degree of variability precluded the detection of any statistically significant effect. The failure to find any effect with the POMS may have also been due to subject reactivity. Although much of the endorphin-related literature has employed this inventory (Farrell et al., 1983, 1986; Markoff et al., 1982) we have found in our research that subjects frequently complain about the lengthy format. In addition, the significant rise in β-EP during the 60% condition (from 19 pg/ml at rest to 58 pg/ml) was associated with the lowest rating of perceived exertion during the workload. This finding is indirectly supportive of identifying the primary role of endorphines as promoters of physiological economy during exercise or any stress (as opposed to a primary role of affective change). To illustrate, Morgan (1985) has postulated that the peripheral effects of β-EP, such as adipolysis and ventilatory restraint, may promote a central psychological effect by way of reduced discomfort during exercise. Interestingly, Farrell et al.'s (1982) results are consistent with such a model, in that the 60% exercise stress as the significant elevation of β-EP was associated with the lowest levels of rated perceived exertion. In any case, it is difficult to draw definitive conclusions from the study because of the failure to actively manipulate β-EP level.

However, the dissociation between β-EP and psychological state may be caused by the singular reliance on subjective self-report methods to assess the latter. To overcome this limitation, Janal et al. (1984) recently employed a number of behavioral measures (thermal, cold pressor, and ischemic pain tolerance), as well as a variety of psychological scales, to investigate responses to intense exercise (i.e., running 6.3 miles "in the field" at approximately 85% of VO_2 max). In addition, an active intervention approach was employed as each of the behavioral variables was assessed after two separate runs involving postexercise saline and naloxone administration. Janal et al. did find evidence for both an analgesic (i.e., ischemic tolerance was reduced after pharmacological intervention) and mood alteration effect of circulating β-EP. Self-reported mood was assessed by means of visual analogue scales, which may represent an improvement over other scales because they allow for the employment of a ratio

---

[6]Studies that examine β-EP and psychometric profiles often incorporate small sample sizes because of the expense involved in analyzing β-EP. Such small sample sizes pose problems for obtaining meaningful results with psychological questionnaires.

scale of measurement. Specifically, joy and euphoria ratings were attenuated upon administration of naloxone. Importantly, the results of the study demonstrated that the behavioral effects of β-EP are highly specific. Both thermal pain tolerance and the cold pressor response were unaffected by the experimental treatment, reinforcing the concept of opioid- and non-opioid-mediated nociceptive or pain pathways. It should be noted too that a number of other self-reported psychological variables were unaffected by naloxone.

Similarly, experimental support for the analgesic effect of exercise was provided by Haier et al. (1981), who found pain tolerance for a weight (or pressure) exerted on the hand to be decreased subsequent to naloxone intervention. However, the demonstration of this effect was dependent on the dosage of opioid antagonist employed. Others (e.g., Morgan, 1985) have pointed out that the dosage used may have been a problem in those studies (e.g., Markoff et al., 1982) that failed to find a relation between β-EP and psychological variables subsequent to exercise. However, a dosage similar to that employed by Markoff (i.e., 8 mg/2 ml of saline) was also used by Janal et al. (1984), who did find positive results. One problem may be the employment of the POMS as the measure of psychological state because it may not be a suitable index of any β-EP-induced effect. The POMS was also used by Farrell et al. (1982, 1983, 1986) in three exercise/β-EP studies. In all of the investigations, no consistent relation was found—in one case (Farrell et al., 1982) no change was observed, in another (Farrell et al., 1983) psychological tension decreased while no concomitant change was seen in enkephalinlike immunoreactivity, and in the third (Farrell et al., 1986), no alteration was seen in POMS profile during naloxone- or saline-treated exercise conditions.

As stated earlier, the psychological effects of β-EP may also accrue indirectly, as a result of a primary physiological role. Recently, evidence has been provided for the economizing effect of circulating β-EP on the hormonal response to exercise (Farrell et al., 1986; Grossman et al., 1984). It has been well established that β-EP is coreleased with adrenocorticotrophic hormone as a response to nonspecific stress. Farrell et al. (1986) and Grossman et al. (1984) have shown that naloxone intervention that blocks β-EP receptor binding resulted in a significant rise in catecholamine levels during exercise. Apparently, an intact β-EP response may arrest such extraordinary sympathetic drive. In addition, Harber and Sutton (1984) and Santiago and Edelman (1985) have discussed the role of circulating β-EP in promoting reductions of ventilatory activity during workload. For example, Grossman et al. (1984) found minute ventilation to increase to 105.7 ± 5.0 l/min from 94.8 ± 4.9 upon administration of the opioid antagonist. In light of the strong association of ventilation to the perceived discomfort of muscular exertion, circulating β-EP may play an important role, psychologically, during the exercise stress. On the basis of this model, one might hypothesize "that an increased opiate activity during exercise in trained subjects (Carr et al., 1981) might be an advantage, as it would demand less ventilation and result in less respiratory muscle fatigue at excessively high levels of work" (Grossman & Sutton, 1985, p. 323). Recent evidence from McMurray, Sheps, and Guinan (1984) failed to support the ventilatory economy effect of β-EP, but the extremely low dosage of naloxone used (i.e., 0.4 mg) may have been problematic.

Thus it seems that there is empirical evidence to support the role of β-EP in the psychological response both during and following exercise. In fact, a number of early studies (Catlin, Gorelick, Gerner, Aui, & Li, 1980; Gerner, Catlin, Gorelick, & Huikk, 1980; Kline et al., 1977) conducted with psychiatric populations showed that intravenous β-EP injections caused psychological alterations of clinical significance, although these effects were pharmacological (i.e., exogenous) rather than exercise induced (i.e., endogenous). Such findings provided rather direct experimental support for the role of β-EP in centrally mediated change, and, according to Catlin et al. (1980), "this suggests that peripherally administered β-endorphin may enter the CNS" (p. 470). However, critics of these studies argue that the dosage levels employed (8.5–10 mg) are several orders of magnitude above the naturally occurring levels in exercising humans. Typically, these values are reported in picograms per millimeter. However, the pharmacological significance or potency of endogenous secretions may be substantially higher than that of exogenously administered substances (K. Hargraves, personal communication, March 1986). In addition, McArthur (1985) has cited unpublished evidence that the permeability of the blood–brain barrier may be altered during exercise. Thus these pharmacological studies provide additional support for the role of β-EP as an agent of change for exercise-induced mood alteration.

Autonomic alterations. The sense of well-being reported by some exercise participants may result "in part from an adjustment of the autonomic nervous system" (Michael, 1957, p. 50). These effects may occur within the sympathetic and parasympathetic nerve branches of the ANS and within the adrenal medulla. According to animal studies, Richter (cited in Michael, 1957) reported hypertrophy of the adrenal glands in exercise-stressed animals and although such an adaption to exercise stress is unknown in humans, such a consequence could result in larger catecholamine secretions in a shorter time period, resulting in faster recovery of adrenal output. Hull, Young, and Ziegler (1983) noted such a model-consistent heart rate patterning response to psychosocial stress in conditioned subjects when contrasted to those who were less fit. In other words, fits subjects showed a fast and stronger heart rate response to psychological stress but a more rapid return to baseline. Of course, heart rate is largely affected by adrenal medullary output. In essence, such adrenal hypertrophy would result in a more temporally efficient stress response and "lessens the duration of the adjusting phase" (Michael, 1957, p. 53). The increased adrenal activity resulting from repeated exercise also seems to cause an increased reserve of cortical steroids that may also be available to counter a given stress.

Alternatively, trained subjects may experience a gradual increase in parasympathetic dominance as a function of repeated exposure to exercise stress. Michael (1957) cited earlier research (Van Liere et al.) with exercised rats that demonstrated increased propulsive motility of the small intestine when compared with that of nonexercised rats. Such a finding suggested a chronic dominance of the parasympathetic nervous system. More recently, Hahner and Rochelle (1968) demonstrated enhanced parasympathetic dominance in 10 aerobically trained athletes compared with 10 power-trained athletes and 16 nonactive controls while using Wenger's test of autonomic balance in the resting state. Therefore, the study supports the possibility that alteration of the ANS by physical conditioning is feasible. However, the correlation nature of this work does not rule out competing explanations for the data (such as the possibility of initial differences in the subjects).

In terms of opponent-process theory Solomon and Corbit (1973) offered speculation that the opponent process to a fear state, in terms of heart rate response, may be mediated by vagal "overshoot" subsequent to the enhanced sympathetic drive. Such a response may be paralleled by a postexercise vagal overshoot subsequent to the sympathoadrenal drive experienced during work or exercise. This would hold particular relevance for the acute response to exercise, but the above discussion also relates to chronic training effects in individuals because it offers an explanation for the differential response of aerobically trained individuals who have been found to experience enhanced emotional responses upon cessation of exercise when compared with sedentary people (Boutcher & Landers, 1988).

It may be that regular aerobic exercise, with its requirements of sympathetic nervous system activation and associated endocrine response, leads to a reduction in the individual's stress responses to other stressors. It may be that by extending the capacity of the adrenal medulla to generate catecholamines by means of exercise may help to reduce the experience of psychosocial stress. It has also been suggested that exercise may promote hypertrophy and lower the threshold of stimulation of the adrenal glands, resulting in greater reserves of antistress steroids and faster response time to stressors. Consistent with this notion, Frankenhauser (1975) demonstrated that school children rated as more emotionally stable and competent than their classmates experienced greater catecholamine responses to classroom challenges than did their less emotionally stable classmates.

Neurotransmitter Changes

Finally, in terms of physiological models, recent evidence supports the role of neuroendocrine responses to acute and chronic exercise as a mediating factor of mood alteration. Specifically, this model relates to possible increases in aminergic synaptic transmission within the CNS (Ransford, 1982). The amines are chemical transmitter substances that enable communication between adjacent neurons; as such, any changes in activity would have a profound effect on central brain processes. Three of these major neurotransmitters are norepinephrine, dopamine, and serotonin; the former two are categorized as catecholamines because of their chemical structure, while the latter is classified as an indoleamine. These aminergic neurons originate primarily in brainstem in and around the midbrain and pontine reticular formation. More precisely, the serotonergic and adrenergic neurons are found within the limbic system (which deals with emotion) and the hypothalamus (which mediates several basic motivational drives), respectively, while dopaminergic neurons are densely populated within the basal ganglia, telencephalic structures that subserve basic motor functions. Urinary metabolites of norepinephrine (i.e., 3-methoxy 4-hyroxyphenylglycol [MHPG]), dopamine (i.e., homovanillic acid), and serotonin (i.e., 5-hydroxyindoleacetic acid) can be used as quantitative indexes of brain aminergic activity. However, caution must be applied to the interpretation of such measurable levels because, for example, only 22–27% of urinary MHPG originates from brain locations. The remainder would be derived from peripheral adrenergic fibers of the sympathetic nervous system throughout the body.

The biogenic amines have been implicated in a number of behavioral processes such as sleep and stress-related states. Ransford (1982) has summarized much of the available evidence that relates the amines to depressive states. For example, decreased levels of urinary metabolites have been observed in clinical populations while patients affected by Parkinson's disease (who suffer from lowered levels of dopamine) often exhibit signs of depressive disorder. In addition, many of the active treatments used to alleviate depression, such as electroconvulsive therapy and REM sleep deprivation, are known to enhance aminergic synaptic transmission. Certain medications (the monoamine oxidase inhibitors) alleviate depression and promote an active inhibition of norepinephrine breakdown within the neurons. Conversely, experimental depletion of the monoamines with pharmacological agents (e.g., reserpine) causes enhancement of depression. This latter effect has been shown with both animal (Ellison, 1977) and human models (Carlsson, 1961).

Because exercise training has been associated with reductions in self-reported depression, it may actively enhance aminergic activity. Convincing evidence, derived from rat model studies, has shown increases in dopamine and serotonin levels in brain tissue consequent to acute exercise. The evidence is somewhat contradictory regarding the effect on serotonin. Furthermore, increased levels of urinary MHPG have been observed in psychiatric patients following a day of heightened physical activity compared with their "normal" hypoactive state. However, simultaneous measurement of aminergic metabolites (i.e., MHPG) and subjective self-report in other clinical samples has shown no relation between the two variables. Although this finding would seem to support the dissociation between physical activity and affective states, recent work by Sothmann and Ismail (1984) has shown that the employment of a sophisticated statistical model did provide support for the association between MHPG and mood state as a function of fitness level.

The relation among exercise stress, aminergic activity, and mood state may be complex. Mood alteration may also depend on interactions between the amines, as opposed to any singular and independent influences promoted by them. In addition, epinephrine has been shown by several investigators to be more sensitive to psychological stressors, whereas peripheral norepinephrine levels may be more indicative of physical stress responses. As such, the measured levels of MHPG may be more indicative of the physical response to exercise stress as opposed to affective outcome.

Ransford (1982) also pointed out the need to consider the role of cognitive factors in this model of psychological change. For example, a time lag of several days is typically observed between the administration of antidepressant medication and self-reported psychological changes, even though "the antidepressant medication enhances adrenergic synaptic transmission almost immediately" (Ransford, 1982, p. 8). Accordingly, Morgan, Roberts, Brand, and Feinerman (1970) found that 6 weeks of exercise training resulted in no change in self-reported depression within normal subjects, whereas significant changes were observed by Brown, Ramirez, and Taub (1978) with such a population after 10 weeks of training. Such discrepant findings may underlie the contribution of several factors, both psychological and physiological, which take time to summate to a significant and reproducible psychological experience.

Although such findings would seem to delimit the neuroendocrine model to chronic or training responses, alterations in monoamine activity subsequent to an acute bout of exercise may provide one of the many psychophysiological inputs that, in concert with other such changes, results in a perceived change in mood state.

Psychological Theories

To further discuss the anxiolytic properties of exercise, the work of Bahrke and Morgan (1978) and the formulation of their distraction hypothesis are important. These authors controlled for the psychological expectancy effect of exercise by contrasting 20 min of treadmill running, at an intensity of 70% maximal heart rate, with an equal amount of noncultic meditation and reading. Running and meditation reportedly yield similar stress reduction consequences. Seventy-five adult males (ages 22–71) were randomly assigned to one of the three groups and completed the STAI-1 prior to, immediately after, and 10 min after each of the treatments. Cardiac frequency, oxygen uptake, skin temperature, and systolic and diastolic blood pressure were also recorded during each condition. Again, exercise participation was associated with a decrease in anxiety; however, an ANOVA revealed that a significant anxiety reduction effect occurred for the other treatments as well. Thus, the outcome of physical exercise, assessed 10 min following exertion, was no more effective in reducing anxiety than was simple rest (quiet reading).

Because of the lack of any unique contribution of exercise to stress reduction, Bahrke and Morgan (1978) hypothesized that simple distraction or a cognitive "time-out" served as the primary mechanism of anxiety alleviation. However, such an explanation was based solely on the self-reported outcomes of exercise and therefore remains incomplete. Although the measured outcomes of exercise and quiet rest may be the same at a given point in time, the process by which they achieve this end may be substantially different. Interestingly, recent evidence (Raglin & Morgan, 1986) has revealed that the temporal duration of exercise-induced anxiety reduction extends significantly beyond that of simple rest when psychophysiological (i.e., systolic blood pressure) and self-reported assessments are employed over a prolonged period (i.e., 3 hr following treatment), and this finding lends further support to the notion that the mechanisms of effect are probably dissimilar.

Few studies have examined both psychological (i.e., outcome) and psychophysiological (i.e., process) measures concurrently. For example, Sime (1977) assigned 48 test-anxious students to three separate treatment groups consisting of 10 min of treadmill exercise, 15 min of Bensonian relaxation, or placebo expectancy control (i.e., pharmacological intervention) to contrast the efficacy of treatment of reducing psychological reactivity to a testing situation. A number of responses were assessed, and the results showed that exercise did produce a greater reduction in heart rate and electrodermal response than the other treatments. However, all three treatments similarly showed a significant decrease in EMG and systolic and diastolic blood pressure. Self-reported anxiety was nonsignificantly lowered for the exercise and meditation groups. Thus, acute exercise promoted a more efficient psychophysiological coping reaction to the threatening situation, compared with pretreatment levels, and this reduction was significantly greater for some responses (i.e., heart rate and electrodermal response) than others (i.e., self-report and systolic and diastolic blood pressure). Sime (1977) concluded that brief, mild exercise can reduce some autonomic responses to psychosocial stress.

In a similar manner Andres, Metz, and Drash (1978) reported a significant reduction in state anxiety following a 20-min treadmill run at 70% of subjects' age-related maximal heart rate, while concurrent measures of urinary catechol-amines showed a significant elevation. Morgan (1979a) also cited such a frac-tionated arousal response while reviewing some of his earlier work (Morgan & Horstman, 1976).

The relative independence (or dissociation) between the self-reported and psychophysiological responses is not unusual when considered in terms of the multidimensional model of arousal advanced by others (Borkovec, 1976; Lacey & Lacey, 1978). Although the finding by Andres et al. (1978) would seem to support a multidimensional arousal state, the "apparent" fractionation may be artifactual in that the appearance of the urinary metabolites would not be reflec-tive of concomitant circulating levels of epinephrine and norepinephrine be-cause a number of factors may affect the temporal onset of their appearance in the urine (Levi, 1972).

Finally, we need to examine the larger picture. Recently, a multimodal as-sessment of postexercise change was conducted by McGowan, Robertson, and Epstein (1985). Twelve male subjects (ages 21–29 years) of moderate physical fitness (VO$_2$ max $= 47.04 + 4.30$ ml/kg-1) were exposed to each of three 15-min exercise periods (i.e., 40%, 55%, and 70% of VO$_2$ max) and a resting attentional control condition. Psychophysiological responsivity was measured by integrated EMG assessment. Measurement sites were individually deter-mined from initial inspection of a number of standard muscle locations, and locations for each subjects were selected on the basis of highest reactivity. The authors subscribed to the principle of individual response specificity (Lacey, Kagan, Lacey, & Moss, 1963), which represented a level of methodological sophistication beyond that of other EMG researchers (Balog, 1983; deVries, 1968). In addition, psychological assessment was accomplished by means of two new subscales contained within the Addiction Research Center Inventory to assess the sedative and euphoric effects of exercise. This inventory appears to represent an especially appropriate scale for exercise-induced mood alteration, in light of the recent findings of Janal et al. (1984) regarding endorphin-mediated euphoria, and also provides an additional measure to the STAI-1 and POMS scales employed in other investigations. The study also employed a randomized posttest-only design to control for any test reactivity associated with repeated test administrations.

CONCLUSION

Both anecdotal reports and empirical evidence support the observation that physical exercise is associated with certain psychological consequences. These outcomes have been examined as a function of both acute and chronic exercise stimuli. The justification for the present emphasis on acute responses seems warranted in light of a recent statement by Dishman (1985) that "it appears that exercise is best viewed as a method for *intermittent* coping with daily events or thoughts that provoke an anxiety response" (p. 124). In other words, if we stop exercising we lose the psychological benefits. Therefore, anxiety did not decrease during the exercise. In fact, it increased. However, this is still unresolved—perhaps the changes are in fact more enduring.

These psychological outcomes have been operationalized in terms of psychometric, psychoendocrine, and neurophysiological terms, although the extent of the literature is not remarkable. Psychometric measurement was typically accomplished with the STAI-1 (e.g., Morgan, 1973), although more recent investigations have used a variety of affective scales (e.g., McGowan et al., 1985) as well as behavioral measures of pain tolerance (e.g., Janal et al., 1984). The employment of a number of assessment strategies seems warranted in light of the degree of specificity of affective change (Janal et al., 1984).

Studies employing different methodologies have supported a similar psychological response by the sexes (Wiese et al., 1983). The use of combined groups (i.e., male and female) in other studies (Balog, 1982; deVries, 1968; deVries & Adams, 1972; deVries et al., 1982, 1982; Nowlis & Greenberg, 1979; Wiese et al., 1983; Wilson, Berger, & Bird, 1981) implicitly subscribes to the notion that males and females respond similarly. Importantly, Anderson and Morgan (1972) (cited in Morgan, 1973) found that high- and low-anxiety females responded similarly with anxiety decrements.

The temporal pattern of self-reported mood change typically revealed a nonsignificant elevation in anxiety immediately upon cessation of the exercise, while decrements began approximately 3–5 min following (and continued at least one-half hour postexercise) (Morgan, 1973). This information was further extended by Morgan and Horstman (1976), who evaluated state anxiety prior to, during, and following exhaustive treadmill exercise at an intensity of 80% of maximal aerobic power. STAI-1 results revealed a linear increase in self-reported anxiety throughout the first half of exercise that reached an asymptote and remained stable for the remainder of the workload. Therefore, anxiety did not decrease during exercise. In fact, it increased. However, consistent with earlier reports, self-reported anxiety returned to preexercise levels within 5 min after exercise.

The evidence provided for the temporal patterning of tension reduction over longer durations is contradictory. For example, Seemann (1978) (cited in Morgan, 1981b) monitored state anxiety over a 24-hr period following exertion and found a gradual decrease followed by a slow return to preexercise baseline. This study provided evidence for the transient or noncumulative effect of exercise on affective state, as held by Dishman. Accordingly, one would have to engage in periodic repetitions of exercise stress. Other reports examined affective consequences over a 48-hr period using the STAI-1 (Bahrke, 1981), and a 3-hr period by means of EMG assessment (Balog, 1983). Neither investigation supported the pattern noted by Seemann. Bahrke (1981) concluded that multiple determinants of psychological states are encountered during an individual's normal or daily routine and these may overshadow any exercise-induced effects. As such, little is known about the duration of the psychological response.

In addition, self-report measures may not be sensitive to some of the subtle alterations that occur. Accordingly, neurophysiological assessments have been operationalized by the EEG, AEP, integrated surface EMG, and Hoffman reflex. Unfortunately, little attempt has been made to obtain concurrent measures of psychological states to determine whether much change is associated with mood alteration. Another limitation of those studies that have used EEG is the exclusive focus on the alpha band. Recent evidence provided by Ray and Cole (1985) indicates that EEG beta band (16–20 Hz) is more indicative of affect and emotion. Future studies would provide a more intensive investigation of such central changes by reporting activity throughout the EEG spectrum. These kinds of development would be further aided by using electrode placements at several regional locations in an attempt to relate such electrophysiological change to neuropsychological theory and the localization of cognitive.

Some investigators who have examined psychoendocrine changes (i.e., β-EP) have extended their assessment of psychological change by obtaining assessments during exercise. The ability to actively manipulate β-EP levels by means of naloxone or naltrexone intervention has contributed to a more definitive understanding of such mechanisms of change. However, one problem with this approach is the lack of receptor specificity for such pharmacological interventions. However, the notion of ventilatory and adrenergic efficiency, as promoted by β-EP, provides a testable model of psychological effect. Although there is conflicting evidence (McMurray et al., 1984), β-EP may promote peripheral changes that are perceived centrally as reductions in perceived exertion.

Our failure to test such models of psychological change prompted Morgan (1979b) to state, "It is unfortunate that exercise scientists have not addressed, at least in a serious and systematic fashion, the question of *why,* relative to tension reduction following vigorous physical activity. While the tacit assumption seems to be that exercise per se causes anxiety to be reduced, there has simply not been evidence to support *causality*" (italics added, p. 147).

Although such a statement is indicative of a significant problem with this literature, more recent experimental evidence is clearly supportive of exercise-induced causal change (Janal et al., 1984). Furthermore, the application of psychological theory in an a priori manner enables specific predictions of psychological change to be tested (Boutcher & Landers, 1988). Attention to individual difference variables and the assessment of interactional effects (i.e., regarding subject characteristics and exercise intensity) should allow a more specific assessment of such change. For example, high-trait-anxiety (Hatfield et al., 1984) and aerobically trained subjects (Boutcher & Landers, 1988) have been shown to respond differently to exercise stimuli. The failure to partition such subject variables, and examine only main affects, would reduce the sensitivity to detect such change.

It would seem that a number of developments have occurred since the early 1960s when the first reports of psychological response to exercise appeared. Although the results are generally positive, a number of methodological concerns limit the conclusions that can be reached. Moreover, few attempts have been made to explain such outcomes. In spite of the progression from largely uncontrolled studies, and the limited attempts to combine process measures (i.e., psychophysiological) along with self-report, the exercise literature offers little guidance regarding the conceptual basis of affective change. A more definitive understanding of the underlying mechanisms requires examination of a number of empirically based models. This was the intent of the present chapter—to propose such mechanisms. In addition, the dependent measures employed by investigators must relate directly to the theoretical mechanisms proposed. For example, examination of the hyperthermic model (Von Euler & Soderberg, 1957) would require appropriate measures of central and peripheral neural activation (i.e., EEG and spinal reflex activation, respectively), as well as verification of central hyperthermia. These assessments should be accompanied by additional measures of subjective self-report. Such an approach represents a methodological and technological challenge, but only by testing such hypotheses in an a priori manner can a more definitive understanding of mechanisms be achieved. As stated earlier in this chapter, even the rejection of testable hypotheses is informative! The advancement of processes (e.g., distraction or time-out) in a post-hoc manner is helpful, but lacks the power of predictive hypothesis testing.

Although the basis for exercise-induced mood alteration in human subjects is speculative, a number of tenable hypotheses do exist. A number of these hypotheses have been discussed at some length as a follow-up to the psychological reports. It is hoped that the mechanisms presented will contribute to the generation of testable hypotheses in future investigations (realizing, of course, that any psychological consequences of acute exercise are probably multifaceted in origin).

REFERENCES

Andres, F. F., Metz, K. F., & Drash, A. L. (1978). Changes in state anxiety and urine catecholamines produced during treadmill running. *Medicine and Science in Sports, 10,* 51 (abstract).

Bahrke, M. S. (1981). Alterations in anxiety following exercise and rest. In F. S. Nagle & H. J. Montoye (Eds.), *Exercise in health and disease* (pp. 291–298). Springfield, IL: Charles C Thomas.

Bahrke, M. S., & Morgan, W. P. (1978). Anxiety reduction following exercise and meditation. *Cognitive Therapy and Research, 2,* 323–333.

Balog, L. F. (1983). The effect of exercise on muscle tension and subsequent muscle relaxation training. *Research Quarterly for Exercise and Sport, 54,* 119–125.

Bonvallet, M., & Bloch, V. (1961). Bulbar control of cortical arousal. *Science, 133,* 1133–1134.

Borkovec, T. D. (1976). Physiological and cognitive processes in the regulation of anxiety. In G. E. Schwartz & D. Shapiro (Eds.), *Consciousness and self-regulation: Advances in research* (Vol. 1, pp. 261-312). New York: Plenum.

Boutcher, S. H., & Landers, D. M. (1988). The effects of vigorous exercise on anxiety, heart rate, and alpha activity of runners and nonrunners. *Psychophysiology, 25,* 696–702.

Brown, R. S., Ramirez, D. E., & Taub, J. M. (1978, December). The prescription of exercise for depression. *The Physician and Sportsmedicine, 6,* 35–45.

Byrd, O. E. (1963). A survey of beliefs and practices of psychiatrists in the relief of tension by moderate exercise. *Journal of School Health, 33,* 426–427.

Carlsson, A. (1961). Brain monoamines and psychotropic drugs. *Neuropsychopharmacology, 2,* 417.

Carr, D. B., Bullen, B. A., Skrinar, G. S., Arnold, M. A., Rosenblatt, M., Beitens, I. Z., Martin, J. B., & McArthur, J. W. (1981). Physical conditioning facilitates the exercise-induced secretion of beta-endorphins and beta-lipotropin in women. *New England Journal of Medicine, 305,* 560–562.

Catlin, D. H., Gorelick, D. A., Gerner, R. H., Aui, K. K., & Li, C. H. (1980). Clinical effects of β-endorphin infusions. In E. Costa & M. Trabucchi (Eds.), *Neural peptides and neural communication* (pp. 465–472). New York: Raven Press.

Colt, W. D., Wardlaw, S. L., & Frantz, A. G. (1981). The effect of running on plasma β-endorphin. *Life Sciences, 28,* 1637–1640.

Davidson, R. J., Horowitz, M. E., Schwartz, G. E., & Goodman, D. M. (1981). Lateral differences in the latency between finger tapping and the heart rate. *Psychophysiology, 18,* 36–41.

deVries, H. A. (1968). Immediate and long term effects of exercise upon resting muscle action potential. *Journal of Sports Medicine and Physical Fitness, 8,* 1–11.

deVries, H. A., & Adams, G. M. (1972). Electromyographic comparison of single doses of exercise and meprobamate as to effects on muscular relaxation. *American Journal of Physical Medicine, 51,* 130–141.

deVries, H. A., Simard, C. P., Wiswell, R. A., Heckathorne, E., & Carabetta, V. (1982). Fusimotor system involvement in the tranquilizer effect of exercise. *American Journal of Physical Medicine, 61,* 111–122.

deVries, H. A., Wiswell, R. A., Bulbulian, R., & Moritani, T. (1981). Tranquilizer effect of exercise. *American Journal of Physical Medicine, 60,* 57–66.

Dishman, R. K. (1985). Medical psychology in exercise and sport. *Medical Clinics of North America, 69,* 123–143.

Duffy, E. (1962). *Activation and behavior.* New York: Wiley.

Ellison, G. D. (1977). Animal models of psychopathology: The low-norepinephrine and low-norepinephrine low-serotonin rat. *American Psychologist, 32,* 1036–1045.

Engel, G. L., Romano, J., Ferris, E. B., Webb, J. P., & Stevens, J. P. (1944). A simple method of determining frequency spectrums in the electroencephalogram. *Archives of Neurology and Psychiatry, 51,* 134–146.

Ewing, J. H., & Scott, D. G. (1984). Effects of aerobic exercise upon affect and cognition. *Perceptual and Motor Skills, 59,* 407–414.

Farmer, P. K., Olewine, P. A., Comer, D. W., Edwards, M. E., Coleman, T. M., Thomas, G., & Homes, C. G. (1978). Frontalis muscle tension and occipital alpha production in young males with coronary prone (Type A) and coronary resistant (Type B) behavior patterns: Effects of exercise. *Medicine and Science in Sports, 10,* 51.

Farrell, P. A., Gates, W. K., Maksud, M. G., & Morgan, W. P. (1982). Increases in plasma β-endorphin and β-lipotropin immunoreactivity after treadmill running in humans. *Journal of Applied Physiology: Respiration Environmental Exercise Physiology,* 1245–1249.

Farrell, P. A., Gates, W. K., Morgan, W. P., & Pert, C. B. (1983). Plasma leucine enkephalin-like radioreceptor activity and tension-anxiety before and after competitive running. In H. G. Knuttgen, J. A. Vogel, & J. Poortmans (Eds.), *Biochemistry of exercise* (pp. 637–644). Champaign, IL: Human Kinetics.

Farrell, P. A., Gustafson, A. B., Garthwaite, T. L., Kalkhoff, R. K., Cowley, A. W., & Morgan, W. P. (1986). Influence of endogenous opioids on the response of selected hormones to exercise in humans. *Journal of Applied Physiology, 61,* 1051–1057.

Frankenhauser, M. (1975). Experimental approaches to the study of rate cholamines and emotion. In L. Levi (Ed.), *Emotions—Their parameters and measurement.* (209–234). New York: Raven Press.

Gerner, R. H., Catlin, D. H., Gorelick, D. A., Huikk, x. x., & Li, C. H. (1980). β-endorphin: Intravenous infusion causes behavioral change. *Archives of General Psychiatry, 37,* 642–647.

Gliner, J. A., Matsen-Twisdale, J. A., Horvath, S. M., & Maron, M. B. (1979). Visual evoked potentials and signal detection following a marathon race. *Medicine and Science in Sports, 11,* 155–159.

Goldfarb, A. H., Hatfield, B. D., Sforzo, G. A., & Flynn, M. G. (1987).

Serum beta-endorphin levels during a graded exercise test to exhaustion. *Medicine and Science in Sports and Exercise, 19,* 78–82.

Graham, C., Cook, M. R., Cohen, H. D., Gerkovich, M. M., Phelps, J. W., & Fotopoulis, S. S. (1986). Effects of variation in physical effort on frontalis EMG activity. *Biofeedback and Self-Regulation, 11,* 135–141.

Greist, J. H., Klein, M. H., Eischens, R. R., Faris, J., Forman, A. S., & Morgan, W. P. (1978). Running through your mind. *Journal of Psychosomatic Research, 22,* 259–294.

Greist, J. H., Klein, M. H., Eischens, R. R., Faris, J., Gurman, A. S., & Morgan, W. P. (1979). Running as treatment for depression. *Comprehensive Psychiatry, 20,* 41–54.

Grossman, A., Bouloux, P., Price, P., Drury, P. L., Lam, K. S. L., Turner, T., Thomas, J., Besser, G. M., & Sutton, J. M. (1984). The role of opioid peptides in the hormonal responses to acute exercise in man. *Clinical Science, 67,* 483–491.

Grossman, A., & Sutton, J. R. (1985). Endorphins: What are they? How are they measured? What is their role in exercise? *Medicine and Science in Sports and Exercise, 17,* 74–81.

Grosz, H. J., & Farmer, B. B. (1969). Blood lactate in the development of anxiety symptoms: A critical examination of Pitts and McClure's hypothesis and experimental study. *Archives of General Psychiatry, 21,* 611–618.

Hahner, R. H., & Rochelle, R. H. (1968). A comparison of autonomic nervous system activity between physically trained and untrained individuals. *Research Quarterly, 39,* 975–982.

Haier, R. J., Quaid, K., & Mills, J. S. C. (1981). Naloxone alters pain perception after jogging. *Psychiatric Research, 5,* 231–232.

Hantas, M. N., Katkin, E. S., & Reed, S. D. (1984). Cerebral lateralization and heartbeat discrimination. *Psychophysiology, 21,* 274–278.

Harber, V. J., & Sutton, J. R. (1986). Endorphins and exercise. *Sports Medicine, 1,* 154–171.

Hatfield, B. D., Goldfarb, A. H., Sforzo, G. A., & Flynn, M. G. (1987). Serum beta-endorphin and affective responses to graded exercise. *Journal of Gerontology, 42,* 429–431.

Hatfield, B. D., Landers, D. M., & Ray, W. J. (1987). Cardiovascular–CNS interactions during a self-paced intentional attentive state: Elite marksmanship performance. *Psychophysiology, 24,* 542–549.

Hatfield, B. D., Vaccaro, P., Brown, E., Moore, T., & Ostrove, S. (1984). Electrocortical (EEG) relaxation response in high and low cognitively anxious persons as a result of cardiovascular exercise stress. In *Motor development—sport psychology and motor learning/motor control scientific program abstracts (proceedings of the Olympic Scientific Congress)* (pp. 65–66). Eugene, OR: Olympic Scientific Congress.

Hull, E. M., Young, S. H., & Ziegler, M. G. (1984). Aerobic fitness affects cardiovascular and catecholamine responses to stressors. *Psychophysiology, 21,* 353–360.

Iwamoto, G. A., & Kaufman, M. P. (1987). Caudal ventrolateral medullary cells responsive to muscular contraction. *Journal of Applied Physiology, 62,* 149–157.

Jacobson, E. (1938). *Progressive relaxation.* Chicago: University of Chicago Press.

Janal, M. N., Colt, E. W. D., Clark, W. C., & Glusman, M. (1984). Pain sensitivity, mood and plasma endocrine levels in man following long-distance running: Effects of naloxone. *Pain, 19,* 13–25.

Jones, G. E., & Hollandsworth, J. G. (1981). Heart rate discrimination before and after exercise-induced augmented cardiac activity. *Psychophysiology, 18,* 252–257.

Kamp, A., & Troost, J. (1978). EEG signs of cerebrovascular disorder using physical exercise as a provocative method. *Electroencephalography and Clinical Neurophysiology, 45,* 295–298.

Kline, N. S., Li, C. H., Lehmann, H. E., Lajtha, A., Laski, E., & Cooper, T. (1977). β-endorphin-induced changes in schizophrenic and depressed patients. *Archives of General Psychiatry, 34,* 1111–1113.

Lacey, J. I., Kagan, J., Lacey, B. C., & Moss, H. A. (1963). The visceral level: Situational determinants and behavioral correlates of autonomic response patterns. In P. H. Knapp (Ed.), *Expression of the emotions of man* (pp. 161–196). New York: International Universities Press.

Lacey, B. C., & Lacey, J. I. (1978). Two-way communication between the heart and the brain. Significance of time within the cardiac cycle. *American Psychologist, 33,* 99–113.

Levi, L. (1972). Methodological consideration in psychoendocrine research. *Acta Medica Scandinavica, 191,* 28–48.

Markoff, R. A., Ryan, P., & Young, T. (1982). Endorphins and mood changes in long-distance running. *Medicine and Science in Sports and Exercise, 14,* 11–15.

McArthur, J. W. (1985). Endorphins and exercise in females: Possible connection with reproduction dysfunction. *Medicine and Science in Sports and Exercise, 17,* 82–88.

McGowan, C. R., Robertson, R. J., & Epstein, L. H. (1985). The effect of bicycle ergometer exercise at varying intensities on the heart rate, EMG and mood state responses to a mental arithmetic stressor. *Research Quarterly for Exercise and Sport, 56,* 131–137.

McMurray, R. G., Sheps, D. S., & Guinan, D. M. (1984). Effects of naloxone on maximal stress testing in females. *Journal of Applied Physiology: Respiration Environmental and Exercise Physiology, 56,* 436–440.

Michael, E. D. (1957). Stress adaptation through exercise. *Research Quarterly, 28,* 50–54.

Montgomery, W. A., & Jones, G. E. (1984). Laterality, emotionality, and heart-beat perception. *Psychophysiology, 21,* 459–465.

Morgan, W. P. (1973). Influence of acute physical activity on state anxiety. In *Proceedings of the National College Physical Education Association for Men* (pp. 113–121). Pittsburgh, PA: National College Physical Education Association for Men.

Morgan, W. P. (1979a). Negative addiction in runners. *The Physician and Sportsmedicine, 7*(2), 56–63, 67–70.

Morgan, W. P. (1979b). Anxiety reduction following acute physical activity. *Psychiatric Annals, 9,* 141–147.

Morgan, W. P. (1981a). Psychophysiology of self-awareness during vigorous physical activity. *Research Quarterly for Exercise and Sport, 52,* 385–427.

Morgan, W. P. (1981b). Psychological benefits of physical activity. In F. S. Nagle & H. J. Montoye (Eds.), *Exercise in health and disease* (pp. 299–314). Springfield, IL: Charles C Thomas.

Morgan, W. P. (1985a). Affective beneficence of vigorous physical activity. *Medicine and Science in Sports and Exercise, 17,* 94–100.

Morgan, W. P. (1985b). Psychogenic factors and exercise metabolism: A review. *Medicine and Science in Sports and Exercise, 17,* 309–316.

Morgan, W. P., & Horstman, D. H. (1976). Anxiety reduction following acute physical activity. *Medicine and Science in Sports, 8,* 62 (abstract).

Morgan, W. P., Roberts, J. A., Brand, F. R., & Feinerman, A. D. (1970). Psychological effect of chronic physical activity. *Medicine and Science in Sports, 2,* 213–217.

Morgan, W. P., Roberts, J. A., & Feinerman, A. D. (1971). Psychologic effect of acute physical activity. *Archives of Physical Medicine and Rehabilitation, 52,* 422–425.

Nowlis, D. P., & Greenberg, N. (1979). Empirical description of effects of exercise on mood. *Perceptual and Motor Skills, 49,* 1001–1002.

Pineda, A., & Adkisson, M. (1961). Electroencephalographic studies in physical fatigue. *Texas Reports of Biological Medicine, 19,* 332–342.

Pitts, F. N., Jr., & McClure, J. N., Jr. (1967). Lactate metabolism in anxiety neurosis. *New England Journal of Medicine, 277,* 1329–1336.

Raglin, J. S., & Morgan, W. P. (1986). Influence of acute exercise and quiet rest on state anxiety and blood pressure. *Medicine and Science in Sports and Exercise, 19,* 456–463.

Ransford, C. P. (1982). A role for amines in the antidepressant effect of exercise: A review. *Medicine and Science in Sports and Exercise, 14,* 1–10.

Ray, W. J., & Cole, H. W. (1985). EEG alpha activity reflects attentional demands and beta activity reflects emotional and cognitive processes. *Science, 228,* 750–752.

Reeves, D. L., Justesen, D. R., Levinson, D. M., Riffle, D. W., & Wike, G. L. (1985). Endogenous hyperthermia in normal human subjects: I. Experimental study of evoked potentials and reaction time. *Physiological Psychology, 13,* 258–267.

Russell, P. O., Epstein, L. H., & Erickson, K. T. (1983). Effects of acute exercise and cigarette smoking on autonomic and neuromuscular responses to a cognitive stressor. *Psychological Reports, 53,* 199–206.

Sackeim, H. A., & Weber, S. L. (1982). Functional brain asymmetry in the regulation of emotion: Implications for bodily manifestations of stress. In L. Goldberger & S. Breznitz (Eds.), *Handbook of stress* (pp. 183–199). New York: Free Press.

Santiago, T. V., & Edelman, N. H. (1985). Opioids and breathing. *Journal of Applied Physiology, 59,* 1675–1685.

Seemann, J. C. (1978). *Changes in state anxiety following vigorous exercise.* Unpublished master's thesis, University of Arizona.

Sime, W. E. (1977). A comparison of exercise and meditation in reducing physiological response to stress. *Medicine and Science in Sports, 9,* 55 (abstract).

Solomon, R. L., & Corbit, J. D. (1973). An opponent-process theory of motivation: II. Cigarette addiction. *Journal of Abnormal Psychology, 81,* 158–171.

Sothmann, M. S., & Ismail, A. H. (1984). Relationships between urinary catecholamine metabolites, particularly MHPG, and selected personality and physical fitness characteristics in normal subjects. *Psychosomatic Medicine, 46,* 523–533.

Surwillo, W. W. (1975). The EEG in the prediction of human reaction time. *Biological Psychology, 3,* 79–90.

Tucker, L. A., Cole, G. E., & Friedman, G. M. (1986). Physical fitness: A buffer against stress. *Perceptual and Motor Skills, 63,* 955–961.

Von Euler, C., & Soderberg, U. (1957). The influence of hypothalamic thermoceptive structures on the electroencephalogram and gamma motor activity. *Electroencephalography and Clinical Neurophysiology, 9,* 391–408.

Walker, B. B., & Sandman, C. A. (1979). Human visual evoked responses are related to heart rate. *Journal of Comparative and Physiological Psychology, 93,* 717–729.

Walker, B. B., & Sandman, C. A. (1982). Visual evoked potentials change as heart rate and carotid pressure change. *Psychophysiology, 19,* 520–527.

Wiese, J., Singh, M., & Yeudall, L. (1983). Occipital and parietal alpha power before, during and after exercise. *Medicine and Science in Sports and Exercise, 15,* 117.

Wilson, V. E., Berger, B. G., & Bird, E. I. (1981). Effects of running and of an exercise class on anxiety. *Perceptual and Motor Skills, 53,* 472–474.

Wood, D. T. (1977). The relationship between state anxiety and acute physical activity. *American Corrective Therapy Association Journal, 31,* 67–69.

3

ANXIETY REDUCTION AND STRESS MANAGEMENT THROUGH PHYSICAL FITNESS

Ronald B. Simono

University of North Carolina at Charlotte

In this chapter we will look at the extent to which we can authoritatively state that physical fitness through exercise is a viable means by which individuals can alleviate the negative consequences of anxiety and stress. Stress and anxiety are considered together because investigators often couple these two concepts in their research and, more important, because anxiety and stress often share the same psychophysiological responses.

Anxiety as defined here encompasses the type of anxiety experienced by people in general as part of normal living and excludes from consideration anxiety more closely associated with categories of behavior seen in such systems as the *Diagnostic and Statistical Manual of Mental Disorders* (Third Edition-Revised) (American Psychiatric Association, 1987). Some of what is included here may have relevance for individuals with traditional anxiety disorders, but that is not an intended result. Anxiety is an unpleasant feeling that has both a psychological and physiological component. Thoughts, feelings, and bodily sensations are all often a part of this negative state. Many of the studies designed to look at the impact of exercise on anxiety differentiate between trait anxiety and state anxiety. Trait anxiety is seen as a consistent personality characteristic that can be observed as a feeling of apprehension or uneasiness across a wide variety of situations. State anxiety is described as a more transitory aspect of an individual's personality that would be seen or observed only in specific situations, such as the worry or dread that an individual might experience at the time of a very important job interview.

Stress can be defined as a response that individuals have when they must deal with demands in the environment that require them to adapt to often novel situations that might be perceived to be beyond their capabilities. When in such situations, individuals commonly report feelings of anxiety; therefore it seems logical to examine the effect of exercise on both of these. The psychological aspects of stress conditions are often immediately available to the individual experiencing them in the form of negative thoughts and uncomfortable feelings. However, the physiological side of these situations is often not immediately in the individual's awareness, although these physiological responses might be equally intense. Psychological stress will generate the same neurophysiological response as actual physical danger. The brain and the neuroendocrine systems translate psychological/physical stress into a physiological response primarily through the involuntary or autonomic nervous system. One challenge is to determine what, if any, role exercise might have with the two parts of the autonomic nervous system involved, the sympathetic and parasympathetic systems. If physical fitness through exercise is therapeutic in dealing with exercise and/ or stress, is this due to a real modification of the neurophysiological responses or is it more simply an alteration in the individual's assessment of the anxiety-inducing or stress-producing experience?

If there are changes that we can associate with physical fitness through exercise, exactly what are these changes, and how stable might they be? Personality is commonly seen as long-standing patterns of perceiving, relating to, and thinking about ourselves and the world in which we live. Is this what is altered though exercise? Or is it more likely to be a change in transient mood variables? Are there identifiable personality characteristics that might be predictive of those individuals who achieve a therapeutic effect through exercise? Any movement to promote exercise as an intervention for anxiety and stress should be founded on evidence developed through controlled studies that would help us to determine whether there is such an association and if so, whether the therapeutic effect of exercise is due to behavioral change, changes in attitude, or biochemical changes in the form of endorphins. Finally, some question needs to be raised about the wholesale prescription of exercise for anxiety reduction and stress management because there is some evidence to suggest that anxiety symptoms might be exacerbated by exercise in a small select population that reacts adversely to the increase of lactic acid resulting from physical exertion (Pitts & McClure, 1967).

Writers addressing this topic approach the subject from a variety of angles and define anxiety in different ways, which makes comparative statements about their results very difficult. For some, the presence of anxiety is obtained from a subject's responses to items on instruments such as the State-Trait Anxiety Inventory (STAI) and the Profile of Mood States (POMS). Others assess anxiety by looking at a variety of psychophysiological measures associated with the autonomic nervous system. Others, in a much less definitive fashion, simply obtain very general self-report survey data on levels of anxiety being experienced and events or life experiences that seem to be associated with the anxiety. In the literature exercise is also a term that, out of the context of the particular work, does not tell us much about what was being considered. For example, some writers are very exact and not only describe the kind of exercise that subjects participated in but also define "moderate" and "heavy" exercise in terms of a certain percentage of maximum heart rate or maximum oxygen uptake measured in quite precise ways. On the other hand, some define exercise as participation in "an aerobics class" without informing the reader about the specifics of the exercise activity or its intensity. Finally, some investigators use the laboratory situation to induce anxiety and/or stress responses in individuals by having them perform a variety of different tasks. This way of looking at the association between autonomic nervous system arousal and exercise is much in contrast with that which simply asks subjects to rate their anxiety in response to a stimulus or set of stimuli.

Folkins and Sime (1981) have written a very comprehensive and useful review of research on the effects of physical fitness training on cognition, perception, behavior, affect, and personality. Included in their work were studies that focused on the actual clinical application of physical fitness training vis-à-vis a range of personal problems often seen in clinical practice. In addition, they looked at five specific studies in which the primary focus was anxiety reduction and concluded that there was clear evidence to support the notion that physical fitness training is beneficial when the goal is anxiety reduction. In another helpful review of the related literature, Browman (1981) concluded that light to moderate exercise was not significant enough to substantially alter mood in a population with clinically significant indices of anxiety, but did acknowledge that exercise would probably have some effect on those with non-pathological symptoms. The speculation that exercise had to be of a very high intensity to affect an anxious state has some support in the literature and is mentioned later in this chapter. Browman suggested that some optimal level of regular exercise is advisable but specifying exactly what program on the basis of the research is difficult. However, "too much" or "too little" exercise is often associated with a disturbance in emotional areas.

Hughes (1984) has written an excellent review of the methodological deficits, including a look at the expectancies with which a person approaches such research projects. It is commonly known that many individuals have an a priori belief that exercise is going to reap some psychological benefits. Hughes reviewed 12 studies on the psychological effects of habitual exercise, and 4 of them were on anxiety. He found exercise to relieve anxiety in 2 of these studies and proposed that (a) cognitive diversion was the agent that lessened anxiety, (b) the experience of mastery gained through exercise was the therapeutic aspect, or (c) exercise improves an individual's accuracy of perception of somatic signals and therefore affects the labeling of something as "anxious." "In summary, the enthusiastic support of exercise to improve mental health has a limited empirical basis and lacks a well tested rationale" (Hughes, 1984, p. 76).

Specific target populations are sometimes the focus of attempts to examine the relation between anxiety reduction and physical fitness. For example, Morgan and Pollock (1976) reviewed a number of studies regarding the association between cardiovascular health and psychological factors. They concluded that the studies strongly supported "psychological gains" including less tension and anxiety from regular exercise.

Other writers have not attempted to establish empirically a relation between anxiety reduction and exercise but instead have taken a more promotional stance in extolling the virtues of exercise. Falkenberg (1987) has developed an intriguing model for those who might be interested in setting up an exercise/ fitness program as a way to reduce anxiety/stress in a business or industrial setting. Others support the development of such a program in a wide variety of settings, including not only business and industry but also social service settings, hospitals, and schools (Freeberg, 1984; Rosenbluh, 1985; Rubin & Feeney, 1986). One such intervention was a combination of aerobic exercise and group psychotherapy aimed at clients who were functioning fairly well in their social and work lives but needed some support (VanDenBergh, 1985). This combination of exercise and group support program met 2 hr once a week for a 10-week period. During the 1-hr exercise period, clients could walk, walk/jog, or jog. This would be followed by a 1-hr session discussing topics related to stress and anxiety, including sharing personal experiences. The population in this program was not described, but the author mentioned that this program worked best in "homogeneous" groups. Although there were no specific evaluations of the pre- and posttreatment changes, this did appear to be the kind of exercise–psychotherapy link that is often supported by anecdotal evidence.

Writers in a number of popular exercise periodicals have often suggested, if not declared, that runners, cyclists, and so forth, often have feelings of euphoria due to various biochemical reactions in their bodies as a result of exercise. Endorphins became the topic of conversation as runners gathered at pre- and postrace events and researchers worked in laboratories. *Endorphin* is a generic name for all native brain peptides that act as opiates. Many have proposed that the euphoria associated with the postexercise period is due to a powerful secretion of endorphins (Cooper, Gallman, & McDonald, 1986). Grossman and Sutton (1985) have written an excellent article particularly useful for those not familiar with this topic. They have written very clearly on the measurement of endorphins, their chemical properties, their role in the cardiovascular and respiratory responses to exercise, as well as their connection to the significant responses to growth hormones to exercise. This work should be required reading for those with a limited background in exercise physiology who still want to have some foundation for understanding what definitely appears to be some biochemical response to exercise even if its affective and cognitive components are unclear at the present time.

Researchers have gone about investigating this issue in a variety of ways. Weingarten, Dlin, and Karlsson (1984) looked at the connection between state anxiety and metabolism at the onset of blood lactate accumulation during exercise. Subjects in this study were 23 Israeli national water polo players, an elite group as far as physical fitness was concerned. The researchers found an increased autonomic nervous system response at the preexercise state in those subjects who had been assessed to be high in state anxiety. They also found that those labeled "high state anxious" rated the level of perceived exertion much higher than those at the other end of the anxiety continuum. Other researchers have used highly conditioned athletes to examine this question. Farrell, Gustafson, Morgan, and Pert (1987) studied 7 experienced male distance runners on treadmill workouts that required the use of 40%, 60%, and 80% VO_2 max. (VO_2 max is the maximum amount and rate of oxygen used when an individual is exercising as hard as he or she can.) Sessions consisted of 80-min runs at 40% or 60% and a 40-min run at 80%. Affective factors were measured by the POMS. In this study, it was found that tension and anxiety decreased after the more strenuous runs at time when Leu-Enk RRA (a native brain peptide) was stable.

This finding supported a previous study that found that peripheral levels of endorphins activated by exercise have no effect on mood alterations consequent to exercise (Farrell, Gates, Morgan, & Maksud, 1982). Farrell et al. (1987) also found that there was no tension/anxiety reduction at 40% VO_2 max, which suggested that exercise had to be of a certain intensity to be associated with changes. The earlier Farrell et al. study (1982) had worked with 6 experienced distance runners, 5 males and 1 female. Their experimental sessions consisted of 30-min runs at 60% and 80% VO_2 max and one freely chosen pace. The POMS was administered before and after each run and included a measure of tension and anxiety. They concluded "that exercise stimulates either an increased production or a decreased degradation of endogenous opiate-like ligands" (Farrell et al., 1982, p. 1248) but no conclusions were drawn as to whether this variable affected a runner's perception of strain during runs. Composite measures of mood compared with the baseline values were found to improve by 15 and 16 raw score points for the 60% and 80% VO_2 max conditions, respectively, following exercise. There also was some slight reduction in the composite measure of mood following the freely chosen pace, but the reduction was not found to be statistically significant.

Instead of highly trained individuals, some researchers have used populations closer to what might be described as "normal." For example, Hull, Young, and Ziegler (1984) chose subject groups with varying degrees of aerobic fitness ranging in age from 21 to 64 (35 males and 20 females). Baseline systolic blood pressure and relative diastolic responses to a film of serious industrial accidents, a word color task, and exercise were lower in fit subjects over age 40 than in less fit subjects of the same age groups. Norepinephrine was lower after 9 min of exercise in fit subjects but was much higher at exhaustion, which reflected a significantly greater amount of work done by fit subjects. Norepinephrine levels fell rapidly and were not different among groups 10 min after exercise. They concluded that there was no "preferential generalization" of the "fitness effect" to the active psychological task (i.e., the Stroop Word Color Task). All the stressors, which included the film, the Stroop Word Color Task, a cold-pressor test, and running to exhaustion, elevated epinephrine responses, but aerobic fitness was not associated with lower epinephrine responses to any stressor.

Another study looked at the tranquilizing effect of high-intensity exercise and contrasted these results with light to moderate exercise previously reported as optimal (Bulbian & Darabos, 1986). In this study, the subjects were a mixture of 10 college students and faculty ages 20–45 (5 males and 5 females). All were described as "experienced runners" and this was specifically defined as a VO_2 max of 55.8. Ten subjects acted as their own control in a crossover design. The treatments included high-intensity exercise defined as 75% VO_2 max for 20 min on a treadmill, low intensity defined as 40% VO_2 max for 20 min on a treadmill, and a nonexercise period during which the subjects sat quietly and read. The researchers used resting muscle electromyogram as an index of muscular tension or stress and the Hoffman reflex as an index of spinal cord alpha motor neuron excitability. Measurements of the direct stimulation of motor nerve fibers and the accompanying motoneuron excitability were made. Statistical interpretations of these measurements demonstrated that both high- and low-intensity exercise resulted in a significant calming effect but that high-intensity exercise was significantly better than low-intensity exercise.

Peronnet, Blier, Brisson, Diamond, Le Doux, and Volle (1986) compared plasma catecholamine concentration at rest and in response to exercise in subjects who were designated as low and high in trait anxiety. One hundred forty-nine subjects were administered a standard measure of trait anxiety, and 6 were identified as low and 6 as high. Plasma norepinephrine and epinephrine were measured at rest and during mild to moderate exercise (i.e., 40% and 60% VO_2 max) on a bicycle ergometer. Plasma epinephrine at rest and exercise was not significantly different in low- or high-trait-anxiety groups. Plasma norepinephrine was not significantly different at rest and mild exercise in low- or high-trait-anxiety groups but was significantly higher in the high-anxiety group than in the low-anxiety group in response to *moderate* exercise. Therefore, plasma catecholamine response to exercise was related to subjects' psychological characteristics.

Grossman, Bouloux, and Price (1984) conducted a double-blind crossover and randomized study with 6 male subjects considered to be normal as far as physical fitness was concerned. They exercised at 40% and 80% VO_2 max on a bicycle ergometer for 20 min under each condition (mild and severe). The subjects exercised with and without a high dose of naloxone, an opiate antagonist. A psychological questionnaire that was not specified suggested very minor mood changes after exercise but no evidence of the runner's high or euphoria. They found that the endogenous opioids seemed to be important in perception of effect at intense levels of effort.

Many investigations have not looked at the biochemical connection. For example, one study contrasted responses of 15 highly trained and 15 untrained individuals ages 20–30 years (Sinyor, Schwortz, Peronnet, Brisson, & Seraganian, 1983). Part of the experimental condition was a stress session that included mental arithmetic problems with exposure to white noise. Also included was the Electrocardiogram Quiz and the Stroop Word Color Task. Measures taken included VO_2 max, aerobic points earned, heart rate, subjective arousal level (SAL), the STAI, and a biochemical analysis. Heart rate and SAL increased significantly during the stress task for both the highly trained as well as the untrained group. However, the highly trained group as we would suspect, showed significantly faster recovery on physiological indices (i.e., heart rate) and on the anxiety measures obtained from the STAI. The biochemical analysis showed that during the stress task peak norepinephrine response occurred significantly earlier in the highly trained individuals than in the untrained.

A similar study (Sinyor, Golden, Steinert, & Seraganian, 1986) looked at 38 males ages 20–30 who were randomly assigned to an aerobic, an anaerobic (i.e., weight lifting), or a wait list control group. The experimental group met three to four times per week in 1-hr sessions and were tested 2 weeks prior to treatment including a STAI. The senior author again used a mental arithmetic task with exposure to white noise, a brief version of the Electrocardiogram Quiz and the Stroop Word Color Task. No group differences were found at pretreatment time on all of the physical measures. *All three groups* showed marked elevations in arousal during stress periods, followed by reductions by recovery. Subjects in all three groups showed reductions in anxiety following the psychosocial stress session and this reduction remained unchanged as a function of treatment.

Roskies, Seraganian, Oseasohn, Hanley, and Coller (1986) also did a comparative study when they looked at aerobic exercise, cognitive–behavioral stress management, and weight training in modifying behavioral and cardiovascular reactivity to psychosocial stressors in a laboratory situation. This research included 33 subjects in the aerobics segment, 37 in the cognitive–behavioral stress management segment, and 37 subjects in the weight training segment. All subjects were male. They were assessed to be "healthy" Type A men as assessed by the Structured Interview. The stress tasks that the subjects performed were again as in the other studies, a mental arithmetic task as well as the Raven's Progressive Matrices task. The aerobic exercise consisted of jogging for 20–25 min at an intensity that was sufficient to attain an individually determined heart rate. The treatment effects were measured by behavioral reactivity changes to the Structured Interview, heart rate changes, and changes in systolic and diastolic blood pressure. The stress management group showed significantly greater changes in behavioral reactivity reductions than did the aerobics group and the weight training group. In addition, the two exercise groups did not differ significantly from each other. Equally important was the finding that changes in physical reactivity were "trivial" for all three treatments.

Another study induced stress with a video game as well as a mental arithmetic task (Perkins, Dubbert, Martin, & Faulstich, 1986). This study included males ages 21–63, 18 of whom were mildly hypertensive and 9 of whom were normotensive. Eleven of the 18 mildly hypertensive subjects did a 10-week aerobic training program. The normotensive subjects did not exercise at all. Measures in response to the stressors in the laboratory situation were systolic and diastolic blood pressure as well as heart rate in order to measure cardiovascular reactivity. The aerobically trained mildly hypertensive subjects reacted to the video game stress task with only half of the diastolic blood pressure increase and two-thirds of the systolic blood pressure increase of comparable but untrained mildly hypertensive subjects. The heart rate reactivity showed no difference between trained and untrained individuals. There was no significant difference on the mental arithmetic task in heart rate or blood pressure.

Some studies have not come from laboratory situations in which stress was actually induced during the course of the treatments. Bahrke and Morgan (1978) took 75 adult males ranging in age from 22 to 71 and randomly assigned 25 each to an exercise program consisting of walking for 20 min on a treadmill at 70% self-imposed maximum heart rate, a meditation group who listened to tape recorded instruction describing Benson's relaxation response, and a control group who simply rested in a recliner. All three groups had decreased anxiety across time as measured by the STAI. There were no significant differences between the three groups. The researchers also combined the three groups and divided subjects into high and low trait anxiety and then did find some decrease in anxiety for both on state anxiety values. The authors concluded that "simply taking time out is as effective" as exercise or meditation. This was certainly a strong piece of data to support the notion that diversion may be as important as anything in alleviating symptoms of anxiety.

Berger and Owen (1983) looked at college students ages 17–50 who were in swimming classes and compared them with individuals in physical education and health science lecture courses. The swim classes met twice a week for 40-min sessions for 14 weeks. The control classes met three times a week for 14 weeks at 50-min periods. The measurement used was the POMS. Swimmers reported significantly greater pre- and postclass changes than did the controls on depression, anger, vigor, and confusion. Within the swim groups there were significant pre- to postclass changes on tension/anxiety, depression, anger, vigor, and confusion. There was no evidence in this study to suggest that the size of the pre- to postclass mood changes was different for males versus females.

One study compared an exercise class with a "hobby or interest" class (Lichtman & Poser, 1983). This study consisted of 64 subjects, 28 of whom were male and 36 were female. Thirty-two were in a YMCA or YWCA exercise class and 32 were in a hobby group. The exercise consisted of 45 min of jogging and other physical activities. Mood was assessed by the Nowlis Mood Scale and the POMS. There were significant pre- to postclass changes on the tension/anxiety scale of the POMS and the depression/dejection, anger/hostility, fatigue/enertia, and confusion scales for the exercise group. However, the hobby and interest group also had significant pre- to postclass changes on tension/anxiety. There were no significant pre- to postclass differences on the Nowlis Mood Scale for anxiety in either the exercise or the hobby and interest group.

Another study using the POMS took 21 sedentary individuals who had volunteered for a fitness program (Hughes, Cosol, & Leon, 1986). The subjects had not exercised in the preceding year and were described as having no "psychiatric or psychological" problems. Subjects were assigned to a control or an exercise group for 12 weeks followed by a 4-week "washout period"; then the subjects switched the last 12 weeks. The exercise was treadmill, walking, and stair climbing, while the other group was involved in watching television, listening to music, or reading. Subjects were asked to abstain from exercise outside the treatment programs. The POMS showed no improvement in exercise in anger, anxiety, confusion, fatigue, vigor, or total mood disturbance. In this study, the authors did speculate that there were no positive outcomes because of the randomized crossover design, the low intensity of the exercise, exercise without a socialization aspect, or the fact that the subjects were free of any significant psychological problems.

A unique study was done with employees in a hospital equipment facility in northwest Pennsylvania (Bruning & Frew, 1987). A group of 350 supervisors, managers, engineers, and technical and other support personnel formed the group from which the subjects were selected. Eighty-six of them volunteered to participate in the study and 65 completed a 6-month study. Their ages were 23–60 and most of them were married. The subjects were randomly assigned to four groups (management skills, meditation, exercise, or control). The exercise group was asked to spend 30 min every other day at some aerobic activity of their choice. They were instructed to raise their heart rate by at least 15% of normal but no more than 75%. All three experimental groups significantly changed heart rate and systolic blood pressure, which were used as physiological measures of stress. One drawback to this research program was the fact that the exercise group was on their own to determine exercise. In addition, Bruning and Frew lost their control group because controls wanted training also and started exercising on their own, therefore invalidating themselves as a control group.

Long (1984) examined 44 females and 17 males ranging in age from 24 to 65 who were volunteers from the community, 80% of whom had previously sought help for stress and anxiety reduction. The subjects were assigned to aerobic exercise (jogging), stress inoculation training, and a control/waiting list. The programs went on for 10 weeks at 1½ hr per week. Both the aerobic exercise and the stress inoculation training were effective in reducing self-reported anxiety. In addition, this was maintained for 3 months after the end of the program. The STAI was used in this research and the differences were found in both the state and trait factors. Long also checked expectations of outcome from all three groups and no group differences were found. An interesting sidelight was the researcher's classification of the subjects into "somatic" or "cognitive" anxiety as determined by the Cognitive–Somatic Anxiety Questionnaire. Subjects did not respond differentially to treatments considered most effective for their type. Finally, because self-efficacy is often considered critical in exercise reduction, this variable was examined and it was found that the performance-based aerobics program did not result in greater perceptions of self-efficacy than the stress inoculation did. Both groups increased perceived self-efficacy. In a follow-up to this study 15 months later, Long (1985) located 45 of the original 61 subjects. Both the jogging and the stress inoculation training groups still equally reported less anxiety on both the trait and state scales of the STAI and greater self-efficacy. However, it was ironic that only 40% of the jogging group were still jogging at this follow-up some 15 months later.

Morgan and Hortsman (1976) used as subjects both "normals" and clinically anxious individuals in an approach that used the STAI during and following exercise at 80% VO_2 max. There were 215 subjects (177 male and 38 female). They found that state anxiety increased during the first half of exercise, reached a plateau, and remained elevated through exercise. Decrements in anxiety commenced immediately following exercise and significant decreases continued. Raglin and Morgan (1987) used the STAI to look at 15 normotensive subjects instructed to rest quietly for 40 min and then perform aerobic exercise on separate occasions. The systolic and diastolic blood pressures as well as state anxiety were reduced on measures following exercise. They also applied the same conditions for 15 pharmacologically controlled hypertensive subjects and found that systolic blood pressure and state anxiety reduced significantly following both conditions. They reported that the antianxiety effects were sustained for a longer period of time following exercise.

In another study, 48 male patients who had had a heart attack or bypass surgery were randomly assigned to either a no-treatment control or a cardiac rehabilitation program (Roviaro, Holmes, & Holmsten, 1984). As in other studies, general anxiety was measured by the trait anxiety scale of the STAI and anxiety specific to the patient's heart problem. There were no differences found on either the trait anxiety scale or the cardiac anxiety questionnaire. One interesting note is that the patients' scores on the trait anxiety scale were well below the 50th percentile for normals at entry.

Steptoe and Cox (1988) looked at 32 female medical students in a single-session experiment in which there were two 8-min trials of high-intensity exercise and two 8-min trials of low-intensity exercise on a bicycle ergometer. One high-intensity and one low-intensity exercise period were accompanied by music, and the other high-intensity and low-intensity periods were accompanied by metronome. For measurement the modified version of the POMS was used at pre- and postexercise for each trial, and the subjects were classified as fit and unfit on the basis of heart rate. Also used was the trait anxiety scale of the STAI. It was found that high-intensity exercise led to *increases* in tension/anxiety.

Wilson, Berger, and Bird (1981) did a quick study using 11 male and 9 female runners, 2 males and 10 females in an organized exercise class, and 6 males and 4 females who were simply eating lunch at a YMCA. They used the STAI to measure state anxiety pre- and postactivity and found that all three groups showed significant decreases in anxiety after the three activities, with no significant differences between groups.

A similar lack of differences was found with 26 males and 26 females recruited from a university community medical center when half of them were assigned randomly to a treadmill group and the other half to a control group that sat at rest (Ewing, Scott, Mendez, & McBride, 1984). In this study, the POMS was used and certain aspects of cognitive functioning were also measured using the Rorschach Ink Blots and Holtzman Blots. Those subjects who were in the exercise group continued on a treadmill to 70% of predicted maximum heart rate. Both the group who sat at rest and the exercise group had significant reductions in tension/anxiety as measured on the POMS.

In a private all-female secondary school, Brown and Lawton (1986) looked at 220 students ages 11–17. Life stress was assessed using the Schedule of Recent Events and students' exercise habits were assessed. There was no correlation between stress events and anxiety and exercise, but the researchers did find that those who "exercised infrequently were more vulnerable to stress induced deteriorations in emotional well-being" (Brown & Lawton, 1986, p. 130). A similar study with 212 students in Grades 7–11 measured the amount of time spent weekly in 14 types of physical activity ranging from jogging and swimming to yoga. Also used was a measure of life events that resulted in a stress score and a modified version of the Seriousness of Illness Rating Scale. This study concluded that "the negative impact of high stress declined as the amount of time spent in vigorous activity increased" (Brown & Siegel, 1988, p. 341). Another group of 83 subjects enrolled in an individual exercise program in a university setting were studied in order to determine whether an exercise program would be associated with an improvement in terms of reduced tension/anxiety as measured by the POMS (Wilfley & Kunce, 1986). Forty-nine of the

83 subjects completed an 8-week exercise program and showed statistically significant improvement in terms of reduced psychological tension/anxiety. When the authors further examined initial levels of fitness and stress, they found that changes in stress following exercise occurred only for those who were below the mean of the sample both physically and psychologically before the start of the program. Continuing the theme of looking at stressful life events, Kobasa, Maddi, and Puccetti (1982) took 137 male middle to upper management personnel selected at random and had them complete a question-naire of life events and illness symptoms as well as a measure of "personality hardiness" and exercise. There were no specific treatments for exercise, and the subjects simply self-reported on their exercise activities. There was no correlation between exercise and "personality hardiness," which was defined as feeling in control, optimistic, and decisive. It was speculated that if an individ-ual is "hardy," he or she doesn't need the stress- and anxiety-reducing effects of exercise.

In an attempt to look at a specific profession in terms of the benefits of exercise, Barrow, English, and Pinkerton (1987) examined 196 North Carolina psychologists who were listed in the *National Register of Health Service Pro-viders in Psychology*. Seventy-one percent of them regularly exercised, and the most positive effect that they associated with exercise was physical stamina/energy level followed very closely by mood and mental stamina/energy level. Ninety-three percent of the psychologists reported that they would recommend exercise as an intervention for anxiety to their clients. A single case example of such an intervention was presented by Muller and Armstrong (1975). They described a single case study of a person with "elevator phobia" whose treat-ment consisted initially of the therapist's jogging with the client to a department store, which resulted in the client's being fatigued and out of breath and having a rapid heart rate as well as weakness in the legs. Of course, all of these symptoms had been associated with her phobia, but in the instance after the initial exercise the patient was calm and agreed to ride the elevator up and down one floor but was unable to take a second ride until the same jogging routine was repeated. Taller and taller buildings were approached and a session was added about information about the actual mechanisms of elevator operation. For example, the client was shown how escape from the elevator was very easy. The authors concluded by saying "the experience of running" made legitimate "high levels of arousal without the need to employ 'panic' as an explanation" (Muller & Armstrong, 1975, p. 386).

There seems to be little doubt from the literature that exercise is an effective way of lessening the negative consequences associated with anxiety and stress for some individuals under some circumstances. Exactly how this occurs, how-ever, is certainly not clear. When a relation exists between exercise and anxiety reduction, it probably is due to a combination of factors and not to one in isolation. That is, the person may perceive events as being less anxiety producing, having an increased sense of self-efficacy, have his or her attention diverted away from anxiety-inducing stimuli, or experience biochemical and physiological changes as a result of strenuous exercise. Because there are little longitudinal data on physical fitness through exercise as a way to alleviate anxiety, there is no support for the notion that long-term personality changes are brought about by exercise. Research has demonstrated that the outcomes of such studies are significantly affected by the anxiety level of the subjects, their initial level of physical fitness, and the intensity of the exercise. The exercise has to be of a certain high level of intensity before effects are witnessed, and decrements in anxiety will probably occur more often in those whose anxiety is elevated and those who have a low level of physical fitness. What we might be seeing when those with elevated anxiety and low fitness show improvement could well be regression toward the mean. There is evidence to suggest that physical fitness might operate as a buffer against anxiety in some individuals and, in addition, be associated with an individual's ability to respond faster to and cope more effectively with anxiety-producing stimuli. However, there are very little data to support the notion that exercise is any more effective in anxiety reduction than other activities such as reading, meditation, or some hobby or special interest that can divert the individual's attention to stimuli that arouse pleasant feelings.

REFERENCES

American Psychiatric Association. (1987). *Diagnostic and statistical manual of mental disorders* (3rd ed., rev.). Washington, DC: Author.

Bahrke, M. S., & Morgan, W. P. (1978). Anxiety reduction following exercise and meditation. *Cognitive Therapy and Research, 2,* 323, 333.

Barrow, J. C., English, T., & Pinkerton, R. S. (1987). Physical fitness training: Beneficial for professional psychologists. *Professional Psychology: Research and Practice, 18,* 66–70.

Berger, B. G., & Owen, D. R. (1983). Mood alteration with swimming—swimmers really do "feel better." *Journal of Psychosomatic Research, 45,* 425–433.

Browman, C. P. (1981). Physical activity as a therapy for psychopathology: A reappraisal. *Journal of Sports Medicine and Physical Fitness, 21,* 192–197.

Brown, J. D., & Lawton, M. (1986). Stress and well-being in adolescence: The moderating role of physical exercise. *Journal of Human Stress, 12*(3), 125–131.

Brown, J. D., & Siegel, J. M. (1988). Exercise as a buffer of life stress: A prospective study of adolescent health. *Health Psychology, 7,* 341–353.

Bruning, N. S., & Frew, D. R. (1987). Effects of exercise, relaxation, and management skills training on physiological stress indicators: A field experiment. *Journal of Applied Psychology, 72,* 515–521.

Bulbian, R., & Darabos, B. L. (1986). Motor neuron excitability: The Hoffman reflex following exercise of low and high intensity. *Medicine and Science in Sports and Exercise, 18,* 697–702.

Cooper, K. H., Gallman, J. S., & McDonald, J. L. (1986). Role of aerobic exercise in reduction of stress. *Dental Clinics of North America, 30* (Supplement), 5133–5142.

Ewing, J. H., Scott, D. G., Mendez, A. A., & McBride, T. J. (1984). Effects of aerobic exercise on affect and cognition. *Perceptual and Motor Skills, 59,* 407–414.

Falkenberg, L. E. (1987). Employee fitness programs: Their impact on the employee and the organization. *Academy of Management Review, 12,* 511–522.

Farrell, P. A., Gates, W. K., Morgan, W. P., & Maksud, M. G. (1982). Increases in plasma β-endorphins/β-lipotropin immunoreactivity after treadmill running in humans. *Journal of Applied Physiology, 52,* 1245–1249.

Farrell, P. A., Gustafson, A. B., Morgan, W. P., & Pert, C. B. (1987). Enkephalins, catecholamines, and psychological mood alterations: Effects of prolonged exercise. *Medicine and Science in Sports and Exercise, 19,* 347–353.

Folkins, C. H., & Sime, W. E. (1981). Physical fitness training and mental health. *American Psychologist, 36,* 373–389.

Freeberg, S. G. (1984). Effortless exercises to balance daily executive stress. *Journal of Rehabilitation Administration, 8,* 128–132.

Grossman, A., Bouloux, P., & Price, P. (1984). The role of opioid peptides in the hormonal responses to acute exercise in man. *Clinical Science, 67,* 483–491.

Grossman, A., & Sutton, J. R. (1985). Endorphins: What are they? How are they measured? What is their role in exercise? *Medicine and Science in Sports and Exercise, 17,* 74–81.

Hughes, J. R. (1984). Psychological effects of habitual aerobic exercise: A critical review. *Preventive Medicine, 13,* 66–78.

Hughes, J. R., Cosol, D. C., & Leon, A. S. (1986). Psychological effects of exercise: A randomized cross-over trial. *Journal of Psychosomatic Research, 30,* 355–360.

Hull, E. M., Young, S. H., & Ziegler, M. G. (1984). Aerobic fitness affects cardiovascular and catecholamine responses to stressors. *Psychophysiology, 21,* 353–360.

Kobasa, S. C., Maddi, S. R., & Puccetti, M. C. (1982). Personality and exercise as buffers in the stress–illness relationship. *Journal of Behavioral Medicine, 5,* 391–404.

Lichtman, S., & Poser, E. G. (1983). The effects of exercise on mood and cognitive functioning. *Journal of Psychosomatic Research, 27,* 43–52.

Long, B. C. (1984). Aerobic conditioning and stress inoculation: A comparison of stress management interventions. *Cognitive Therapy and Research, 8,* 517–541.

Long, B. C. (1985). Stress management interventions: A fifteen-month follow up of aerobic conditioning and stress inoculation training. *Cognitive Therapy and Research, 9,* 471–478.

Morgan, W. P., & Hortsman, D. H. (1976). Anxiety reduction following acute physical activity. *Medicine and Science in Sports, 8,* 62.

Morgan, W. P., & Pollock, M. L. (1976). *Physical activity and cardiovascular health: Psychological aspects.* Paper presented at the International Congress of Physical Activity Science, Quebec City.

Muller, B., & Armstrong, H. E. (1975). A further note on the "running treatment" for anxiety. *Psychotherapy: Theory, Research, and Practice, 12,* 385–387.

Perkins, K. A., Dubbert, P. M., Martin, J. E., & Faulstich, M. E. (1986). Cardiovascular reactivity to psychological stress in aerobically trained versus untrained mild hypertensives and normotensives. *Health Psychology, 5,* 407–421.

Peronnet, F., Blier, P., Brisson, G., Diamond, P., Le Doux, M., & Volle, M. (1986). Plasma catecholamines at rest and exercise in subjects with high and low trait anxiety. *Psychosomatic Medicine, 48*(1–2), 52–58.

Pitts, F. N., & McClure, J. N. (1967). Lactate metabolism in anxiety neurosis. *New England Journal of Medicine, 277,* 1329–1336.

Raglin, J. S., & Morgan, W. P. (1987). Influence of exercise and quiet rest on state anxiety and blood pressure. *Medicine and Science in Sports and Exercise, 19,* 456–463.

Rosenbluh, E. S. (1985). Exercise, body chemistry and stress. *Emotional First Aid, 2,* 33–43.

Roskies, E., Seraganian, P., Oseasohn, R., Hanley, J. A., & Coller, R. (1986). The Montreal Type A intervention project: Major findings. *Health Psychology, 5,* 45–69.

Roviaro, S., Holmes, D. S., & Holmsten, R. D. (1984). Influence of a cardiac rehabilitation program on the cardiovascular, psychological, and social functioning of cardiac patients. *Journal of Behavioral Medicine, 7,* 61–81.

Rubin, D. C., & Feeney, C. (1986). A multicomponent stress management program for college students. *Journal of Counseling and Development, 64,* 531.

Sinyor, D., Golden, M., Steinert, Y., & Seraganian, P. (1986). Experimental manipulation of aerobic fitness and the response to psychosocial stress: Heart rate and self-report measures. *Psychosomatic Medicine, 48,* 334–337.

Sinyor, D., Schwortz, S. G., Peronnet, F., Brisson, G., & Seraganian, P. (1983). Aerobic fitness level and reactivity to psychosocial stress: Physiological, biochemical, and subjective measure. *Psychosomatic Medicine, 45*, 205–217.

Steptoe, A., & Cox, S. (1988). Acute effects of aerobic exercise on mood. *Health Psychology, 7*, 329–340.

VanDenBergh, N. (1985). Aerobic therapy: A feminist/wholistic approach in time-limited group practice. *Social Work with Groups, 8*(2), 125–130.

Weingarten, G., Dlin, R. A., & Karlsson, J. (1984). The relationship between state anxiety, muscularity, and metabolic responses at the "OBLA point." *International Journal of Sport Psychology, 15*(2), 110–116.

Wilfley, D., & Kunce, J. T. (1986). Differential physical and psychological effects of exercise. *Journal of Counseling Psychology, 33*, 337–342.

Wilson, V. E., Berger, B. G., & Bird, E. I. (1981). Effects of running and of an exercise class on anxiety. *Perceptual and Motor Skills, 53*, 472–474.

4

STEROID AND DRUG USE BY ATHLETES

Linda L. Weinhold

National Institute on Drug Abuse Addiction Research Center

Beginning on the play grounds and continuing through grade school, high school, college, and the amateur elite and professional ranks, athletics provides a common bond in American culture. People from all walks of life share the joys and pain of competition, as participants and as spectators. Illicit drug use among athletes is shocking to Americans who feel admiration for sports figures, both amateur and professional. . . . While acknowledging the limits of the mandate of the Conference, the Drug-Free Sports Committee of the White House Conference also considered the problem of legal drugs and certain medical practices being used to unfairly increase an athlete's competitive advantage. These include anabolic steroids, stimulants, diuretics and pain-masking drugs and practices such as blood doping and detection avoidance. (White House Conference for a Drug Free America, 1988, p. 105)

PREVALENCE OF DRUG USE BY ATHLETES

There are approximately 20,000 professional athletes in the United States (Cowart, 1986). The prevalence of legal and illicit drug use among professional athletes is not known. Deaths of athletes from illicit drug use—for example,

The opinions expressed herein are those of the author and do not necessarily reflect the official position of the National Institute on Drug Abuse or any part of the U.S. Department of Health and Human Services.

those of Len Bias, University of Maryland star basketball player, and Don Rogers, professional football player, who died from cocaine—make front-page news and raise questions about the magnitude of illicit drug use by athletes. It is estimated, however, that the prevalence of illicit use among athletes is no greater than in the general population.

The use of ergogenic aids—performance-enhancing drugs such as steroids, stimulants, diuretics, and pain-masking drugs, commonly referred to as doping substances—is banned for use by the International Olympic Committee (IOC) and the U.S. Olympic Committee (USOC). Urine specimens provided by elite athletes who participate in international events serve as a measure of compliance with the committees' antidoping regulations. A study of such urine samples conducted in 1985 revealed,

> Of the 825 specimens analyzed for doping substances [during the 1983 Pan American Games in Caracas], 19 (including two from American athletes) were declared positive for banned substances. Fifteen of those declared positive showed testosterone and/or anabolic steroids in the specimen. Two were positive for stimulants (ephedrine) and two for fencanfamine [a psychomotor stimulant]. (Bergman & Leach, 1985, p. 169)

The prevalence of anabolic steroid use by athletes is not known. According to a 1972 report,

> Between 10 and 25 percent of weight lifters use steroids according to Russell Wright, president of the medical committee of the International Federation of Weight Lifting. But Donald Cooper, medical committee chairman of the National Collegiate Athletic Association (NCAA) says that 80 to 90 percent of all weight lifters in the world are taking steroids. The weight of opinion seems to favor the higher estimate. (Wade, 1972, p. 1400)

Although the prevalence of anabolic steroid use among professional, elite amateur, and collegiate athletes is not known, a study by Buckley et al. (1988) revealed that of the high school male seniors ($N = 3,403$) who completed their questionnaires, 6.6% had used anabolic steroids and two-thirds of this group began using steroids at age 16 or younger. The results quickly generated a great deal of public interest in the issue of steroid abuse among high school athletes.

A report by the *Los Angeles Times* (Scott, 1988) reemphasized the findings of Buckley et al. (1988) that health care professionals were the primary source of steroids for about 20% of the male seniors and that 26.7% of high school users said they used steroids primarily for cosmetic reasons. Yesalis (1988) informed readers that

The Anti Drug Abuse Act of 1988 makes the distribution of anabolic steroids to minors without a prescription a felony punishable by a six-year prison term (distribution to adults is punishable by up to three years in prison). In addition, at least 10 states have passed laws designed to curtail the non-medical use of steroids. (p. 1)

Physicians, however, are not the only source of doping agents. A report by the *Washington Post* (Berkowitz, 1989) indicated that an estimated $400 million to $500 million worth of steroids are trafficked in a national black market that is becoming increasingly more fraternal with the traffic in controlled substances, such as cocaine. In addition, Dr. Frank Young, commissioner of the U.S. Food and Drug Administration, estimates that approximately 10% of all high school students in the United States use anabolic steroids for cosmetic reasons. Finally, Buckley et al. (1988) reported that in their study that there was a group of high school students who habitually used steroids and were psychologically addicted to the steroids.

Public concern about the use of anabolic–androgenic steroids has been reflected in the recent proliferation of scientific publications about the effects of steroid use by athletes. Also, new random urine testing programs have recently been initiated. Cowart (1988) reported in the *Journal of the American Medical Association (JAMA)* on the National Football League's (NFL's) new testing program for anabolic–androgenic steroids begun during the 1988 preseason. The NFL urinalyses returned a 6% user rate, which Cowart felt was an underestimate. Cowart (1989c) reported for *JAMA* that the Pentagon plans to start a pilot program to test some of its military personnel for the use of anabolic steroids— the first time any federal agency will have tested its employees for steroid use.

Most of the effort to curtail steroid use by athletes has been directed toward detection of use through urine-testing programs. Many sports governing bodies issue penalties when steroid use is detected. The last section of this chapter provides details about programs that monitor and invoke penalties for the use of drugs by athletes. Control of the black market in steroids was enacted in 1986 by a task force of the Justice Department, the Federal Bureau of Investigation, and the Food and Drug Administration (Cowart, 1987). Educational programs to prevent the use of steroids are provided in colleges and high schools.

The results from the urine specimen analyses collected during international competition, the estimated prevalence of steroid use by high school students, the recent proliferation of scientific papers on the effects of anabolic steroids, and the recent increase in urine assays for anabolic steroid use clearly indicate that blood doping is a serious problem of great international concern in the sports community. Therefore, the main focus of this chapter is on the use of anabolic–androgenic steroids by athletes. However, the use of other drugs by athletes, especially the stimulants, is also discussed.

The use of steroids by athletes continues to be a controversial issue. Information in this chapter is presented to help the readers draw his or her own conclusions. I offer no opinion about the use of steroids by athletes.

MOTIVATION FOR THE USE
OF ERGOGENIC AIDS

Think about how small the differences usually are between first and second place, between winning and losing (in high level competition). And keep in mind the drive and ambition and the competitive spirit of someone competing at that level. Think about the time, the energy and the pain invested. . . . The financial rewards are, in most cases, minimal, . . . I hate to admit it, but an obsessive–compulsive personality is practically a requirement (for success at these levels). . . . The advice I value most is from people who've been there. . . . The average guy on the street, and even lots of people in sports obviously don't understand the pressures. . . . It's like everything else in life, when it all gets down to the nitty-gritty, you grab anything you can that might give you a winning edge. (A world class athlete during a personal interview with James Edward Wright; Wright, 1978, p. 109)

THE ANABOLIC–ANDROGENIC STEROIDS

Shortly after the synthesis of testosterone from cholesterol by Butenandt and Hanisch in 1935 and Ruzicka and Wettstein in 1935, commercial production of testosterone and its esters began and clinical treatment of endocrine deficiencies was initiated. Kenyon (1938) conducted one of the first clinical investigations in which testosterone and testosterone propionate were administered by injection to treat 4 adult males for eunuchoidism, in which the symptoms were testicular deficiency. Treatment with testosterone propionate resulted in the reversal of androgenic deficits and hence eunuchoidism was treated. However, the anabolic effects of weight gain during treatment also occurred. The weight gain was, in part, attributed to fluid retention caused by a positive shift in the sodium balance. Although 2 subjects also increased food intake during treatment, cessation of the treatment resulted in rapid weight loss for 3 subjects that was attributed to loss of fluids. For the 4th subject, insignificant weight loss accompanied the discontinuance of treatment, thereby suggesting that weight gain may have occurred through changes in the tissue.

Subsequently, a second experiment was conducted by Kenyon, Sandiford, Bryan, Knowlton, and Koch (1938) to investigate whether changes in tissue may have been a treatment side effect. The 4 patients continued on steroid treatment, but dietary intake was controlled. During treatment, a striking drop in total urinary nitrogen and a positive shift in nitrogen balance occurred. These complementary conditions accompany increased protein synthesis and new tissue formation. The authors concluded that although new tissue formation resulted in the treatment of eunuchoidism, the magnitude of the positive shift in nitrogen balance indicated that new tissue was being formed elsewhere. The authors speculated that the site of new tissue formation in eunuchoids undergoing treatment with testosterone propionate probably occurs in muscle.

Since that time, numerous structural variations of testosterone have been produced synthetically; these are the *anabolic–androgenic steroids*. The synthetic derivatives of testosterone that held promise for clinical applications were further tested in the animal laboratory to determine their anabolic : androgenic ratios. The ratios were determined by observing where increases in muscle tissue weight occurred following administration of the steroid, usually to castrated male rats. The comparisons of increase in muscle weight usually were the levator ani muscle (anabolic) versus the ventral prostrate (androgenic). The ratios, therefore, are simply measures of the relation between multiples of weight gain in different muscles. Another indicator of anabolic activity is a temporary positive shift in the nitrogen balance which is usually brought under homeostatic control after 1–2 months of the steroid regimen.

Although the different clinical applications (e.g., hereditary angioneurotic edema and hypogonadism) require different anabolic:androgenic ratios from the steroids to obtain optimal clinical results, it was, and remains, desirable to produce synthetic derivatives of testosterone that show less androgenic activity. To date, the structural variations of testosterone have not resulted in the production of any pure anabolic steroids. Therefore, most authors refer to the synthetic derivatives of testosterone as the anabolic–androgenic steroids, rather than as the anabolic steroids.

In human males, actions of the endogenous androgens are the stimulation of (a) development of the male reproductive tract in utero; (b) growth of the male accessory sex organs, penis, and scrotum at puberty; and (c) long bone growth and subsequent induction of epiphyseal plate closure at puberty. Endogenous androgens also maintain male secondary sex characteristics, increase libido, and perhaps aggravate aggressive behavior in males. Anabolic actions of the anabolic–androgenic steroids are the stimulation of (a) erythropoiesis (production of red blood cells in peripheral blood) and (b) muscle development (Keenan, 1988). The anabolic–androgenic steroids have been prepared for administration by mouth or by injection, usually intramuscularly.

Many of the anabolic–androgenic steroids were prepared for oral use by alkylation of the testosterone molecule at the 17 alpha position and are referred to as the *17 alpha-alkylated androgens*. The 17 alpha-alkylated androgens are more resistant to inactivation by the liver, which increases their half-life. Also, the 17 alpha-alkylated androgens have less affinity for human sex hormone binding globulin (SHBG) and hence are more likely to travel through the circulatory system in a free-active form that allows the steroids greater access to receptor sites. The 17 alpha-alkylated androgens readily bind to their receptors, activate the hormone–receptor complex, and seem to have the anabolic advantage of readily enhancing protein synthesis in muscle cells (Colby & Longhurst, 1988).

Most of the injectable anabolic–androgenic steroids were prepared by esterification of the 17 beta-hydroxyl group of the testosterone molecule, which makes these steroids more lipid soluble. Lipid solutions are absorbed from injection sites into general circulation more slowly than are aqueous solutions. However, drugs vary in their degree of solubility in lipid solutions. In general, there is a positive relation between lipid solubility and duration of action for the anabolic–androgenic steroids. Plasma testosterone levels may be used to monitor the effectiveness of therapy with the 17 beta-hydroxyl androgens because the esters are hydrolyzed back into testosterone before the hormone action begins (Murad & Haynes, 1985).

Table 1 shows some of the anabolic–androgenic steroids that athletes have self-administered. The information has been adapted from tables previously presented by Colby and Longhurst (1988) and Murad and Haynes (1985). Generic and brand (in capital letters) names, the doses prescribed in clinical settings, the route of administration, the dominant function in terms of the anabolic–androgenic ratio, and the structural variation that produced the synthetic derivative are presented for each drug.

Athletes are known to use more than one steroid at a time—a phenomenon known as *stacking*. The anabolic–androgenic steroid mixtures are also at times supplemented by mixtures of the testosterone injectables. An example of a stacking regimen (see Alen, Rahkila, & Marniemi, 1985; Alen, Rahkila, Reinila, & Vihko, 1987; Alen, Reinila, & Vihko, 1985; Kiraly, 1988; Kiraly, Alen, Rahkila, & Horsmanheimo, 1987; Kiraly, Collan, & Alen, 1987; Ruokomen, Alen, Bolton, & Vihko, 1985) is as follows:

Methandienone 5–26 mg/day (orally),
Nandrolone phenpropionate 50 mg/week (intramuscularly),
Stanozol 50 mg/week (intramuscularly), and
Testosterone 250 mg (consisting of:
   testosterone decanoate 100 mg,
   testosterone isocaproate 60 mg,
   testosterone phenylpropionate 60 mg, and
   testosterone propionate 30 mg) once–twice/month (intramuscularly).

Effects of Steroids on Female Athletes' Performances

Only one report (Strauss, Liggett, & Lanese, 1985) is available on the use of anabolic–androgenic steroids by women athletes. Ten women weight lifters were interviewed to assess whether they thought that the anabolic–androgenic

TABLE 1 Characteristics of some anabolic–androgenic steroids

Generic (brand) name	Clinical dose and route	Dominant function	Structural variation
Testosterone (Testoject-50)	10–50 mg 3 times/wk i.m.[a]	Androgenic	None
Testosterone propionate (Testex)	10–25 mg 2–3 times/wk i.m.	Androgenic	17 beta-ester
Testosterone enanthate (Delatestryl)	50–400 mg every 2-4 wks i.m.	Androgenic	17 beta-ester
Testosterone cypionate (Depo-Testosterone)	50–400 mg every 2-4 wks i.m.	Androgenic	17 beta-ester
Nandrolone decanoate (Deca-Durabolin, Androlone-D)	50–100 mg every 3-4 wks i.m.	Anabolic	17 beta-ester
Nandrolone phenpro-pionate (Durabolin, Androlone, Nan-drolin)	15–50 mg once/wk i.m.	Anabolic	17 beta-ester
Methyltestosterone (Metandren, Oren-ton Methyl)	10–40 mg daily p.o.[b]; buccal tablets 5-20 mg/day	Androgenic	17 alpha-alkylated
Oxandrolone (Anavar)	5–10 mg daily p.o.	Anabolic	17 alpha-alkylated
Stanozolol (Winstrol)	6 mg daily p.o.	Anabolic	17 alpha-alkylated
Methandrostenolone (Dianabol[c])	2.5–5 mg daily p.o.	Anabolic	17 alpha-alkylated

[a]Intramuscular.
[b]By mouth.
[c]Dianabol is no longer produced by CIBA-Geigy; however, methandrostenolone is still available and widely used.

steroids, which they had reported taking, enhanced their athletic performances. The women athletes claimed that the anabolic–androgenic steroids produced a significant increase in their muscle strength and muscle size that supported enhanced athletic performances. No objective measures of strength were obtained from the female weight lifters.

Effects of Steroids on Male Athletes' Performances

In contrast to the literature on female athletes using steroids, for male athletes, numerous review articles have been published in which the results of original research are evaluated to determine whether anabolic–androgenic steroids enhance athletic performance.

Effects of Anabolic–Androgenic Steroids on Aerobic Capacity

According to Wright (1978), aerobic capacity is muscle endurance of the entire body, which is the same as the body's ability to use oxygen during work. There is general agreement that anabolic–androgenic steroids do not enhance the aerobic capacity of athletic performance in athletes. Such agreement among scientific reviewers, however, is not apparent on the issue of the effects of the anabolic–androgenic steroids on muscle size, muscle strength, and the performance of strength tasks.

Effects of Anabolic–Androgenic Steroids on Athletic Strength

> On the one hand, the testimonial evidence obtained in the gymnasium and on the field is nearly unanimous that steroids produced marked gains in performance; whether these gains are caused by improvement in muscle mass or by psychologically induced improvements in capacity for weight training is of little concern to the athlete. On the other hand, the results of scientific experiments are about evenly divided between positive and negative results. (Lamb, 1984, p. 35)

What does concern athletes, and scientists, however, are what seem to be contradictory findings about the effects of anabolic–androgenic steroids on athletic tasks of strength. How is it possible to draw any convincing conclusions about the effects of steroids on performance from contradictory scientific findings? Indeed, the contradiction in scientific findings serves to fuel the controversy between the majority opinions of athletes who believe that steroids enhance performance in strength tasks and the officials of sports governing bodies and physicians who claim that steroids have no effect on the performance of strength tasks.

Scientific review of discrepant results usually raises questions about what might have been systematically different in how the information was obtained, which may explain the difference in the results. The usual questions concern research design and data analysis and focus on (a) How many subjects participated in the studies? (b) Did the subjects and/or researchers know which drug the subjects received (i.e., how "blind" was the study?)? (c) Was an inactive drug (i.e., placebo) used? (d) Were the data analyzed properly? (e) Were the conclusions based on the results? And (e) was the dependent variable, in this instance muscle strength, accurately measured?

Upon considering the various reasons why the scientific studies could yield different results about the effectiveness of anabolic–androgenic steroids, Lamb (1984) could not detect any systematic differences in the research designs of studies reporting positive results compared with studies reporting negative results. He concluded that individual differences in the athletes' potential to enhance their strength explained the differences in results.

Wright (1978) proposed that the scientific results were in conflict because the research question of steroid efficacy—that is, Do steroids enhance performance?—limited the scientific investigations. Scientists could only use human subjects because no adequate way of inducing a stable muscular hypertrophy, which is a type of muscle expansion, in laboratory animals was established. The exclusive reliance on results from human subjects to answer a research question is more limiting, in part, because human subjects may show a placebo effect. That is, when subjects are administered placebo, but believe they have received active drug (in this instance steroid), their belief alone may enhance performance. In addition, the problems of limited budgets, subject recruitment, and institutional approval are exacerbated when the effects of controversial drugs, such as anabolic–androgenic steroids, are studied. Recently, prominent drug expert Jerome H. Jaffe, M.D., explained that

> *researchers are caught in a "Catch-22." They cannot say anything about the effects of using steroids at high doses without conducting an investigation, and they cannot investigate because it would be unethical to do so. (Marshall, 1988, p. 184)*

Wright (1978) also questioned whether the amount of athletic training before participation in the experiments influenced performance gains by the athletes during the experiments. He observed that

> *As of early 1978, eleven of twelve English language reports which used subjects accustomed to weight training (i.e., individuals with a minimum of one year and many with competitive training experience) indicate that therapeutic doses of steroids enabled the individuals to gain muscle size, strength, or both more rapidly than training alone. (Wright, 1978, p. 60)*

Wright concluded that anabolic–androgenic steroids can effectively assist in the gain of muscle mass, strength, and power by athletes who are intensively trained and also maintained on adequate protein and calorie diets. Williams (1974) reviewed the relevant scientific literature and concurred with Wright. From his review, Williams concluded that steroids will increase levels of strength if taken by athletes who are in proper training and maintained by adequate diets. He cautioned, however, that the research results were inconclusive and added that athletes should take drugs when under the care of a physician and only if allowed by the rules and regulations of the sports governing bodies.

In contrast, Ryan's (1981) review of the scientific experiments revealed, from his perspective, a blatant systematic set of differences between studies that reported positive effects of anabolic–androgenic steroids and muscle strength and those that reported no anabolic–androgenic steroid advantage. He observed that studies in which steroids were reported to enhance performance were flawed because (a) there were too few subjects, (b) subjects and/or researchers knew which drugs were given, (c) an error was observed in calculation of the results, (d) conclusions were not supported by the data, and (e) gains in strength were merely marginal. Ryan stated, in effect, that false-positive results were reported and concluded that no substantial evidence was presented to indicate that anabolic–androgenic steroids enhance performance in progressive weight training. Mellon (1984) in large part agreed with Ryan's conclusions, but added that the doses administered by the researchers were much less than what athletes self-administer and thus the results from the experiments are not necessarily applicable to athletes.

Wilson and Griffin (1980) concurred with Ryan's (1981) and Mellon's (1984) criticisms of the scientific experiments and added that reported weight gain with anabolic–androgenic steroids consisted of fluid retention rather than gain in muscle mass, thereby adding structural mass to the argument against efficacy of the steroids. They concluded that if enhanced performance was observed with anabolic–androgenic steroids, it was probably the result of enhanced training that the steroids psychologically motivated, rather than by any direct pharmacological effect on muscle mass.

Haupt and Rovere (1984) argued that the discrepant scientific results regarding the efficacy of anabolic–androgenic steroids could be explained by considering how muscle strength was measured. They contended that when researchers measured muscle strength of the weight lifters by using strength tasks that were typically performed in competition (e.g., the 1-RM technique, which is a measurement of the maximal weight lifted in a single repetition of the weight lifting exercise using bench press and squat), more positive results of steroid efficacy were obtained. However, they observed that the 1-RM technique was not the only necessary condition that differentiated studies that yielded positive results from studies that yielded negative results.

Haupt and Rovere (1984) proposed that the following conditions are required to obtain enhancement of muscle strength by anabolic–androgenic steroids: (a) Subjects must be trained in weight lifting before anabolic–androgenic steroid treatment is initiated, and (b) muscle strength should be measured by observing relevant strength performance tasks, such as the 1-RM technique.

Recently, the Council on Scientific Affairs of the American Medical Association recognized that steroids may enhance athletic performance by the growth of lean muscle mass in some persons who are weight trained and on a high-protein diet (Marshall, 1988).

Ferner and Rawlins (1988) concurred with Haupt and Rovere (1984), noting that

> Methandienone has been shown to increase muscle bulk. . . . Indeed, no negative trial is likely to be as convincing to athletes as Ben Johnson's performance in the Olympic 100 m final. . . . Doctors cannot, with real confidence, claim that anabolic steroids have no effect on athletic performance. (Ferner & Rawlins, 1988, pp. 877–878)

Haupt (1989) updated his remarks about the efficacy of the anabolic–androgenic steroids, adding a further necessary condition: that athletes should maintain diets adequate in carbohydrates and protein. He also extended the range of athletic activities that may benefit from the use of anabolic–androgenic steroids to include sprinters.

Although the latter article by Haupt (i.e., 1989) added more credibility to the argument that anabolic–androgenic steroids can enhance the performance of strength tasks in trained athletes, it also expanded on the dangers encountered in using anabolic–androgenic steroids. While describing the often cited physiological side effects accompanying steroid use, Haupt also discussed the potential for steroids to induce adverse psychological effects and the potential for steroid use to result in addiction.

Side Effects of the Anabolic–Androgenic Steroids

According to *Dorland's Illustrated Medical Dictionary* (1988), a side effect is

> a consequence other than the one(s) for which an agent or measure is used, as the adverse effects produced by a drug, especially on a tissue or organ system other than the one sought to be benefited by its administration. (p. 1519)

Anabolic–androgenic steroids are taken by athletes to increase muscle mass and muscle strength and enhance the performance of tasks requiring strength. However, much of the evidence about the side effects of anabolic–androgenic steroids offered in the literature was obtained from observations of patients undergoing treatment for medical abnormalities. Side effects by definition are additional bodily or psychological effects reported by, or observed in, a target population.

The present discussion therefore is limited to considerations of the side effects as they were reported by or observed in athletes who took anabolic–androgenic steroids. Side effects include dermatological (skin) problems; gynecological disorders; feminization; gastrointestinal (digestive) problems; endocrine (hormone) disruptions; sexual disorders; hepatic (liver) disorders; cardiovascular effects due to metabolic changes; psychological/psychiatric effects including moderate to severe changes in motivation, mood, perception, cognition, and behavior; and potential for addiction.

Drug Preparation and Occurrence of Side Effects

An additional question that demands consideration when examining scientific evidence about the side effects from anabolic–androgenic steroids is, Does the way in which steroids were prepared for administration affect the occurrence of side effects? Do ingestions of the oral steroids result in side effects different from those observed with injectable steroids? Wright (1978) wrote that oral steroids are more dangerous than the injectable ones:

> *The point I wish to emphasize is that oral steroids (because they have been chemically altered in order to slow down their deactivation by the liver), to a greater extent than the injectables, normally do cause symptomless alterations in liver function. Injectable steroids are also modified to prolong their lifespan in the body. However, because the modifications are different and because they are released into the blood stream more slowly, they appear not to stress the detoxifying system of the liver to the same extent as the oral compounds. (pp. 86–87)*

Where appropriate, the differential side effects of the oral and injectable steroids are noted in the following sections.

Side Effects of Steroids in Female Athletes

Strauss et al. (1985) prepared the only published report on the use of anabolic–androgenic steroids by women athletes. They interviewed 10 female weight lifters who described the side effects associated with their steroid use. Primarily, the female athletes described the signs that are contained in the clinical definition of verilization (Berkow, 1982). Thus, the women athletes described increases in acne, facial hair, body hair, and size of clitoris, and decreases in body fat. Temporal balding, which has been observed in women who are prescribed steroids to correct medical problems, however, was not reported. Additional gynecological signs reported by the female athletes were decreases in breast size and diminution of menses.

An increase in libido was the only change in sexual behavior mentioned by the women athletes. The sole gastrointestinal change observed by the female athletes was an increase in appetite. In general, the women claimed that their side effects were not too bothersome. An exception was the onset of a lowered voice, which the women athletes cited as the most annoying cost of the anabolic–androgenic steroids. Also, annoying to spouses and significant others of the athletes and of concern to the athletes themselves, was an increase in aggressiveness; however, the women felt this provided a positive psychological edge in athletic competition. No objective measures of the side effects of the anabolic–androgenic steroids were obtained.

Side Effects of Steroids in Male Athletes

For male athletes, three review articles and a number of original research papers contain information about the side effects of steroids. Therefore, most of the information about the side effects of anabolic–androgenic steroids in this chapter is based on observations of male athletes.

Dermatological side effects are those changes that occur in the skin, sebaceous glands, and hair while taking anabolic–androgenic steroids. Observations of side effects in the scientific literature include increases in acne of the face and torso, male pattern baldness, and skin rash or local irritations at injection sites (Haupt, 1989; Haupt & Rovere, 1984; Wright, 1978). Also, increased serum excretion rate and enlarged sebaceous glands have been observed with steroid use (Kiraley, Alen, et al., 1987; Kiraly, Collan, et al., 1987). In addition, according to the review authors, steroid use by male athletes infrequently resulted in gynecomastia, which is enlargement of the breasts. Wright (1978) observed that the self-administration of oral anabolic–androgenic steroids may result in reduced appetite, diarrhea, and constipation.

Endocrinological effects. Endocrinological side effects of the anabolic–androgenic steroids are usually monitored by measurement of general changes in the plasma levels (i.e., blood) of testosterone and the gonadotropins (i.e., follicle-stimulating hormone [FSH] and interstitial cell-stimulating hormone [ICSH]). More complex hormone profiles that monitor the effects of anabolic–androgenic steroids on testicular and thyroid functions have also been obtained.

Haupt and Rovere (1984) and Wright (1978) observed that each of the anabolic–androgenic steroids produced characteristic changes in the plasma levels of testosterone and the gonadotropins. Methandrostenolone and mesteralone reduced plasma testosterone to castrate levels, but the plasma levels of FSH and ICSH were not changed. Deca-Durabolin reduced plasma levels of testosterone, FSH, and ICSH. Neither naldrone nor norethandrolone affected the plasma levels of testosterone, FSH, and ICSH. All anabolic–androgenic-steroid-induced changes in the plasma levels of testosterone, FSH, and ICSH were reversed after steroid use was discontinued. Therefore, it appears that the use of anabolic–androgenic steroids by athletes results in either no changes of plasma testosterone levels or a reduction in serum testosterone levels.

Recently, an Olympic athlete's testosterone level became public information. Ben Johnson's world record in the 1988 Olympic 100-m race was disqualified because his urine sample tested positive for stanozol. Also,

There was a second damning piece of evidence in this case, Dugal says. Normally the Olympic Committee does not release information about an athlete's testosterone level, but in this case it made an exception because Johnson claimed his drink had been spiked. Analysis showed that his testosterone was 15% of the normal value, a fact that would be consistent with long-term steroid use, not a single incident of sabotage. (Marshall, 1988, p. 184)

The relation between anabolic–androgenic steroid use and testosterone levels appears to be useful in resolving controversy, but is it possible to conclude that all factors in the Ben Johnson incident were considered? What is the scientific evidence about how running exercises affect testosterone levels in male athletes?

Wheeler, Wall, Belcastro, and Cumming (1984) compared the serum testosterone levels of 31 males who ran at least 64 km each week with the serum testosterone levels of 18 sedentary males who served as matched controls. They reported the serum testosterone showed no relation with (i.e., they could not be correlated with) the height, weight, age, or ponderal index (height [cm] × weight [kg] − 1/3). However, there was a strong relation between activity levels (e.g., runners vs. sedentary controls) and testosterone levels. Only 4 of the 31 runners had testosterone levels that were higher than the mean testosterone level for the sedentary males. The average value of testosterone levels in the runners was 83.3% of the average value of testosterone levels in the sedentary males. One male runner's testosterone level was 29% of that of the sedentary males, but nonetheless, it is improbable that a testosterone level of 15% of the normal value, as was Ben Johnson's, could be solely attributable to the effects of running exercises.

For power athletes who supplement their self-administration of the anabolic–androgenic steroids with injections of testosterone, serum testosterone levels increase while taking the drug mixtures (Alen et al., 1987; Alen, Reinila, et al., 1985; Ruokonen et al., 1985), but drop rapidly following withdrawal from the steroid/testosterone mixtures, remaining low at 12 weeks postdrug (Alen, Reinila, et al., 1985). Steroid testosterone levels recover to predrug testosterone levels 16 weeks following withdrawal (Ruokonen et al., 1985).

In contrast, leutinizing hormone (LH) and FSH levels of the male athletes decreased during self-administration of the anabolic–androgenic and testosterone mixtures (Alen et al., 1987; Alen, Reinila, et al., 1985). SHBG also decreased during self-administration of the steroid mixtures (Alen et al., 1987; Ruokonen et al., 1985). Following discontinuance of the steroid mixtures, FSH and LH returned to predrug levels (Alen et al., 1987; Alen, Reinila, et al., 1985), but SHBG did not return to predrug levels (Alen et al., 1987; Ruokonen et al., 1985).

The effects of anabolic–androgenic steroid and testosterone mixtures on thyroid gland function were examined by Alen et al. (1987). They observed that the use of anabolic–androgenic steroid and testosterone mixtures by 7 power athletes led to significant decreases in serum levels of thyroid-stimulating hormone (TSH), thyroxine (T_4), triiodothyronine (T_3), free thyroxine (FT_4), and calculated free thyroxine index (FT_{4-1}), but T_3 uptake increased. Dramatic depletion in serum levels of thyroid-binding globulin (TBG) was also observed. The results indicated that the steroid mixtures affected the thyroid gland primarily through TBG. All thyroid gland indicators returned to baseline following steroid cessation.

Sexually related disorders. Sexually related disorders are characterized by the physiological and psychological factors that reduce reproductive potential. Examples of anabolic–androgenic steroid-induced sexually related disorders in male athletes include changes in libido and changes in spermatozoa that reduce the reproductive potential.

Wright (1978) observed that the effects of anabolic–androgenic steroids on sexually related disorders in male athletes vary widely across drugs. Nilevar (norethandrolone) reduced (a) sperm output and motility for 24–26 weeks after drug use, (b) libido for 2–3 weeks following drug use, and (c) testicular size and potentia for 2–3 weeks following drug use. Dianabol (methandrostenolone) reduced sperm count and motility, but had mixed effects on libido. Neither mesterolone nor Deca-Durabolin affected changes in the indices of reproductive potential. Wright concluded,

> The chances of steroids inducing major or irreversible changes seems rather remote in view of the fact that newly developed oral and injectable steroids are currently being tested for possible use as "reversible" male contraceptives. (1978, pp. 93–94)

Haupt (1989) concurred with Wright (1978) and observed that, in general, anabolic–androgenic steroid use by male athletes may induce increases or decreases in libido, testicular atrophy, and transient infertility.

Hepatic effects. Hepatic effects are changes in the function or condition of the liver that occur with the self-administration of the anabolic–androgenic steroids. The liver is a multifaceted organ that influences practically all metabolic processes. It is a filtering system that attends to substances arriving by the gastrointestinal tract and circulating through the bloodstream. The liver coordinates intricate enzyme systems that detoxify toxic substances, conjugate hormones, and release other waste products into bile for excretion by the urinary and gastrointestinal tracts. The liver also contributes enzymes that assist in the transformation of food molecules into essential cellular building blocks.

Whether steroids were prepared for oral use or for use by injection is a critical determinant of hepatic side effects. A high percentage of orally administered drugs enter the liver and undergo metabolism during their first pass from the small intestine to the liver. It is thought that the first pass of megadoses of anabolic–androgenic steroids that were chemically altered to increase their resistance to hepatic inactivation may enhance liver tissue damage. In addition, the self-administration of other drugs such as alcohol, amphetamines, or cocaine magnifies the possibility of liver tissue damage.

Changes in the liver's inactivation, detoxification, and elimination of harmful substances from the body are assessed by the BSP (Bromsulphalein, sulfobromophthalein sodium) retention/excretion rate test. BSP is a white, odorless, crystalline, water-soluble dye that competes with bile salts for excretion by the liver. An increase in BSP retention rate indicates reduced efficiency in the liver's inactivation, detoxification, and elimination of harmful substances. Wright (1978) reported that during the 1st through 4th weeks of steroid treatment, BSP retention rates increased and were somewhat dependent on the steroid's dose. However, BSP retention rates returned to normal with continued steroid use.

Nonspecific evaluation of liver function is assessed through serum levels of SGOT (serum glutamic-oxaloacetic transaminase; currently ASAT, aspartate transferase) and SGPT (serum glutamic-pyruvic transaminase; currently ALAT, alanine transferase). Increased serum levels of SGOT and SGPT usually indicate that the enzymes had leaked from damaged body tissue, such as the liver, kidney, heart, and skeletal muscle. Increases in serum SGOT and SGPT levels were occasionally reported for weight lifters who were not taking steroids (Haupt & Rovere, 1984). The typical pattern reported, however, was two- to threefold increases in SGOT and SGPT serum levels during the first 4 weeks of steroid use, with return to normal levels following continued steroid use (Wright, 1978). In contrast, Lenders et al. (1988) observed elevated ASAT and ALAT serum levels in male athletes during an 8-week course of multiple anabolic–androgenic steroid mixtures that remained elevated 5 months after cessation from steroids.

Haupt and Rovere (1984) argued that specific tests of liver function, such as serum elevations of alkaline phosphatese and LDH (L-lactic dehydrogenase), in conjunction with SGOT and SGPT levels may provide more accurate information about liver function. They reported that of the 149 male athletes (the subject pool from 11 studies) who took anabolic–androgenic steroids, the following proportions showed serum elevations of SGOT (18%), SGPT (20%), LDH liver enzyme (7%), and alkaline phosphatase (1%). They observed a strong relation between the steroid used and increases in serum levels of LDH liver enzyme and alkaline phosphatase. For those athletes who took methandrostenolone and presented with elevated serum levels of SGOT or SGPT, only 2 of 30 athletes also had elevated serum levels of LDH liver enzyme or alkaline phosphatase. In contrast, for athletes who took oxandrolone and presented with elevated serum levels of SGOT or SPGT, 11 of 11 athletes also had elevated serum levels of LDH liver enzyme or alkaline phosphatase.

At a recent meeting sponsored by the National Institute on Drug Abuse (see Cowart, 1989b), Friedl observed that since 1960 only three cases of liver tumors in athletes have been reported. Two of the cases were noncancerous, in which one patient recovered following surgery. The third case was cancerous and the athlete died within 3 months of diagnosis. Haupt and Rovere (1984), Lenders et al. (1988), and Wright (1978) concluded that although the use of anabolic–androgenic steroids may result in some disturbance of liver function and a few instances of serious liver damage, the most serious physiological complications from the use of steroids probably involve increased risks of cardiovascular disturbances.

Cardiovascular effects.   Cardiovascular effects are those changes in the function or condition of the heart and blood vessels that occur with the self-administration of the anabolic–androgenic steroids. Of particular interest are changes in the plasma high-density lipoprotein:low-density lipoprotein (HDL:LDL) ratio and changes in the plasma high-density lipoprotein:total cholesterol (HDL:total cholesterol) ratio.

The liver packages cholesterol in LDLs that are delivered to the cells by the cardiovascular system. Cholesterol is used by the cells to produce their membranes and by the glands to produce steroids. Excess cholesterol is released by the cells into the cardiovascular system where it is absorbed by HDLs. HDL is synthesized in the liver and intestines. When the plasma contains more LDL than can be absorbed by HDL, then macrophages consume the excess LDL and become the "foam cells" that have been observed in atherosclerotic lesions (Ganong, 1987).

Depending on other conditions of the cardiovascular system, atherosclerotic lesions may lead to myocardial infarction (heart attack), stroke, and coronary heart disease. Of much concern, therefore, is the amount of foam cells in the cardiovascular system. The plasma HDL:LDL or HDL:total cholesterol ratios are measures of the efficiency of the cardiovascular cholesterol transport system and so indirectly measure the accumulation of foam cells. Ganong (1987) concluded that the HDL:total cholesterol ratio is an index of risk of the development of atherosclerosis.

Epidemiological studies indicated that the risks of myocardial infarction are reduced in the subpopulations who have higher HDL levels. Women have higher HDL levels than men, and, hence, women are at lower risk of myocardial infarction than men. Persons who exercise and drink alcohol moderately (1–2 glasses/day), have higher HDL levels than sedentary individuals who do not consume alcohol, and hence persons who exercise are at lower risk of myocardial infarction than the sedentary individuals.

Investigations into the effects of anabolic–androgenic steroids on the plasma HDL:LDL and HDL:total cholesterol ratios in male athletes began to appear in the literature during the middle 1980s. The early—and some of the later—reports, however, published their findings from the perspective of LDL:HDL and total cholesterol:HDL ratios. To simplify the present discussion, all previous findings are reported from the perspective of HDL:LDL and HDL:total cholesterol ratios. The original meaning of the reported findings has not been altered.

All investigators reported that the use of anabolic–androgenic steroid and testosterone mixtures by trained weight lifters, power athletes, and body-builders resulted in significant decreases in the plasma HDL:LDL ratios or significant decreases in plasma HDL:total cholesterol ratios, depending on which ratio was measured. In contrast, no significant changes in plasma HDL:LDL ratios or plasma HDL:total cholesterol ratios were observed in trained weight lifters, power athletes, and bodybuilders who did not take steroids. The time course for changes in the plasma lipoprotein ratios during regimens of anabolic–androgenic steroid self-administration and cessation is as follows.

After 4–6 weeks' use of the anabolic–androgenic steroid and testosterone mixtures by bodybuilders and power lifters, significant decreases in the plasma HDL:LDL ratios were detectable (Hurley et al., 1984). With continued use of the anabolic–androgenic steroid and testosterone mixtures by power athletes, significant decreases in the plasma HDL:total cholesterol ratios were maintained from 4 weeks through 12 weeks of steroid use (Kiraly, 1988), at which time the study ended. Unlike elevated serum levels of SGOT and SPGT, plasma ratios of HDL:LDL and HDL:total cholesterol do not recover during steroid use.

After 8 weeks of taking anabolic–androgenic steroid and testosterone mixtures during training, the HDL:total cholesterol ratios significantly decreased in power athletes, remained low through 14 additional weeks of steroid use, and recovered to presteroid HDL:total cholesterol ratios 12 weeks after discontinuance of steroid use (Alen, Rahkila, et al., 1985). Similarly, for power athletes who had taken anabolic–androgenic steroid and testosterone mixtures for 1 month, a threefold increase in HDL:LDL ratio was obtained, but following discontinuance of the anabolic–androgenic steroid and testosterone mixtures, plasma HDL:total cholesterol and HDL:LDL ratios slowly recovered to presteroid levels (Webb, Laskarzewski, & Glueck, 1984).

Significant increases in the plasma HDL:total cholesterol and HDL:LDL ratios were also achieved by formerly sedentary subjects (6 women and 8 men) who had undergone 16 weeks of weight training exercises (Goldberg, Elliot, Schutz, & Kloster, 1984). However, McKillop and Ballantyne (1987) observed no differences in the plasma HDL:LDL ratios of sedentary men and body-builders who did not take steroids. Hurley et al. (1984) observed that for athletes who abstained from anabolic–androgenic steroids, the plasma HDL:LDL ratios were lower in power lifters than in bodybuilders and runners of comparable age and body fat.

Haupt (1989) concluded from the literature that the use of anabolic–androgenic steroids can cause a significant decrease in the plasma HDL:LDL ratios that, however, returns to normal after steroid use is discontinued. The long-term effects of significant decreases in plasma HDL:LDL and HDL:total cholesterol ratios are unknown, but two reports of stroke in bodybuilders who had taken anabolic–androgenic steroids were recently published (Frankle, Eichberg, & Zachariah, 1988; Mochizuki & Richter, 1988). Also unknown is whether the use of anabolic–androgenic steroids can result in long-term compromise of cardiovascular function. At a recent meeting sponsored by the National Institute on Drug Abuse (Cowart, 1989b), Bardin said that a research priority is to investigate the occurrence of heart disease in steroid users. However, of greater concern to Haupt (1989) was the potential for steroids to induce adverse psychological effects and the potential for steroid use to result in addiction.

Psychological/Psychiatric Effects

Psychological/psychiatric effects are those moderate to severe changes in motivation, mood, perception, cognition, and behavior that occur with the self-administration of the anabolic–androgenic steroids. Haupt (1989) commented,

> The most disturbing adverse effect of androgenic steroids may be their psychological effects. A high percentage of athletes who take anabolic–androgenic steroids will suffer some degree of personality change that may range from increased irritability to a toxic psychosis that may require hospitalization. Athletes taking anabolic steroids often become extremely intense, aggressive, and sometimes violent individuals. These characteristics allow the athlete to train in a much more strenuous and focused manner. However, these aggressive side effects carry over into everyday life as well. The athletes assume a Jekyll and Hyde personality where even a slight provocation can cause them to react in a violent and sometimes uncontrolled manner. They can become virtual sociopaths who can no longer maintain effective relationships with friends, family, or loved ones. Their only release is in the weight room or playing field where violent behavior may be more acceptable. These individuals not uncommonly lose girlfriends, suffer divorces, move away from family, and frequently find themselves in trouble with the law. . . . Ultimately, personality alterations return to normal following discontinuance of the steroids. Unfortunately, scars on relationships between friends, family, loved ones, and any arrest records will remain with the athlete for the rest of their life. (p. 572)

Wright (1978) acknowledged early reports of increases in nervous tension by athletes who had taken anabolic–androgenic steroids and occasional reports of increased or decreased feelings of aggression. Haupt and Rovere (1984) reported that 52 of the 155 male athletes (the subject pool from 13 studies) complained of at least one subjective side effect that occurred with their anabolic–androgenic steroid use. They observed that the complaints of the 52 athletes were of the following proportions: euphoria (4%), aggression (31%), irritability (6%), and nervous tension (6%).

Pope and Katz (1988) used structured interviews and criteria from the *Diagnostic and Statistical Manual of Mental Disorders* (Third Edition-Revised) (*DSM-III-R;* American Psychiatric Association, 1987) to measure the occurrence of psychiatric symptoms in 39 men and 2 women who had histories of anabolic–androgenic steroid use. During periods of steroid abstinence, subjects were asymptomatic and offered no reports of psychotic symptoms or manic episode, even at subthreshold levels. In contrast, while taking anabolic–androgenic steroids the subjects' reports met *DSM-III-R* criteria in the following proportions: psychotic symptoms (12%), mild or equivocal psychotic symptoms (10%), manic episode (12%), and subthreshold manic episode (20%).

Fifty-four percent of those interviewed in Pope and Katz's (1988) study complained of psychiatric symptoms while taking anabolic–androgenic steroids. The psychiatric symptoms were quite disturbing, as, for example, the following descriptions of psychotic symptoms: auditory hallucinations of voices lasting 5 weeks, the paranoid delusion that friends were stealing from the athlete, and the grandiose delusion of one athlete that he could pick up a car and tip it over.

No less disturbing were the descriptions of the behaviors of subjects who were scored as manic or subthreshold manic. For example, Pope and Katz (1988) reported,

> *One 23-year-old man bought a $17,000 sports car while taking methandrostenolone. When he stopped the drug, he realized that he could not afford the payments and sold the car; a year later, during another cycle, he impulsively bought a $20,000 sports car. Another subject bought an old car and deliberately drove it into a tree at 40 miles per hour while a friend videotaped him. Another became enraged when the driver in front of him inadvertently left his directional signal flashing at the next stoplight, he jumped out and smashed the offender's windshield. (p. 489)*

In a recent report in *Science* magazine, the Council on Scientific Affairs of the American Medical Association declared a neutral position about reports on the reputed power of anabolic–androgenic steroids to make users aggressive (Marshall, 1988). However, during a recent meeting sponsored by the National Institute on Drug Abuse (see Cowart, 1989a), Katz reported that the psychiatric side effects of the anabolic–androgenic steroids may be more serious than physical alterations of body chemistry. Bardin (see Cowart, 1989a) and Katz concluded that study of the psychiatric effects of the anabolic–androgenic steroids should be expanded.

Potential for Addiction

The anabolic–androgenic steroids can be classified as drugs because they do not occur naturally in the body. Hence, the potential for addiction to the anabolic–androgenic steroids may be evaluated through the criteria cited in a definition of drug addiction. A definition of the term *drug addiction* was referenced by Kolb (1962) as follows:

> According to the United Nations World Health Organization (World Health Organization Technical Report Series No. 21, 1950), "Drug addiction is a state of periodic or chronic intoxication detrimental to the individual and to society, produced by the repeated consumption of a drug (natural or synthetic). Its characteristics include: (1) an overpowering desire or need (compulsion) to continue taking the drug and to obtain it by any means; (2) a tendency to increase the dose; (3) a psychic (psychological) and sometimes, a physical dependence on the effects of the drug." This definition is inclusive and scientifically accurate, but it applies not only to drugs designated in narcotic statutes but also to drugs which are not specifed. (p. 3)

Only one investigation in the literature was designed to measure the addictive potential of the anabolic–androgenic steroids. Therefore, the potentially addictive properties of the anabolic–androgenic steroids are at best a proposal. Haupt (1989) proposed that the addiction potential of the anabolic–androgenic steroids is probably the most devastating side effect of steroid self-administration.

According to Haupt (1989), upon discontinuance of the anabolic–androgenic steroids, athletes lose (a) the steroid euphoria, (b) the psychological capability for maintaining high-intensity in training, (c) the size and strength improvements in muscles, (d) the sexual drive, and (e) the positive admiration of peers. Most athletes cannot tolerate these temporary losses and hence compulsive self-administration of the anabolic–androgenic steroids resumes. Haupt (1989) concluded that the athletes' obsessions with body image and the compulsive behaviors to obtain the distorted body image may be similar to the obsessions of anorexia nervosa sufferers and their compulsive behaviors to obtain their distorted body image.

Haupt's model of the addictive behaviors occurring with the self-administration of anabolic–androgenic steroids includes two of the three characteristics in the World Health Organization's definition of drug addiction. Haupt's model may be relevant for some athletes, but at this time none of the model's elements or assumptions have been empirically tested. The proposal that chronic self-administration of the anabolic–androgenic steroids results in addiction requires further study.

Operational definitions (i.e., detailed specifications of how a concept may be measured) of tolerance and physical dependence provide more guidelines to examine the addictive potential of the anabolic–androgenic steroids. According to Kalant (1978), there are no universal definitions for tolerance and physical dependence; however,

> *For the present purposes* [of examining the hypotheses of tolerance and the relation of tolerance to physical dependence], *tolerance refers only to* acquired functional tolerance, *a change in response to repeated or prolonged administration of a drug, such that the concentration-effect curve is shifted to the right, and the initial maximum effect can usually be re-evoked by raising the drug concentration sufficiently.* Physical dependence *refers to an altered state in the chronically drug-treated subject, recognizable by the appearance of functional disturbances on sudden withdrawal of the drug or administration of an antagonist, alleviated rapidly by renewed administration of the original or a pharmacologically related drug, and disappearing gradually if the drug is withheld. (p. 200)*

Indirect evidence of acquired functional tolerance to the anabolic–androgenic steroids with chronic self-administration was provided by Alen, Reinila, et al. (1985). They monitored the stacking regimen—that is, the mixture of steroids—used by athletes during a 26-week period. The athletes completed medication diaries. Accuracy of the diaries was confirmed through analyses of random urine specimens by gas chromatography—mass spectrometry. The medication diaries revealed that over time, the athletes showed a tendency to increase the dose of methandieone and/or the frequency in injections of nandrolone, stanozolol, and the testosterone combination.

Employing similar criteria of steroid self-administration behaviors, Yesalis et al. (1989) recently examined data from a national survey on anabolic–androgenic steroid use by senior high school males to determine if the responses to survey items systematically varied with the different dose regimens used to self-administer the anabolic–androgenic steroids. Of the senior high school males who reported anabolic–androgenic steroid use (7%), two-thirds initiated their use before age 16. A subgroup of the early-initiating subjects (approximately 60%) was identified as "hard core" users because they reported the self-administration of steroid stacking regimens for five or more cycles. This hard core group of anabolic–androgenic steroid users also reported predominant use of the injectables, greater than average athletic strength, a desire to continue using anabolic–androgenic steroids regardless of the side effects, and the opinion that anabolic–androgenic steroid use in sports should not be stopped. It was concluded that the self-administration patterns and response sets of the hard core users were consistent with habituation to the anabolic–androgenic steroids.

Indirect evidence of physical dependence on the anabolic–androgenic steroids was provided by Pope and Katz (1988). During structured interviews, Pope and Katz observed that of the athletes who described their experiences following cessation from the anabolic–androgenic steroids, 12.2% described symptoms that met the *DSM-III-R* criteria for major depression. Therefore, these athletes showed recognizable functional disturbances when their steroid regimens were suddenly withdrawn.

Direct evidence of physical dependence on the anabolic–androgenic steroids was provided by the sole investigation in the literature that was designed to measure the addictive potential of the steroids. Tennant, Black, and Voy (1988) examined a 23-year-old bodybuilder who complained of depression and fatigue when he attempted to stop taking steroids. The bodybuilder also presented with dilated pupils (8.0 mm), enlarged liver, small testicles, and an altered testosterone:epitestosterone ratio. These signs indicated that the bodybuilder had been taking steroids and that he was not presently taking opioids. A naloxone challenge (0.2 mg) was administered and within 15 min, the bodybuilder had nausea, chills, headache, dizziness, and other signs and symptoms of naloxone-precipitated withdrawal from opiates which lasted for 4 hr following the administration of naloxone. The subject therefore showed signs of physical dependence with the sudden appearance of functional disturbances following the administration of an opioid antagonist. Additional research is needed to test the proposal that chronic self-administration of the anabolic–androgenic steroids may result in addiction.

USE OF STIMULANTS BY ATHLETES

From the urine samples taken at the 1983 Pan American Games in Caracas, stimulants were second to steroids as doping agents abused by athletes. Williams (1974) reported that of the stimulants, amphetamines were more frequently abused by athletes. Results from studies about use of amphetamines by athletes were similar to results of studies about steroid use by athletes. In his literature review, Williams (1974) observed the following of amphetamines: (a) that results were conflicting about whether amphetamines enhanced athletic performance, (b) that, according to survey results, 14- and 15-year-old athletes were taking amphetamines, (c) that an estimated 40% of major league baseball and football players were taking amphetamines, and (d) that public outcry was raised. Williams suggested that more effective legislation be enacted to prevent the use of amphetamines by athletes.

Since the 1970s, the use of amphetamines to treat clinical conditions (i.e., obesity, narcolepsy, hyperkinesis, and depression) has declined, while other drugs with less abuse potential are currently being prescribed for these conditions (Lombardo, 1987a). For athletes, the abuse of amphetamines has also declined—but the abuse of other stimulant drugs has increased. Haupt (1989) proposed that cocaine abuse surpasses amphetamine abuse by athletes. In contrast, Nuzzo and Waller (1988) proposed that caffeine abuse in megadoses surpasses amphetamine abuse by athletes.

Cocaine

Cocaine hydrochloride (HCL) is the active drug that is produced from the *Erythroxylon coca* plant. The clinical use for cocaine HCL is as a local anesthetic. Cocaine HCL self-administration is accomplished either by snorting through the nares or by intravenous injection. Cocaine HCL decomposes with burning. Crack cocaine, or freebase, is produced by treating the HCL with an alkali such as sodium bicarbonate, ammonia water, or sodium hydroxide. Crack cocaine is self-administered by inhaling the smoky air into the lungs.

Cocaine stimulates the central nervous system, cardiovascular, and respiratory functioning by blocking the reuptake of the neurotransmitters dopamine and norepinephrine. Cocaine constricts peripheral vessels, which increases core body temperature and increases peripheral resistance to blood transport. Cocaine-induced arrhythmias (muscle spasms) of the cardiovascular system have occurred at sites that are critical to the movement of blood from the heart (i.e., cardiac ventricles and coronary artery). Also, when an individual is under cocaine-induced stress, respirations increase.

In the general U.S. population in 1985, only 613 deaths due to cocaine were reported, whereas 100,000 alcohol-related deaths were reported (Nuzzo & Waller, 1988). The hazardous side effects of cocaine, however, can be life threatening to athletes. During cocaine intoxication the cardiovascular system may be maximally stressed. Myocardial infarction (heart attack), cerebral vascular accident (stroke), coronary thrombosis (collapse of the coronary artery), or status epilepticus (multiple convulsions appearing as pulsating, intense, repetitive cycles of musculoskeletal hyperextension and collapse) may occur. Death following multiple convulsions is usually attributed to hypoxia, which is diminished oxygen supply to brain cells.

Giammarco (1987) provided a different hypothesis of the mechanisms that result in fatalities from cocaine-induced multiple seizures in athletes. Lactate is produced when glycogen stores in the muscles are used for fuel. Skeletal white muscles, as compared with red muscles, primarily use glycogen stores for energy, are more highly developed in sprinter athletes (i.e., basketball players), and are predominantly fast-twitch muscles that are inducted during convulsions. Therefore, sprinters' muscles have a high capacity to produce lactate during cocaine-induced seizure activity.

Cocaine also induces peripheral vasoconstriction, which diminishes the reuptake of lactate by muscles and increases plasma lactate levels. High plasma levels of lactate are readily absorbed by neurons (brain cells), which are abundantly supplied with capillaries that are not constricted with cocaine use. As neurons absorb greater amounts of lactate, neuronal hypertrophy (brain swelling) occurs as fluid is drawn into the cells and concentrations of lactate increase. The intracellular increases in fluid and lactate may result in lactic acidosis and death (Giammarco, 1987).

With chronic use, cocaine HCL is highly addictive. Physical dependence can occur if an individual consumes five "lines of cocaine" (each containing about 25 mg of cocaine HCL) per day for 10 consecutive days (Haupt, 1989). Tolerance to cocaine HCL may also develop, but heightened responsiveness to cocaine has also been observed. Addiction to crack cocaine develops much more quickly.

Athletes have used cocaine as either a performance-enhancing drug or a recreational drug. The prevalence of cocaine HCL use by athletes is not known, but the user patterns among athletes are thought to be similar to user patterns in the general population. Recent surveys estimated that 16% of high school seniors and 28% of adults 20–40 years old have tried cocaine HCL at least once (Haupt, 1989). In contrast, it has been proposed that the prevalence of crack cocaine use seems to be rising in the general population. Cocaine use is banned by the National Collegiate Athletic Association (NCAA) and the USOC (Haupt, 1989).

Caffeine

Caffeine is a methylated xanthine. Caffeine occurs naturally in coffee, tea, kola nuts, and cocoa beans. No special extraction processes, other than boiling water, are required to prepare caffeine for self-administration from ground coffee or tea leaves. Chocolate and many commercially prepared sodas contain caffeine. Caffeine may also be purchased in over-the-counter preparations in which it may be the sole ingredient; mixed with other stimulants, such as phenylpropanolamine and ephedrine; or contained in some aspirin preparations (Nuzzo & Waller, 1988).

Caffeine is self-administered by mouth and placed into general circulation through the gut. Peak blood levels are reached within 30–60 min. Caffeine is usually taken to obtain mild stimulation of the central nervous system. Caffeine readily crosses the blood–brain barrier and causes excitation of the central nervous system by blocking adenosine's binding to receptors. Adenosine functions to inhibit the release of dopamine and norepinephrine. To maintain homeostasis, the cardiovascular system works in opposition to caffeine's stimulatory effect on the autonomic control centers of the central nervous system. Maintenance of the cardiovascular–central nervous system homeostatic mechanisms results in few life-threatening side effects from caffeine use (Blum, 1984).

Caffeine affects the musculoskeletal system by increasing the permeability of muscle tissue to calcium, thereby causing muscle contraction. Contracted muscle tissue is less likely to use its glycogen stores as a primary source of energy during exercise. An alternative energy source is provided by a caffeine-induced increase in plasma levels of free fatty acids, which provide energy through lipid metabolism. Although caffeine may provide the conditions that enhance the performance of endurance tasks, it also acts as a mild diuretic that serves to interrupt endurance tasks (Haupt, 1989).

A strong tolerance to caffeine does not develop. Caffeine-induced central nervous system stimulation is especially resistant to the development of tolerance. Two to three cups of coffee are sufficient to induce mild central nervous system stimulation. If tolerance to caffeine does occur, it can be eliminated either by increasing the dose two- to fourfold, or by complete abstinence. Physical dependence on caffeine, however, does develop and withdrawal symptoms may occur upon cessation of caffeine (Blum, 1984).

To discourage athletes' use of megadoses of caffeine as a performance enhancer, the NCAA and USOC have set upper limits for acceptable caffeine concentration in urine. The maximum acceptable levels of caffeine in urine are 15 μg/ml for the NCAA and 12 μg/ml for the USOC (Nuzzo & Waller, 1988). Haupt (1989) observed that to achieve the maximum acceptable levels, an individual would have to consume 6–10 cups of coffee in one sitting and provide a urine sample 2–3 hr after consuming the dose.

Amphetamines

Amphetamine, the racemic mixture, was first synthesized in 1927. During the 1940s, the *l*- and *d*-isomers of amphetamine were manufactured (Blum, 1984). Generic and brand (in capital letters) names of some of the amphetamines are as follows: racemic amphetamine sulfate (Benzedrine), dextroamphetamine sulfate (Dexedrine), methamphetamine hydrochloride (desoxyephedrine hydrochloride) (Desoxyn and Methampex), and amphetamine complex (amphetamine and *d*-amphetamine resin) (Biphetamine) (Lombardo, 1987a). Clinically, amphetamines are prescribed to treat hyperkinesis and narcolepsy and for epileptic individuals who take phenobarbitol.

Amphetamines have been self-administered by mouth, by the intravenous route, and by snorting through the nares, with subsequent increases in plasma levels of the drug. Amphetamines activate the central and peripheral sympathetic nervous systems. Although amphetamines indirectly activate the sympathetic neurons through affecting dopamine, norepinephrine, and epinephrine, the stimulant effects of amphetamines result primarily from the release of dopamine in the brain (Iversen & Iversen, 1981).

Activation of the sympathetic nervous systems serves to psychologically and physiologically alert bodily systems into a state of heightened arousal. Mental vigilance is enhanced, pupils dilate, and the emphasis of the cardiovascular system shifts toward moving blood supplies (i.e., oxygen) to the musculoskeletal system. Thus, the heart rate increases, contractions of the heart muscle become more pronounced, and arterial pressure increases to push blood supplies to the muscles, where, under sympathetic conditions, the blood vessels are dilated to receive more blood. Peripheral vasoconstriction also occurs, which causes increased peripheral resistance and increased core body temperature.

The amphetamines, therefore, may enhance athletic performance by enhancing mental vigilance during exercise and by increasing blood flow to the muscles. However, exercise also activates blood flow into skeletal muscles through sympathetic vasodilator nerves and through an autoregulator mechanism that is activated by metabolism within skeletal muscles. The amphetamines provide a small margin in enhancing athletic performance in activities that require acute bursts of strength and in activities that require prolonged endurance (Laties & Weiss, 1981).

Amphetamine-induced cardiovascular fatalities, however, have occurred as the result of cerebrovascular hemorrhage and cardiac failure. Also, amphetamine-induced hyperthermia can lead to fatalities for athletes who perform prolonged intensive exercises on hot sunny days. The complications for hyperthermia that can be fatal are hyperpyrexia (extremely high body temperature), cardiovascular shock, and convulsions (Nuzzo & Waller, 1988).

Tolerance and physical dependence to the amphetamines can occur. Prevalence in the use of amphetamines by athletes is not known. It has been estimated that within the general population several million Americans are involved with oral abuse of stimulants (Blum, 1984). Amphetamines are banned by the NCAA and the USOC (Haupt, 1989).

USE OF DEPRESSANTS BY ATHLETES

If central nervous system depressants (i.e., alcohol and marijuana) are used by athletes, they are typically used as recreational drugs. The exception is for athletes who participate in rifle sports, in which performance may be enhanced by alcohol use. Hence, alcohol use in rifle sports is banned by the NCAA. For other sports, alcohol use is not banned by the NCAA or USOC (Haupt, 1989). Marijuana use disqualifies athletes from competition if the concentration of tetrahydrocannabinol (THC) in the urine exceeds 25 ng/ml (Haupt, 1989).

Ethanol

Two-thirds of all American adults drink ethanol-containing beverages (Morgan, 1985). Ethanol is an aliphatic hydrocarbon that contains a hydroxyl group (alcohols). Ethanol is the product of fermenting naturally occurring carbohydrates (i.e., grapes, potatoes, and rye) with yeast. Wine is produced by the natural fermentation process, which will continue until the maximum ethanol concentration (12–14%) is obtained. Beer incorporates carbon dioxide from the fermentation process and contains 3.2–6% ethanol. Ethanol concentrations above 14% (i.e., whiskey and vodka) are obtained through distilling processes in which the more volatile ethanol is collected (Morgan, 1985). Although ethanol-containing beverages are legal to consume and may be easily purchased, ethanol distribution and sales are controlled by state laws.

Ethanol is self-administered by mouth and is absorbed by the circulatory system through the alimentary tract, especially the small intestine. The absorption rate of ethanol into general circulation increases with increasing doses of ethanol and increases with decreasing amounts of food. Blood alcohol levels reach maximum from one-half to 2 hr following self-administration. Very low percentages of ethanol are excreted by the kidneys or lungs. After a moderate dose of ethanol, 2% may be excreted, and after a large dose of ethanol 10% may be excreted. Blood alcohol levels increase with increasing doses of ethanol, and through diffusion ethanol is slowly distributed to other bodily tissues and fluids until equilibrium is reached. Ethanol undergoes complete oxidation in bodily tissues and fluids. The products of oxidation are water, which is excreted by the kidneys, and carbonic acid gas, which is excreted by the lungs (Starling, 1923).

The slow diffusion of ethanol from plasma allows ethanol greater exposure to liver enzymes (i.e., alcohol dehydrogenase) that can oxidize 10 ml of pure ethanol per hour in a person weighing 160 pounds. Higher doses of ethanol are oxidized by a microsomal mixed-function oxidase system that also aids in metabolizing other sedative drugs. Ethanol also affects the liver by interfering with the metabolism of carbohydrates, thereby allowing fat to accumulate in the liver, which during chronic ethanol consumption may result in liver cirrhosis (Morgan, 1985).

Brain tissue and blood alcohol levels reach equilibrium rapidly as a result of the large number of blood vessels in brain tissue. Ethanol markedly affects brain tissue by altering the flow of sodium and potassium ions of the neurons and by altering neuroamine metabolism. Of all the sedative euphoriants, ethanol is the only one whose use results in observable tissue toxicity in the central nervous system. Ethanol interferes with motor function and judgment simultaneously. The American Medical Association and the National Safety Council consider an individual intoxicated with 150 mg of alcohol per 100 ml blood (0.15%) or its equivalent in urine, saliva, or breath (Nuzzo & Waller, 1988).

Ethanol has been found to differentially affect hormone secretion in males and females. Mendelson and Mello (1988) observed that for women, ethanol (2.2 ml of 100-proof vodka per kilogram of body weight) ingestion did not acutely affect plasma levels of leutinizing hormone and estradiol. Although prolactin levels did rise as plasma levels of ethanol fell, the prolactin levels were within normal range for healthy, nonlactating females. In contrast, ethanol (2.4 ml of 100-proof vodka per kilogram of body weight) ingestion acutely affected hormone levels in males. For males, as blood alcohol levels rose, testosterone levels fell and leutinizing hormone levels increased (Mendelson & Mello, 1988).

Also, ethanol intake may result in an increase of the testosterone/epitestosterone (T/E) weight ratio in the urine that may continue for up to 22 hr following the ingestion of ethanol. The average urinary T/E weight ratio achieved by the men who self-administered ethanol (1.0–2.0 grams per kilogram body weight) was approximately 1.50 and the maximum urinary T/E weight ratio value achieved following ethanol drinking was 2.45. Urinary T/E weight ratios are used to detect exogenous testosterone self-administration by athletes; however, a urinary T/E weight ratio value greater than 6 is required to consider evidence for doping (Falk, Palonek, & Bjorkhem, 1988).

Tolerance and physical dependence to ethanol can occur. When exposed to ethanol, central nervous system cells may undergo adaptational changes that result in cellular or pharmacological tolerance to ethanol. If tolerance to ethanol is established, cross-tolerance to other central nervous system depressants also occurs. Physical dependence on ethanol may develop and profound withdrawal syndromes may occur 24–48 hr following abstinence from ethanol-containing beverages (Morgan, 1985).

Ethanol usually has adverse effects on athletic performance. Following the ingestion of ethanol, impairment has been observed in reaction time, hand–eye coordination, accuracy, balance, and complex coordination of gross motor skills (Lombardo, 1987b). Survey estimates indicated that 60% of college athletes were regular users of alcohol. If athletes use recreational drugs, ethanol-containing beverages are the most widely used recreational drug (Nuzzo & Waller, 1988).

Marijuana

Marijuana, hashish, and all varieties of cannabis are derived from the plant *Cannabis salita*. Δ^9-tetrahydrocannabinol (THC) is the main active ingredient in marijuana (Braude, 1972). Although marijuana can be taken by mouth and absorbed by the alimentary tract, in the United States, marijuana is usually self-administered by inhaling the smoky air into the lungs. It is estimated that the smoking process delivers 15–40% of the available Δ^9-THC to pulmonary circulation for absorption (Szara, 1972).

Δ^9-THC is pumped from pulmonary circulation into general circulation by the heart. A reliable dose-dependent physiological effect of Δ^9-THC is an increase in pulse rate and systolic blood pressure. It is not known whether Δ^9-THC affects cardiac function by direct action on the heart muscle or through effects on the autonomic nervous system. Chronic marijuana smoking has not resulted in cardiovascular disease (Szara, 1972).

Δ^9-THC is rapidly converted to 11-hydroxy-THC metabolites by the liver and lungs. In an unusual process, the metabolic products of Δ^9-THC are recirculated between the liver and gastrointestinal tract where metabolites are reabsorbed and either directed back toward the liver or expelled in feces. Marijuana commonly stimulates the appetite by undefined biological mechanisms. Plasma levels of glucose and free fatty acids are not affected by marijuana use. However, glucose in glucose tolerance tests deteriorates more rapidly following the administration of Δ^9-THC (Ramsey, 1972).

Inconclusive and conflicting evidence about the effects of chronic marijuana use on plasma levels of testosterone, estradiol, leutinizing hormone, and prolactin have been reported. Similarly, the effects of marijuana on spermatozoa count and spermatozoa motility have not been conclusively determined. Reports of gynecomastia and reduced spermatozoa count following chronic marijuana use have occasionally appeared in the literature (Ramsey, 1972).

Marijuana affects performance by interfering with attention. External stimuli are responded to more slowly. The maintenance and coordination of behaviors that are required to perform prolonged tasks are temporarily distracted with marijuana use. Some behavioral tolerance to marijuana's disruption of performance in prolonged tasks was observed in chronic marijuana users, who made fewer mistakes than marijuana initiates did. However, tolerance to other effects of marijuana have not been reported, and in some instance diminution of motivation to do work has been exacerbated with chronic marijuana use. Physical dependence on Δ^9-THC has not been observed; however, a mild "withdrawal" syndrome has been reported and attributed to psychological dependence on the effects of marijuana (Ramsey, 1972).

The prevalence of marijuana use by athletes is estimated to be comparable with the prevalence of marijuana use by the general population. Surveys conducted during the 1970s revealed that approximately 9% of the adult population had used marijuana at some time and of the 9% who ever used marijuana, 5% were daily users (Richards, 1972). Meer (1987) reported that marijuana use was the largest drug problem for athletes, for whom more sports careers were terminated by marijuana use than from using all of the other drugs, including alcohol, combined.

MONITORING THE USE
OF DRUGS BY ATHLETES

During the 1960s, two cyclists died during competition and their deaths were attributed to the use of psychomotor stimulants. The International Cycling Federation was the first international organization to issue rules about athletes' drug use and to institute mandatory monitoring of drug use through the analyses of urine specimens. Comprehensive monitoring of drug use during the Olympic Games was initiated at the 1972 summer games in Munich (Catlin, 1987).

Implementation of programs that monitor drug use by athletes, however, continues to be under discussion. Meer (1987) reported poll results of the Houston Oiler football players in which 57% of the players said they favored random drug testing, while 43% said they opposed it. Boswell (1988) interviewed collegiate and professional basketball coaches, some of whom have monitored their athletes for drug use. The five coaches interviewed endorsed mandatory monitoring of their athletes for drug use. In general, the coaches wanted their athletes to be free from drug use because public trust in sports would be enhanced, athletes enjoy a leadership role, athletes' behaviors receive extensive press coverage, and athletes' performances are compromised by drugs.

What does the public want from its athletes? Burnwell (1988) cited Padwe's (1986) observations from a *Sports Illustrated* poll of 2,000 adults in which 73% of the respondents indicated that they favored monitoring athletes' drug use. Haupt (1989) observed that mandatory monitoring of drug use is a fact of life for many athletes, especially nonprofessionals. The NCAA, the USOC, and the IOC require mandatory monitoring of drug use by athletes who compete in events governed by their sanctioning organizations. A well-managed drug monitoring program consists of the following characteristics.

Written consent is obtained from all athletes. Athletes are selected for monitoring by a random system, by player position or player sport, or by reasonable cause or suspicion. The selected athletes provide urine specimens (100–200 ml) on demand and under supervision. The specimens are evaluated for integrity and accepted if they are acidic and if the specific gravity is above 1.010. To maintain confidentiality and control during analyses, athletes observe as their urine specimens are poured into coded containers. Urine specimens are screened by either chromatography or enzyme multiplied immunoassay technique (EMIT). Confirmations of drug-related contents in the urine specimens are obtained by a gas chromatography/mass spectrometry (GC/MS) study. The GC/MS is the only legally admissible analysis of drug-related contents in urine specimens. If drug-related contents are detected, then the athlete is invited to observe a second set of analyses that are performed within 24 hr (Haupt, 1989).

Consequences for the athletes whose urine specimens indicate drug use depends on the sanctioning body's rules about the type and amount of drug detected in the urine specimens. For example, if one of the approximately 300 substances banned by the USOC is detected in an athlete's urine specimen during Olympic trials, the USOC rules that the athlete is disqualified from competition. Under IOC rules, if a Level 1 drug (i.e., anabolic steroid, amphetamine-related and other stimulants, caffeine, diuretics, beta-blockers, narcotic analgesics, and "designed" drugs) is detected in an athlete's urine specimen, then the athlete is banned from competition for 2 years for the first offense and for life with the second offense (Haupt, 1989).

An alternative system of monitoring drug use by athletes has been proposed by Forest Tennant. Griffin (1988) recently restated Tennant's position that drug use by athletes may be crudely evaluated by performing rapid eye screening tests. Tennant, drug advisor to the NFL, observed that dilated pupils may indicate cocaine or amphetamine use; constricted pupils may indicate heroin or opiate use; red glazed eyes, nonconvergence, and a pupil that reacts slowly to light may indicate marijuana use; and a retracted upper eyelid that projects the image of a blank stare may indicate phencyclidine (PCP) use.

On March 21, 1989, Pete Rozelle, Commissioner of the NFL, announced that the four-game suspension rule, which is invoked after detection of illegal drug use by NFL players, would also be applied when steroids or masking agents are detected. The NFL players union tested the steroid suspension rule in court and lost the decision. On August 28, 1989, the NFL players union was unable to obtain a court order to prevent the NFL management from initiating press releases about the players' use of steroids or masking agents. The following day, 13 NFL players were identified in the press as users of anabolic–androgenic steroid or masking agents ("Eagles' Solt, 12 others suspended for steroid use," August 30, 1989).

REFERENCES

Alen, M., Rahkila, P., & Marniemi. (1985). Serum lipids in power athletes self-administering testosterone and anabolic steroids. *International Journal of Sports Medicine, 6,* 139–144.

Alen, M., Rahkila, P., Reinila, M., & Vikhko, R. (1987). Androgenic–anabolic steroid effects on serum thyroid, pituitary and steroid hormones in athletes. *American Journal of Sports Medicine, 15,* 357–361.

Alen, M., Reinila, M., & Vihko, R. (1985). Response of serum hormones to androgen administration in power athletes. *Medicine and Science in Sports and Exercise, 17,* 354–359.

American Psychiatric Association. (1987). *Diagnostic and statistical manual of mental disorders* (3rd ed., rev.). Washington, DC: Author.

Bergman, R., & Leach, R. E. (1985). The use and abuse of anabolic steroids in

Olympic-caliber athletes. *Clinical Orthopaedics and Related Research, 198,* 169–172.

Berkow, R. (1982). *Merck manual of diagnosis and therapy* (14th ed.). Rathway, NJ: Merck & Co.

Berkowitz, S. (1989, January 15). Locally and nationally, high schools are at a pressure point. *The Washington Post,* pp. D–1, D–2.

Blum, K. (1984). *Handbook of abusable drugs.* New York: Gardner Press.

Boswell, T. (1988). Athletes should be tested for drugs. In J. S. Bach (Ed.), *Drug abuse: Opposing viewpoints* (pp. 145–150). St. Paul, MN: Greenhaven Press.

Braude, M. (1972). The material and analytic methodology. In R. C. Peterson (Ed.), *Marihuana and health: Second annual report to Congress* (pp. 133–156). Washington, DC: Department of Health, Education and Welfare.

Buckley, W. E., Yesalis, C. E., III, Friedyl, K. E., Anderson, W. W., Streit, A. L., & Wright, J. E. (1988). Estimated prevalence of anabolic steroid use among male high school seniors. *Journal of the American Medical Association, 260,* 3441–3445.

Burnwell, B. (1988). Testing athletes is unfair. In J. S. Bach (Ed.), *Drug abuse: Opposing viewpoints* (pp. 151–156). St. Paul, MN: Greenhaven Press.

Catlin, D. H. (1987). Detection of drug use by athletes. In R. H. Strauss (Ed.), *Drugs and performance in sports* (pp. 103–120). Philadelphia: W. B. Saunders.

Colby, H. D., & Longhurst, P. A. (1988). Fate of anabolic steroids in the body. In J. A. Thomas (Ed.), *Drugs, athletes, and physical performance* (pp. 11–30). New York: Plenum.

Cowart, V. (1986). Road back from substance abuse especially long, hard for athletes. *Journal of the American Medical Association, 256,* 2645–2649.

Cowart, V. (1987). Some predict increased steroid use in sports despite drug testing, crackdown on supplies. *Journal of the American Medical Association, 257,* 3025, 3029.

Cowart, V. (1988). Accord on drug testing, sanctions sought before 1992 Olympics in Europe. *Journal of the American Medical Association, 260,* 3397–3398.

Cowart, V. (1989a). National Institute on Drug Abuse may join in anabolic steroid research. *Journal of the American Medical Association, 261,* 1855–1856.

Cowart, V. (1989b). If youngsters overdoes with anabolic steroids, what's the cost anatomically and otherwise? *Journal of the American Medical Association, 261,* 1856–1857.

Cowart, V. (1989c). Athlete drug testing receiving more attention than ever before in history of competition. *Journal of the American Medical Association, 261,* 3510, 3511, 3516.

Dorland's illustrated medical dictionary (27th ed.). (1988). Philadelphia: W. B. Saunders.

Eagles' Solt, 12 others suspended for steroid use. (1989, August 30). *Baltimore Evening Sun,* p. B-7.

Falk, O., Palonek, E., & Bjorkhem, I. (1988). Effect of ethanol on the ratio between testosterone and epitestosterone in urine. *Clinical Chemistry, 34,* 1462–1464.

Ferner, R. E., & Rawlins, M. D. (1988). Anabolic steroids: The power and the glory? *British Medical Journal, 297,* 877–878.

Frankle, M. A., Eichberg, R., & Zachariah, S. B. (1988). Anabolic andro-

Keenan, E. J. (1988). Anabolic and androgenic steroids. In J. A. Thomas (Ed.), *Drugs, athletics, and physical performance* (pp. 91–103). New York: Plenum.

Kenyon, A. T. (1938). The effect of testosterone propionate on the genitalia, prostate, secondary sex characteristics, and body weight in eunuchoidism. *Endocrinology, 23*(2), 121–134.

Kenyon, A. T., Sandiford, I., Bryan, A. H., Knowlton, K., & Koch, F. C. (1938). The effect of testosterone propionate on nitrogen, electrolyte, water and energy metabolism in eunuchoidism. *Endocrinology, 23*(2), 135–153.

Kiraly, C. L. (1988). Androgenic-anabolic steroid effects on serum and skin surface lipids, on red cells and on liver enzymes. *International Journal of Sports Medicine, 9,* 249–252.

Kiraly, C. L., Alen, M., Rahkila, P., & Horsmanheimo, M. (1987). Effect of androgenic and anabolic steroids on the sebaceous gland in power athletes. *Acta Dermatologica Venereology, 67,* 36–40.

Kiraly, C. L., Collan, Y., & Alen, M. (1987). Effect of testosterone and anabolic athletes on the size of sebaceous glands in power athletes. *American Journal of Dermatopathology, 9,* 515–519.

Kolb, L. (1962). *Drug addiction: A medical problem.* Springfield, IL: Charles C Thomas.

Lamb, D. R. (1984). Anabolic steroids in athletes: How well do they work and how dangerous are they? *American Journal of Sports Medicine, 12,* 31–38.

Laties, V. G., & Weiss, B. (1981). The amphetamine margin in sports. *Federation Proceedings, 40,* 2689–2692.

Lendes, J. W. M., Demecker, P. N. M., Vos, J. A., Jansen, P. L. M., Hoitsma, A. J., van't Laar, A., & Thien, T. (1988). Deleterious effects of anabolic steroids on serum lipoproteins, blood pressure, and liver function in amateur body builders. *International Journal of Sports Medicine, 9,* 19–23.

Lombardo, J. A. (1987a). Stimulants. In R. H. Strauss (Ed.), *Drugs and performance in sports* (pp. 69–86). Philadelphia: W. B. Saunders.

Lombardo, J. A. (1987b). Depressants. In R. H. Strauss (Ed.) *Drugs and performance in sports* (pp. 87–102). Philadelphia: W. B. Saunders.

Marshall, E. (1988). The drug of champions. *Science, 242,* 183-184.

McKillop, G., & Ballantyne, D. (1987). Lipoprotein analysis in bodybuilders. *International Journal of Cardiology, 17,* 281-286.

Meer, J. (1987). *Drugs and sports.* New York: Chelsea House.

Mellon, M. B. (1984). Anabolic steroids in athletes. *American Family Physician, 30,* 113-119.

Mendelson, J. H., & Mello, N. K. (1988). Acute and chronic effects of alcohol on the hypothalamic-pituitary-gonadal axis in men and women. In R. H. Rose & J. E. Barrett (Eds.), *Alcoholism: Origins and outcome* (pp. 175-208). New York: Raven Press.

Mochizuki, R. M. & Richter, K. J. (1988). Cardiomyopathy and cerebral vascular accident associated with anabolic-androgenic steroid use. *Physician and Sportsmedicine, 16,* 108-114.

Morgan, J. P. (1985). *Alcohol and drug abuse curriculum guide for pharmacology faculty* (DHHS Publication No. (ADM) 85-1368). Rockville, MD: U.S. Department of Health and Human Services.

Murad, F., & Haynes, R. C., Jr. (1985). Steroids. In A. Goodman Gilman, L. S. Goodman, T. W. Rall, & F. Murad (Eds.), *Goodman and Gilman's: The pharmacological basis of therapeutics* (7th ed.) (pp. 1440-1458). New York: Macmillan.

Nuzzo, N. A., & Waller, D. P. (1988). Drug abuse in athletics. In J. A. Thomas (Ed.), *Drugs, athletics, and physical performance* (pp. 141-168). New York: Plenum.

Padwe, S. (1986, September 27). Unfair attitudes. *The Nation.*

Pope, H. G., & Katz, D. L. (1988). Affective and psychotic symptoms associated with anabolic steroid use. *American Journal of Psychiatry, 145,* 487-490.

Ramsey, A. (1972). Effects in Man. In R. C. Peterson (Ed.), *Marihuana and health: Second annual report to Congress* (pp. 199-258). Washington, DC: Department of Health, Education and Welfare.

Richards, L. (1972). Extent, patterns and social context of use in the United States. In R. C. Peterson (Ed.), *Marihuana and health: Second annual report to Congress* (pp. 31-53). Washington, DC: Department of Health, Education and Welfare.

Ruokonen, A., Alen, M., Bolton, N., & Vihko, R. (1985). Response of serum testosterone and its precursor steroids, SHBG and CBG to anabolic steroid and testosterone self-administration in man. *Journal of Steroid Biochemistry, 23,* 33-38.

Ryan, A. J. (1981). Anabolic steroids are fool's gold. *Federation Proceedings, 40,* 2982-2988.

Scott, J. (1988, December 16). Boys cite athletic performance, "looks": Use of steroids by youths widespread, study finds. *Los Angeles Times,* pp. 1, 45.

Starling, E. H. (1923). *The action of alcohol on man.* New York: Longmans, Green.

Strauss, R. H., Liggett, M. T., & Lanese, R. R. (1985). Anabolic steroid use and the perceived effects in ten weight-trained women athletes. *Journal of the American Medical Association, 253,* 2871–2873.

Szara, S. (1972). Effects in man. In R. C. Peterson (Ed.), *Marihuana and health: Second annual report to Congress* (pp. 199–258). Washington, DC: Department of Health, Education and Welfare.

Tennant, F., Black, D. L., & Voy, R. O. (1988). Anabolic steroid dependence with opioid-type features. *New England Journal of Medicine, 319,* 578.

Wade, N. (1972). Anabolic steroids: Doctors denounce them, but athletes aren't listening. *Science, 176,* 1399–1403.

Webb, O. L., Laskarzewski, P. M., & Glueck, C. J. (1984). Severe depression of high-density lipoprotein cholesterol levels in weight lifters and body builders by self-administered exogenous testosterone and anabolic-androgenic steroids. *Metabolism, 33,* 971–975.

Wheeler, G. D., Wall, S. R., Belcastro, A. N., & Cumming, D. C. (1984). Reduced serum testosterone and prolactin levels in male distance runners. *Journal of the American Medical Association, 252,* 514–516.

White House Conference for a Drug Free America. (1988). *Final report.* Washington, DC: U.S. Government Printing Office.

Williams, M. H. (1974). *Drugs and athletic performance.* Springfield, IL: Charles C Thomas.

Wilson, J. D., & Griffin, J. E. (1980). The use and misuse of androgens. *Metabolism, 29,* 1278–1295.

Wright, J. E. (1978). *Anabolic steroids and sports: A complete report on the controversial drugs used to increase muscle size and strength.* Natick, MA: Sports Science Consultants.

Yesalis, C. E. (1988, December 4). Steroid use is not just an adult problem. *New York Times,* Section 8, S, p. 1.

Yesalis, C. E., Streit, A. L., Vicary, J. R., Friedl, K. E., Brannon, D., & Buckley, W. (1989). Anabolic steroid use: Indications of habituation among adolescents. *Journal of Drug Education, 19,* 103–116.

5

THE INFLUENCE OF AEROBIC EXERCISE ON ILLNESS

Stephen H. Boutcher

University of Wollongong, Australia

A commonly held belief of runners is that regular aerobic exercise promotes resistance to respiratory infection such as colds and influenza (Mackinnon & Tomasi, 1986; Pederson et al., 1989). Does aerobic exercise effectively prevent illness, and can activities such as running, cycling, and swimming play major roles in preventative health strategies? Interestingly, there is also anecdotal support for the notion that too much exercise can have negative health consequences (Ryan, 1983). Does too much exercise actually suppress the immune system and result in greater incidence of illness?

These questions form the focus of this chapter, which is directed to a general audience. After a brief review of the immune system, the research examining the positive and negative health consequences of exercise is reviewed. Then strategies to optimize the health benefits of exercise and techniques to offset the deleterious effects of intense training are outlined, after which recommendations for future research are discussed.

THE IMMUNE SYSTEM

Billions of microorganisms consisting of bacteria, viruses, parasites, and fungi abound in the environment and on the body's surface and can, if unchallenged, cause disease and fatal affliction. Luckily, the immune system exists to recognize and repel foreign invaders. The immune system is an immensely complex and multifaceted integration of a number of physiological mechanisms whose functioning is only beginning to be understood. The focus of inquiry has been largely undertaken by immunologists, but recent subdisciplines such as psycho-neuroimmunology represent a shift from viewing the immune system as being isolated and autonomous. This development is exciting because there is a clear need to examine and understand the relation between the nervous, endocrine, and immune systems and their effect on health (Jemmott, 1985).

The immune system can be viewed as comprising both innate and acquired immune defenses (Guyton, 1986). Innate defenses include the skin, nose, mucosa lining of the respiratory tract, digestive juices of the stomach, and the triggering of the inflammatory response. Also the activation of proteins (the complement complex) to destroy bacteria and the phagocytosis (destruction of microbes) of invading bacteria and viruses by the macrophage system are part of the innate defense system. *Complement* is a term used to describe the substances in blood serum or plasma that in combination with antibodies cause the destruction of bacteria and foreign blood corpuscles. The phagocytes are part of a family of white blood cells termed *leukocytes* and are most sensitive to any initial disruption of the cellular environment. They are the first line of defense and consume invading microbes that may enter the body through the lungs or open wounds. However, the phagocytes cannot cope with any large-scale microbe invasion such as rhinovirus (common cold); if the phagocytes start to be outnumbered, a macrophage, which is a specialized form of phagocyte, arrives at the site of invasion.

One of the major roles of the macrophage is to alert the acquired immune defenses. The two basic types of acquired immune defenses are cell-mediated immunity and humoral immunity (Guyton, 1986). Both cell-mediated and humoral immunity involve approximately one trillion specialized white blood cells called *lymphocytes* that exist to counteract viruses or bacteria that may enter cell membranes. The white cells of the cell-mediated defense, which are mainly created in the thymus, are T cells (thymus dependent), whereas the white cells of the humoral immune defense involve B cells (bone marrow).

The macrophage alerts the T and B cells of the lymphocytes, which in contrast to phagocytes, reside in the lymph nodes that are scattered throughout the body. The lymph nodes act as sites where B cells produce antibodies. The macrophage captures an invading microbe and attaches it to its body. Helper T cells circulating throughout the blood then recognize the displayed antigen (microorganisms that invoke some form of immune response) and in turn communicate chemically to killer T cells, which multiply rapidly and destroy the viruses before they have time to multiply. Suppressor T cells turn off both killer and helper T cells and, by regulating the activity of other cells, circumvent unnecessary damage to the body.

The helper T cells also play an important role by exciting the B cells of the humoral defense system. Antibodies produced by the B cells can attach themselves to the surface of any invading microbe, slowing their activity and making them easier targets for phagocytes. There are five classes of antibody (IgA, IgD, IgE, IgG, and IgM) that collectively are called *immunoglobulins* (Lentner, 1984). The majority of immunoglobulins consist of IgG, which provides a defense against viruses, toxins, and bacteria. IgA are mainly found in nasal mucosa and saliva. These and the other different immunoglobulins generate antibody accumulation in a variety of sites such as cell surfaces, blood, and exocrine glands (e.g., the pancreas).

Over days and weeks the cell-mediated and humoral defenses are called into action and eventually the invading bacteria or virus is defeated. The invading virus is not forgotten, however, because specialized T and B cells remember the structure of the antigen, and should it reappear a second time it will be defeated far more quickly.

Certain viruses such as those involved in acquired immune deficiency syndrome (AIDS) and hepatitis B are only dangerous if they enter directly into the bloodstream, whereas other viruses such as cold and flu are airborne and can enter the body through the respiratory tract. Autoimmune disorders involve the immune system's failing to recognize the body's cells and attacking its own body. For instance, in rheumatic fever the heart is attacked, whereas in rheumatoid arthritis the joints are affected.

Factors that modify immune function include genetics, age, metabolism, anatomy, environment, stress, and exercise (Bellanti, 1985). Young and old individuals generally have lower levels of immunity and thus are more prone to contract infection and disease. In a young person the immune system is underdeveloped, whereas in an elderly person the immune system is weakened through constant exposure to antigens. For more in-depth descriptions of the immune system, see Guyton (1986); Keast, Cameron, and Morton (1988); and Boggs and Winklestein (1983).

The Effect of Exercise on Immunity Enhancement

Anecdotal evidence (Nash, 1986) and results of surveys (Jorgenson & Jorgenson, 1979; McCutcheon & Hassini, 1981) indicate that runners perceive that exercise promotes resistance to infection. Although the buffering effect of aerobic exercise on illness and disease seems to be a widespread view among exercisers, data to support this belief are equivocal. Even though many biochemical studies have shown that exercise changes certain immune parameters, it has not been conclusively demonstrated that exercise increases resistance to illness.

Generally, the majority of studies examining the effect of exercise on biochemical parameters of the immune system have indicated that moderate exercise can enhance certain immune parameters (Mackinnon & Tomasi, 1986). The most consistent changes in immune function after exercise are an increase in white blood cells (Hanson & Flaherty, 1981; Landmann et al., 1984; Soppi,

Varjo, Eskola, & Laitinen, 1982), an increase in antibodies (Hedfors, Biber-feld, & Wahren, 1978; Hedfors, Holm, & Ohnell, 1976) and natural killer cells (Edwards et al., 1984; Pederson et al., 1989; Targan, Britvan, & Dorey, 1981), and a redistribution of circulating lymphocytes (Tomasi, Trudeau, Czerwinski, & Erredge, 1982).

For instance, Pederson et al. (1989) examined the concentration of natural killer cells in highly trained racing cyclists and age-matched untrained controls. Subjects' blood was sampled at rest after which maximal oxygen uptake was assessed 1 week later. Subjects were not allowed to exercise 20 hr prior to blood sampling. Natural killer cell activity was measured through use of a release assay. The authors found that the trained cyclists possessed increased natural T-cell killer function and suggested that highly trained aerobic athletes may have greater resistance against infectious diseases.

Whereas Pederson et al. (1989) examined elite athletes at rest, Hanson and Flaherty (1981) measured the concentration and activity of leukocytes, immu-noglobulins, and complement in 6 elite runners before and after an 8-mile training run. The only immune parameter found to change was an increase in lymphocyte cytotoxic activity after exercise, which the authors suggested may provide an enhanced immune response to viral infection. For more in-depth reviews of these and other studies, see Keast et al. (1988), Simon (1984), and Mackinnon and Tomasi (1986).

The Effects of Intense Training on Immune Function

In aerobic sports such as swimming, physiological reactions to heavy training are a constant concern to coaches. Swim coaches typically use "overreaching" as an essential part of their training programs. Overreaching involves intensive bouts of swimming, usually lasting about 5–10 days at intensities well above the normal training intensity. These programs are usually followed by rest or taper-ing periods. Swimmers whose performance is negatively affected by this type of intensive training are usually termed "stale" or "overtrained." From the swimmers' and coaches' standpoint this is a highly undesirable state because the general remedy is immediate cessation of training or significantly reduced workloads. Because recovery from staleness or overtraining can vary from weeks to 3 months (Ryan, 1983), staleness could have drastic effects on the athlete's career (e.g., missing the Olympic Games). Furthermore, anecdotal and clinical evidence suggests that intense training may have the potential to increase susceptibility to illness (Ryan, 1983), which may further prevent sports participation and exacerbate the recovery process.

The negative effects of intense training are not exclusive to swimming, however. For instance, both competitive and recreational runners (Dressendor-fer, Wade, & Scaff, 1985) and speed skaters (Gutmann, Pollock, Foster, &

Schmidt, 1984) have also reported negative health consequences as a result of being involved in intense training regimens. More psychologically oriented forms of high-intensity training (burnout) have also been recorded in coaching (Smith, 1986) and athletic training (Gieck, Brown, & Shank, 1982).

The literature examining the effects of intense training on health and performance has examined a greater variety of variables compared with that investigating immune enhancement. For instance, biochemical markers, mood, infection rates, and performance have been investigated.

Studies have indicated that excessive exercise can reduce salivary IgA and IgM following exercise (Tomasi et al., 1982), decrease natural killer cell activity (Brahmi, Thomas, Park, & Dodeswell, 1985), increase cortisol and creatine kinase levels (Kirwan et al., 1988), and lower complement and immunoglobulin levels (Nieman, Tan, Lee, & Berk, 1988). In addition, a decrease in mood (Morgan, Brown, Raglin, O'Connor, & Ellickson, 1987) and an increase in incidence of respiratory infection rates after exercise (Peters & Bateman, 1983) have been found.

Tomasi et al. (1982) examined the secretory IgA levels in nationally ranked Nordic skiers before and after a national cross-country race. Skiers, compared with age-matched controls, exhibited significantly lower levels of salivary IgA before and after the race. The authors speculated that the mechanism underlying the lower IgA levels may be the depletion of nasal fluid together with the disruption of the mucosal plasma cells as a result of decreased temperature in the mucous membranes. The authors further suggested that this temporary antibody deficiency on the mucosal surface may be the precursor to the acquisition of viral and bacterial infections following vigorous exercise. Thus, exercising in cold environments may result in a temporary antibody deficiency of mucosal immunoglobulins. If this indeed were the case, then individuals who exercise in cold environments may be more susceptible to acquiring bacterial and viral infection immediately after finishing exercise. Barnes (1989) also found that male and female collegiate swimmers involved in an intensive swimming bout recorded declined IgA secretion levels in response to acute and long-term training stimuli.

Cortisol and creatine kinase levels were investigated by Kirwan et al. (1988), who examined the effects of swim training on 12 collegiate swimmers who swam for 10 days building up to more than 8,000 m per day at an intensity of 95% of aerobic capacity. These swimmers did not experience reduced aerobic capacity but did show enhanced serum cortisol and creatine kinase levels to the exercise stimulus. The authors concluded that increased cortisol and creatine kinase levels were a normal response for athletes in these kinds of training programs. Because corticosteroids have been shown to depress immune function (Cupps & Fauci, 1982), it is feasible that increased plasma cortisol levels accompanying intensive exercise such as swimming can depress certain immune parameters.

Complement and immunoglobulin levels after a graded exercise test have been examined by Nieman et al. (1988). Data from 11 marathon runners were collected at rest, during a treadmill test, and 45 min into recovery. Results indicated that complement levels but not immunoglobulin levels were significantly lower in marathon runners during rest, exercise, and recovery. The authors suggested that the lower complement levels in marathoners may represent a normal response to chronic running.

Morgan et al. (1987) summarized the results of 10 years of research examining mood changes associated with swimming and wrestling. For both groups it was found that a mood scale called the Profile of Mood States (POMS; McNair, Lorr, & Droppleman, 1971) was sensitive to negative psychological changes brought by hard exercise. Prior research by Morgan (for an overview see Morgan et al., 1987) has indicated that elite athletes in a variety of sports exhibit the "iceberg" profile when the six subscores of the POMS (tension, depression, anger, vigor, fatigue, and confusion) are plotted. When suffering from the effects of overtraining, however, their scores reflect an "inverted-iceberg" profile, which Morgan suggested is indicative of disturbed mental health. This profile has been found for both wrestlers and swimmers during chronic overtraining over a season (Morgan et al., 1987) and after acute bouts of hard exercise (Morgan, Costill, Flynn, Raglin, & O'Connor, 1988).

Epidemiological evidence also exists suggesting that excessive aerobic exercise in the form of ultramarathon running may decrease host resistance to infection. For instance, Peters and Bateman (1983) carried out a prospective study of the incidence of respiratory infection in randomly selected ultramarathon runners. Responses of runners to questions before and after the race were compared with those of individually matched controls. Results indicated that symptoms of respiratory infection occurred in more than 33% of runners compared with 15% in the controls. Higher incidence of respiratory infection and more musculoskeletal pain during and after the race were found in those runners who achieved the faster race times. The authors suggested that the higher incidence of respiratory infection in the faster runners may have been due to impairment of resistance to infection resulting from the stress of ultramarathon running or to the effects of cold and dry air on local mucosal defenses.

Summary

Despite methodological and conceptual problems, the majority of studies examining the relation between exercise and illness indicate that moderate aerobic exercise is associated with certain immune parameter enhancement, whereas intensive aerobic exercise is associated with a depression of certain immune functions. The ability of exercise to actually prevent illness, however, has not been conclusively demonstrated.

THE USE OF EXERCISE AS A PREVENTATIVE HEALTH STRATEGY

Although the negative and positive effects of exercise on illness have still not been clearly identified, the general suggestion that moderate exercise is more health efficacious than intensive exercise is in accordance with data found in other health areas. For instance, moderate exercise as opposed to heavy exercise is associated with less cardiovascular disease (Paffenberger, 1985). Injuries have also been found to substantially increase after runners increase their weekly mileage (Dressendorfer & Wade, 1983). Too low a level of exercise, however, will not bring about physiological adaptations, and thus establishing the optimal amount of exercise for any given individual is crucial. The amount of exercise for any individual will be a function of medical background, fitness status, age, and exercise goals (Cundiff, 1979). For individuals who are more concerned with health factors than with increasing performance levels, the minimum amount of exercise recommended by the American College of Sports Medicine (1978) is a regimen of three to five aerobic sessions per week, at an intensity of 60–75% of aerobic capacity, for a duration of longer than 20 min. However, considering that the dropout rate of exercisers from programs has been estimated at more than 50% (Dishman, 1988), it is important that both psychological as well as physiological factors are considered. Thus, exercise leaders designing fitness programs should be aware of motivational factors, group dynamics, the influence of attainable goals, and the effect of feedback systems rather than only setting objectives that focus exclusively on immediate gains in fitness or strength. Rejeski and Kenney (1988) have described a variety of motivational strategies and psychological factors that need to be considered when attempting to increase exercise adherence.

STRATEGIES TO OFFSET THE NEGATIVE EFFECTS OF INTENSE TRAINING

Athletes and participants in aerobic sports who are concerned with increasing performance will involve themselves in intensive aerobic activity. Thus, the thin line between an optimal training program and one that results in physiological and psychological duress is a balancing act that most exercisers have to endure. Because the remedy for coping with the negative effects of intense training is usually cessation of training, strategies to recognize and prevent staleness and overtrained states would be preferable.

Interestingly, it has been found that reduced training does not affect performance but can change psychological factors in runners. Wittig, Houmard, and Costill (1989) studied the effects of reduced training in 10 well-trained male runners. Runners underwent a 3-week period that involved a 70% reduction in training volume. Psychological factors and performance measures were collected weekly. The results indicated that even though training was significantly reduced running performance was not affected. In addition, overall global mood state was improved for all weeks of the reduced training period. The authors suggested that reduced training during a season may help prevent mood disturbance associated with overtraining.

Even if the most appropriate regimens are used, however, intense aerobic training will still place tremendous physiological and psychological demands on the athlete. Thus, strategies need to be developed to help individuals involved in intensive aerobic regimens to offset or ameliorate negative performance and health effects. Techniques to counter overtraining appear to have largely been ignored by Western coaches but have been developed by their Eastern counterparts. For instance, Crampton and Fox (1987) have described how a whole range of techniques have been used by Eastern Bloc athletes to counter deleterious aspects of demanding training regimens. For instance, recovery time between exercise bouts can be scheduled into the exercise regime to allow athletes more time to recover from training. Crampton and Fox also suggested that a range of regenerative techniques be built into the athlete's daily schedule. Regeneration measures may include massage, sauna, hydrotherapy, physiotherapy, flotation/relaxation tanks, and stress management.

In addition, methods to identify the onset of the negative effects of heavy training need to be available to athletes and coaches. Potential acute symptoms (during or immediately after exercise) and chronic symptoms (during resting states between exercise) that may be useful for this purpose are illustrated in Table 1. For example, monitoring the heart rate immediately after exercise and during rest has been identified as one of the easiest and most effective ways of identifying the onset of overtrained states (Dressendorfer et al., 1985). Dres-

TABLE 1 Chronic and acute psychological, physiological, and behavioral symptoms of overtraining

Psychological	Physiological	Behavioral
Depression	Increased resting heart rate	Decreased performance
Decreased motivation	Elevated training heart rate	Disrupted sleep
Depressed mood	Elevated blood pressure	Change of eating patterns
Change of attitude	Loss of weight	Lethargy
Helplessness	Increased injuries	Withdrawal
Emotional swings	Increased illness	Communication difficulties
Overload	Fatigue	
Increased training exertion	Muscle soreness	

sendorfer et al. suggested that overtrained athletes' heart rate recovery from exercise is prolonged, whereas resting heart rate can be severely elevated. Also weight loss may be experienced together with a change in eating and sleeping patterns. Psychological markers that have been found to change with training include increased perceived effort during training, and depressed mood state after and between training periods.

RECOMMENDATIONS FOR FUTURE RESEARCH

Some of the major issues confronting future research in this area concern the past use of single measures of immune function, lack of standardization of the exercise stimulus, lack of exploration of the role of individual differences, failure to examine the role of anaerobic and aerobic energy systems, the need to integrate the numerous adaptations that accrue through regular aerobic exercise, the dearth of clinical studies, and the lack of a suitable conceptual framework for the relation between exercise and illness.

Mackinnon and Tomasi (1986) suggested that researchers need to adopt an integrated approach when examining the immune system. Thus, attempts to integrate the effect of immunoregulatory factors such as prostaglandins, and lymphokines on subsets of leukocytes and lymphocytes and other immune cells may reveal a more complete picture of this complex system. In addition, a phenomena such as exercise hyperthermia, which resembles the fever response (raising of inner core temperature), should also be examined. For instance, Cannon and Kluger (1983) found that plasma taken from exercising humans and injected into rats elevated the rat's rectal temperature. The authors suggested that endogenous pyrogen, a protein mediator of fever, is released during exercise. Simon (1984) speculated that the heating effects of exercise may have the potential to influence immune function because exercise hyperthermia may depend on both heat production by skeletal muscle and the production of interleukin-1. Because interleukin-1 promotes immunological responsiveness, heating the body through exercise may enhance immune function. Furthermore, the increases in catecholamines and opiate peptides associated with exercise and their effect on immune function need to be explored. For instance, increases in epinephrine, norepinephrine, cortisol, and opiate peptides accompany exercise, and all these hormones have been shown to affect the immune system (Keast et al., 1988). The effects of other hormones that change with training (e.g., insulin, aldosterone, sex hormones, and antidiuretic hormone) also need to be examined. Thus, the role of hormonal modification to exercise and its consequent effect on the immune system are deserving areas for future research.

Lack of standardization of exercise refers to control of the type, duration, and intensity of the exercise stimulus. Past researchers have used a variety of exercise modalities ranging from stair climbing to ultramarathon running. Similarly, the length of time exercising has varied from 5 min to more than 3 hr. Clearly, there is a need to accurately measure the work output of the exercise stimulus. This can be accomplished by using calibrated bicycle ergometers and treadmills to control work (American College of Sports Medicine, 1986).

Some important individual differences that may affect the relation between exercise and illness are age, gender, physical fitness, heredity, and psychological factors. Because immune efficiency appears to decrease with age, the effect of exercise on the immune response of elderly individuals warrants more research. Gender factors (e.g., the relation among exercise, the menstrual cycle, and immune function) may also play an important role in the female immune response to exercise. In addition, because the ability to perform aerobically is largely genetic (Boutcher, 1990), the role of high genetic aerobic capacity versus high trained aerobic capacity needs to be explored. Linked to this last factor are the fitness level and training history of subjects. Thus, the effects of exercise on the immune system may be affected by training history. Psychological factors such as stress in the form of bereavement (Bartrop, Lazarus, Luckhurst, Kiloh, & Penny, 1977; Schleifer, Keller, Camerino, Thornton, & Stein, 1983), examination stress (Kiecolt-Glaser et al., 1984), and hardy-type disposition (Kobasa, Maddi, Pucetti, & Zola, 1985) should also be examined. Although the methodological weaknesses of these studies have been illustrated by Cohen (1985), the overall conclusion reached by Cohen and other researchers in this area (Schindler, 1985; Tecoma & Huey, 1985) is that there is enough evidence to show that psychological factors can affect immune function. Because exercise can influence psychological states (Boutcher & Landers, 1988), it is also feasible that exercise has the potential to indirectly affect immune function by alleviating psychological stress. Thus, those individuals who use exercise as a timeout to get away from a stressful environment may be indirectly decreasing the effect of stress on their immune system by using the distractive qualities of exercise.

The lack of systematic research examining the relation between immune system function and immediate (adenosine triphosphatecreatine phosphate system), short-term (lactic acid system), and long-term (aerobic system) energy systems has led to a lack of identification of underlying biochemical and physiological mechanisms (Keast et al., 1988). The major physiological adaptations in aerobic energy pathways as well as adaptations in the immediate and glycolytic energy systems should be examined. Thus, training studies assessing all three energy systems need to be conducted in which changes in fitness and immune function are monitored simultaneously.

Other nonbioenergetic changes that accompany regular aerobic exercise may also be important. For instance, a decrease in body fat (Dempsey, 1964); increased strength in muscles, bones, and ligaments involved in the activity (Wilmore, 1974); and a favorable influence on the ratio of high-density lipoprotein to total cholesterol (Martin, Haskell, & Wood, 1977) can happen through regular aerobic exercise. Thus, the effect of the whole host of adaptations to aerobic and anaerobic exercise may be directly or indirectly involved in affecting immune function.

Finally, the clinical importance of changes in immune parameters needs to be assessed. Unfortunately, it is not known if the exercise-induced immune changes previously mentioned have any effect on overall immune function. In fact, Simon (1984) suggested that these changes are short-lived, saying "it seems unlikely that these phenomena alter host defense to an important extent." Furthermore, biochemical data do not answer the question of whether exercise increases resistance to infection. Clinical studies are required, but at present very few epidemiological studies have examined this issue.

Considering that many interrelated systems are involved in both the enhancing or depressing of immune function by exercise, it seems that a systems approach can provide a suitable framework from which to study this phenomenon. Systems theory (Schwartz, 1984) provides a way of organizing interactionary systems into a conceptual framework. The key concepts of system theory include part, whole, interaction, level, and behavior. Briefly, a system is viewed as a whole, composed of a number of subsystems and parts whose interactions form the unique properties of the system interacting with its environment (for further discussion of systems theory see Schwartz, 1982, 1984). An interactionary model encapsulating some of these previously mentioned suggestions is illustrated in Figure 1. As can be seen, a variety of interacting physiological and psychological mechanisms together with the influence of individual differences and the kind of exercise stimulus need to be considered if the relation between exercise and illness is to be more fully understood.

SUMMARY

This chapter has provided a brief review of the effects of aerobic exercise on illness. Research examining both the enhancing and depressing effects of exercise on the immune system has been described. Because methodological and conceptual problems exist, it is not possible to make definitive conclusions regarding the positive and negative effects of exercise on immunity. However, the majority of studies suggest that moderate levels of exercise can enhance certain immune parameters, whereas intensive exercise can depress certain immune functions. Unfortunately, clinical evidence to support either the enhancing or depressing immune effects of exercise is not available. Ideas for the implementation of exercise programs and the development of effective preventive and regenerative strategies have been described. Finally, a model providing an interactionary view of the relation between health and exercise has been outlined. This model emphasizes the need to examine multiple interacting physio-

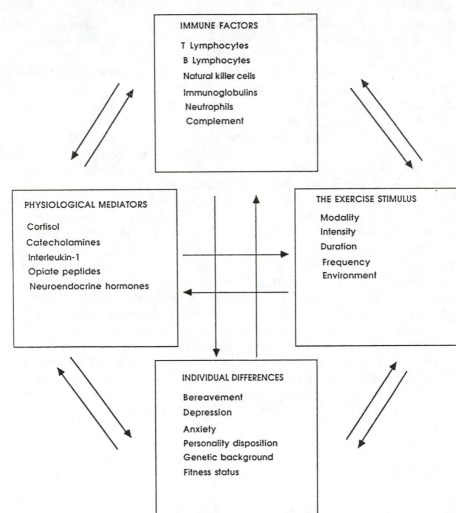

FIGURE 1   The interaction of physiological, individual, and exercise factors with various immune parameters.

logical and psychological systems to develop a better understanding of the relation between exercise and illness.

REFERENCES

American College of Sports Medicine. (1978). Position statement on the recommended quantity and quality of exercise for developing and maintaining fitness in healthy adults. *Medicine and Science in Sports and Exercise, 10,* vii–x.

American College of Sports Medicine. (1986). *Guidelines for exercise testing and prescription.* Philadelphia: Lea & Febiger.

Barnes, M. W. (1989, June). *A psychobiological approach to the prediction of athletic performance and the relationship between the predictors.* Paper presented at the annual meeting of the North American Society for the Psychology of Sport and Physical Activity Conference, Kent, OH.

Bartrop, R. W., Lazarus, L., Luckhurst, L. G., Kiloh, L. G., & Penny, R. (1977). Depressed lymphocyte function after bereavement. *Lancet, 1,* 834–836.

Bellanti, J. A. (1985). *Immunology III.* Philadelphia: W. B. Saunders.

Boggs, D. R., & Winklestein, A. (1983). Lymphocytes and the immune system. In D. Boggs (Ed.), *White cell manual* (pp. 61–97). Philadelphia: F. A. Davies.

Boutcher, S. H. (1990). Aerobic fitness: Issues and measurement. *Journal of Sport and Exercise Psychology, 12,* 235–247.

Boutcher, S. H., & Landers, D. M. (1988). The effects of vigorous exercise on anxiety, heart rate, and alpha activity of runners and nonrunners. *Psychophysiology, 6,* 110–117.

Brahmi, Z., Thomas, J. E., Park, M., & Dowdeswell, I. R. G. (1985). The effect of acute exercise on natural killer-cell activity of trained and sedentary human subjects. *Journal of Clinical Immunology, 5,* 321–328.

Cannon, J. G., & Kluger, M. J. (1983). Endogenous pyrogen activity in human plasma after exercise. *Science, 220,* 617–619.

Cohen, J. J. (1985). Stress and the human immune response: A critical review. *Journal of Burn Care and Rehabilitation, 6,* 167–173.

Crampton, J., & Fox, J. (1987, April). Regeneration vs. burnout: Prevention is better than cure! *Sports Coach, 7*–11.

Cundiff, D. (1979). *Implementation of aerobic programs.* Washington, DC: American Alliance for Health, Physical Education, Recreation, and Dance.

Cupps, T. R., & Fauci, A. S. (1982). Corticosteroid-mediated immunoregulation in man. *Immunological Reviews, 65,* 133–155.

Dempsey, J. A. (1964). Anthropometrical observations on obese and nonobese young men undergoing a program of vigorous physical exercise. *Research Quarterly, 35,* 275–287.

Dishman, R. K. (1988). *Exercise adherence.* Champaign, IL: Human Kinetics.

Dressendorfer, R. H., & Wade, C. E. (1983). The muscular overuse syndrome in long-distance runners. *Physician and Sportsmedicine, 11,* 116–126.

Dressendorfer, R. H., Wade, C. E., & Scaff, J. H. (1985). Increased morning heart rate in runners: A valid sign of overtraining? *The Physician and Sportsmedicine, 13,* 77–86.

Edwards, A. J., Bacon, T. H., Elms, C. A., Verardi, R., Felder, M., & Knight, S. (1984). Changes in the populations of lymphoid cells in human peripheral blood following exercise. *Clinical Experimental Immunology, 58,* 420–427.

Gleck, J., Brown, R. S., & Shank, R. H. (1982, August). The burnout syndrome among athletic trainers. *Athletic Training,* pp. 36–41.

Gutmann, M. C., Pollock, M. L., Foster, C., & Schmidt, D. (1984). Training stress in Olympic speed skaters: A psychological perspective. *The Physician and Sportsmedicine, 12,* 45–57.

Guyton, A. C. (1986). *Textbook of medical physiology.* Philadelphia: W. B. Saunders.

Hanson, P. G., & Flaherty, D. K. (1981). Immunological responses to training in conditioned runners. *Clinical Science, 60,* 225–228.

Hedfors, E., Biberfield, P., & Wahren, J. (1978). Mobilization to the blood of human non-T and K lymphocytes during physical exercise. *Journal of Clinical Laboratory Immunology, 1,* 159–162.

Hedfors, E., Holm, G., & Ohnell, B. (1976). Variations of blood lymphocytes during work studied by cell surface markers, DNA synthesis and cytotoxicity. *Clinical Experimental Immunology, 24,* 328–335.

Jemmott, J. B. (1985). Psychoneuroimmunology. *American Behavioral Scientist, 28,* 497–509.

Jorgenson, C. B., & Jorgenson, D. E. (1979). Effect of running on perception of self and others. *Perceptual and Motor Skills, 48,* 242.

Keast, D., Cameron, K., & Morton, A. R. (1988). Exercise and the immune response. *Sports Medicine, 5,* 248–267.

Kiecolt-Glaser, J. K., Garner, W., Speicher, G. M., Penn, G. M., Holliday, J., & Glaser, R. (1984). Psychosocial modifiers of immunocompetence in medical students. *Psychosomatic Medicine, 46,* 7–14.

Kirwan, J. P., Costill, D. L., Flynn, M. G., Mitchell, J. B., Fink, W. J., Neufer, P. D., & Houmard, J. A. (1988). Physiological responses to successive days of intense training in competitive swimmers. *Medicine and Science in Sports and Exercise, 20,* 255–259.

Kobasa, S. C., Maddi, S. R., Pucetti, M. C., & Zola, M. A. (1985). Effectiveness of hardiness, exercise, and social support as resources against illness. *Journal of Psychosomatic Research, 29,* 525–533.

Landmann, R. M., Muller, F. B., Perini, C., Wesp, M., Erne, P., & Buhler, F. R. (1984). Changes in immunoregulatory cells induced by psychological and physical stress: Relationship to plasma catecholamines. *Clinical Experimental Immunology, 58,* 127–135.

Lentner, C. (1984). Giegy scientific tables: Physical chemistry, composition of blood, haematology, somatometric data (Vol. 3). Basle: Ciba Giegy. *Ciba Giegy, 3.*

Mackinnon, L. T., & Tomasi, T. B. (1986). Immunology of exercise. *Annals of Sports Medicine, 3,* 1–4.

Martin, R. P., Haskell, W. L., & Wood, P. D. (1977). Blood chemistry and lipid profiles of elite distance runners. *Annals of the New York Academy of Sciences, 310*, 346–352.

McCutcheon, L. E., & Hassini, K. H. (1981). Running away from illness. *Journal of Sports Behavior, 4*, 151–156.

McNair, D. M., Lorr, M., & Droppleman, L. F. (1971). *Profile of Mood States manual*. San Diego: Educational and Industrial Testing Service.

Morgan, W. P., Brown, D. R., Raglin, J. S., O'Connor, P. J., & Ellickson, K. A. (1987). Psychological monitoring of overtraining and staleness. *British Journal of Sports Medicine, 21*, 107–114.

Morgan, W. P., Costill, D. L., Flynn, M. G., Raglin, J. S., & O'Connor, P. J. (1988). Mood disturbance following increased training in swimmers. *Medicine and Science in Sports and Exercise, 20*, 408–414.

Nash, H. L. (1986). Can exercise make us immune to disease? *The Physician and Sportsmedicine, 14*, 250–253.

Nieman, D. C., Tan, S. A., Lee, J. W., & Berk, L. S. (1988). Complement and immunoglobulin levels in athletes and sedentary controls. *International Journal of Sports Medicine, 10*, 124–129.

Paffenberger, R. S. (1985). Physical activity as a defense against coronary heart disease. In W. E. Connor & J. D. Bristow (Eds.), *Coronary heart disease: Prevention, complications and treatment* (pp. 135–155). Philadelphia: Lippincott.

Pederson, B. K., Tvede, N., Christensen, L. D., Klarlund, K., Kragbak, S., & Halkjr-Kristensen, J. (1989). *International Journal of Sports Medicine, 10*, 129–131.

Peters, E. M., & Bateman, E. D. (1983). Ultramarathon running and upper respiratory tract infections. *South African Medical Journal, 64*, 582–584.

Rejeski, J. W., & Kenney, E. A. (1988). *Fitness motivation*. Champaign, IL: Human Kinetics.

Ryan, A. J. (1983). Overtraining of athletes. *The Physician and Sportsmedicine, 11*, 93–110.

Schindler, B. A. (1985). Stress, affective disorders, and immune function. *Medical Clinics of North America, 69*, 585–597.

Schleifer, S. J., Keller, S. E., Camerino, M., Thornton, J. C., & Stein, M. (1983). Suppression of lymphocyte stimulation following bereavement. *Journal of the American Medical Association, 250*, 374–377.

Schwartz, G. E. (1982). Testing the biopsychosocial model: The ultimate challenge facing behavioral medicine? *Journal of Consulting and Clinical Psychology, 50*, 1040–1053.

Schwartz, G. E. (1984). Psychobiology of health: A new synthesis. In B. Hammonds & C. Schierer (Eds.), *Psychology and health* (pp. 149–193). Washington, DC: American Psychological Association.

Simon, H. B. (1983). The immunology of exercise. *Journal of the American Medical Association, 19,* 2735–2738.

Smith, R. R. (1986). Toward a cognitive-affective model of athletic burnout. *Journal of Sport Psychology, 8,* 36–50.

Soppi, E., Varjo, P., Eskola, J., & Laitinen, P. A. (1982). Effect of strenuous physical stress on circulating lymphocyte function before and after training. *Journal of Clinical and Laboratory Immunology, 8,* 43–46.

Targan, S., Britvan, L., & Dorey, F. (1981). Activation of human NKCC by moderate exercise: Increased frequency of NK cells with enhanced capability of effector-target lytic interactions. *Clinical and Experimental Immunology, 45,* 352–360.

Tecoma, E. S., & Huey, L. Y. (1985). Psychic distress and the immune system. *Life Sciences, 36,* 1799–1812.

Tomasi, T. B., Trudeau, F. B., Czerwinski, D., & Erredge, S. (1982). Immune parameters in athletes before and after strenuous exercise. *Journal of Clinical Immunology, 2,* 172–178.

Wilmore, J. H. (1974). Alterations in strength, body composition and anthropometric measurements consequent to a 10-week weight training program. *Medicine and Science in Sports, 6,* 133–138.

Wittig, A. F., Houmard, J. A., & Costill, D. L. (1989). Psychological effects during reduced training in distance runners. *International Journal of Sports Medicine, 10,* 97–100.

6

ATHLETIC COMPETITION: STRESS AND PERFORMANCE

Louis Diamant

University of North Carolina at Charlotte

This story is from the Associated Press, July 19, 1989:

> *Former California Angel and Atlanta Braves Pitcher Donnie Moore shot his wife several times and then fatally shot himself in the head Tuesday in an apparent murder-suicide attempt, police said. Moore's wife, Tonia, was hospitalized in critical condition. Moore, a reliever, was released last month from Kansas City's Class AA Team in Omaha, Neb. He had been plagued by injury during his recent years in the majors. He was released from the Angels in 1988, two years after he carried California to within one strike of the 1986 World Series. His agent, Dave Pinter, said Moore, 35, was still tortured by the thoughts of that series. Moore had also played for the Chicago Cubs, Saint Louis Cardinals, and Milwaukee Brewers during eight years in the Major Leagues. ("Ex-Angels Pitcher Dies in Shooting," 1989, p. 1C)*

There are a number of ways to open a chapter on stress and athletic competition. Most are not this dramatic, coming to grips with anxiety—the demon that haunts the world of sports. Cratty (1989) has said that it is not surprising that sport psychology literature is replete with studies of anxiety, together with strategies for reducing it, controlling it, and eliminating it. He added, however, that the anxiety literature is tangled and a major cause of that is the imprecise and interchangeable use of the words *arousal, stress,* and *anxiety.*

It would not be strange to say that Moore's horrible acts of destruction and self-destruction were "stress" related. We can only conjecture what, along with that obsessive thought of failure described by his manager, exacerbated the behavior of an elite athlete.

This tragic episode is not intended to represent a common reaction to the pressures of big-time sports. But it strengthens a notion that there may be, at least for some in highly competitive athletics, reactions and results that are antagonistic to both sports competition and well-being.

A review of the sports psychology literature indicates that a considerable number of studies deal with the problems faced by the stress of competition, with major themes being the study of and reduction of stress (anxiety, or heightened activation and drive levels) in competitive athletes. But Moore's story at least hints that the failure to detect sport-connected stress could also become the problem of the clinician.

FRUSTRATION AND STRESS

Because there is sometimes a problem in clarifying psychological terminology, there is often confusion in the mind of the reader, supported by a writer's avoidance of clarification. For example, Moore's possible obsession with his loss may have been followed by a related frustration that grew increasingly worse. Frustration, which is experienced by everyone and is a key ingredient in much maladaptive behavior, is also an elusive concept. Is Indiana Basketball coach Bobby Knight's converting a chair into a missile a manifestation of frustration? What about Billy Martin, kicking dust on a world of umpires? Or the "Honeymooners" fist-clenching Ralph Cramden: "One of these days, Alice!"? Because most of us associate frustration with not having our way we equate it with irritation, annoyance, or rage.

One of the best known hypotheses in psychology is the Dollard, Doob, Miller, Mower, and Sears (1939) frustration–aggression postulate. It is linked in adjustment psychology to blocked goals and aggressive behavior. Worchel and Goethals (1989) stated that frustration occurs when an important need or routine is not satisfied. Frustration, according to Worchel and Goethals, is virtually always initiated when there is a barrier to a motive-satisfying goal. Barker, Dembo, and Lewin (1941) hypothesized that there is a relation between frustration and regression (the pathological return to an earlier and infantile behavioral and emotional response to stress). This of course could lead to meaningless striking out at others, temper tantrums, and other maladaptive non-problem-solving activity. They noted such behavior in their experiments with young children in which the children were thwarted in their desire to reach desirable toys.

The thwarting of goals can lead to other mental and emotional states. Although the picture of one football coach deprived of victory trying to punch out a player from the opposing team after that Bowl game loss may prove a classic example of the frustration–aggression hypothesis in sports history, the other, not so newsworthy, image of the dejected, depressed athlete, head in hands, is another.

The literature that deals with symptomatic reactions to adversity, especially current or ongoing adversity, is commonly found under the rubric of stress. Frustration is commonly thought of as one of these symptomatic reactions. Saying that Moore may have suffered from frustration that brought on stress could also be seen as a case of the cart before the horse. According to Worchel and Goethals (1989), frustration is one cause of stress, and the one that seems most likely to produce infantile and aggressive responses. Conflict and decision making also produce stress—even a decision that is to be made between the two kinds of satisfaction. Other causes of stress according to Worchel and Goethals are physical change, ambiguous situations, and fears about loss of self-esteem or integrity. Their selection of fear provocation appears to be largely cognitive; that is, the persons could, it seems, review consciously all the social and physical agents with which they were dealing. This would leave an athlete open to a cognitive or behavioral–cognitive approach to change. The sports literature contains a number of studies in which remediation of anxiety is attempted by cognitive measures after the work of Meichenbaum (1977).

At this point, I'd like to mention a personal predilection to emphasize frustration as a general producer of psychological stress with a number of psychopathological consequences, with psychopathology here meaning mental and emotional malfunctioning that may or may not be intense enough to be determined a mental disorder. Mental disorder may be defined as mental and emotional malfunctioning psychopathology intense enough to be classified a mental disorder within the *Diagnostic and Statistical Manual of Mental Disorders* (Third Edition-Revised) (*DSM-III-R*; American Psychiatric Association [APA], 1987). When we discuss stress related to athletic competition we ordinarily are referring to disturbances that interfere with competitive performance and perhaps secondarily some worry and depression that may affect social and academic life. For college athletes academic survival is no small matter because grades are important to athletic survival, and athletic survival in terms of scholarships is also related to grades.

For a minute let's assume that frustration is what people mostly assume it to be, an unpleasant, usually irritable regressive (and/or aggressive) reaction to a thwarting and undesired occurrence. You cannot sink a putt, hit a jump shot, get a serve in, complete a pass. All of this may be followed by fighting, arguing, swearing, and further deteriorating competence, which are obviously angry, poorly controlled behaviors. Most regressive, angry, poorly controlled behavior is thought virtually synonymous with frustration and only an assumption of thwarting is necessary to distinguish it from an identical display, the source of which is not so easily discerned. This unfortunately would eliminate as symptoms of frustration much of its other true spawn such as fear, anxiety, head pain, back pain, and even nonclinical paranoia (Diamant, 1990).

Let me now put forward a non-cognitive-behavioral and non-radical-behavioral notion, since it postulates a mind (including an unconscious) that states that a great part of frustration is structured for all of us and therefore no athlete is immune from the infectious principle that there is unconscious, hidden, and early fantasy projected upon the athletic contest. Freud and later psychoanalysts used the concept of frustration with major importance in the thwarting of satisfaction, but did not develop the construct as a prominent internal mechanism, as they did other constructs, but more or less used the term in a conventional sense even within the context of the unconscious (Fenichel, 1945; Fine, 1986).

In their explanation of learning theory, some psychologists assume something going on between the stimulus and response. To radical behaviorists the study of these in-between things, such as intelligence between a mathematics question and a correct answer, means little or nothing. To the more mind-oriented and cognitive–perceptual scholars, it of course means a great deal. What lies in between, if such a concept fits your theoretical framework, is often called an *intervening variable* or *hypothetical construct.* There are countless of these in-betweens that have been used to account for variations in responses to stimuli, and the distinction between them as intervening variables or hypothetical constructs has done little to help psychology (Bugelski, 1956). Thus, I call frustration an intervening variable (or hypothetical construct). It is the point at which repressed and therefore unconscious fantasies are called into oppositional conflict by external stimuli. It is an unconscious avoidance/approach conflict, which is like trying to be in two places at the same time. Miller (1944) elaborated on the conscious type of approach/avoidance situation. The concept of an unconscious conflict based on psychological theory of development and fantasy is more obfuscated. The key ingredient is the fantasy of power and vulnerability of childhood that performs a service to defense and emotional survival in children (Diamant, 1977) and that if used too long becomes maladaptive in later life. Being both vulnerable and manipulative (a baby) and the conquering hero (a giant or a daddy) are fine for the fantasy of childhood omnipotence but disturbing for the reality and decision making of the adult stage of life.

How we arrived at this conflicted state, and how we can change it, I leave to work in progress. Depending on the omnipotence of childhood fantasies of magically being in two places at once when one is an adult is frustrating. It is this point of ambivalence that destroys clear action and decision making, replacing the original survival drive with symptoms. An athlete who is afraid of the game as ego syntonic (strengthening) behavior regardless of score and who does not rise above the primitive symbolism of victory and defeat, life, death, and manhood or castration gives up the decision to play the game and pathologically lives much of it in its most primitive context. Players who are highly conflicted may feel they can or should disregard rules, especially if they have had bullying parenting, and when caught and penalized may become overtly surly or assaultive and even sent to the bench or showers (to become cleansed). They are then in the role of the chastened child. This may be the end of the behavior for a while—but what an awful pattern should it continue. Freud (1924) recognized that unconscious ambivalence could lead to inhibition of performance that could affect play. A case study on a 9-year-old (Diamant, 1971) indicated that strong ambivalence related to identity could produce stuttering as well as disturbance in games, play, and sports ability. The patient's projected ambivalence could be seen on the Rorschach ink blots: "On card IV Bobby's first response was 'a wild animal or huge monster,' but he abandoned this response quickly and said, 'No, it's a flower.'" (Diamant, 1971, p. 262)

It is possible though that if an individual gives up the aggressive–regressive behavior while the fantasy that caused the conflict is still strong, the frustration may bring on anxiety, depression, and other performance (reality and action) failure. Then what? Consider an outstanding ball player who after an excellent season followed it with a season not at all up to his expected level. He appeared depressed by it and looked depressed. Who wouldn't be, following a great season with a poor one? Some observant people noticed his depression, and commented that it was due to the poor season. In my encounter with this superb athlete I came away with the idea that the attitude-and-performance relation was reversed. He was having a poor season because he was depressed. A brief analysis pointed out the possibility that he was torn between failure and success, basically on a symbolic level. At the point of frustration he had developed hostility, which converted to anxiety, and then to depression to mask and squelch aggressive impulses. The player might have been open to relief by analysis, but time, his style, and the exigencies of a short playing season required techniques to reduce anxiety that were more practical and readily available. Because anxiety and stress are thought of as lacunae from which many disorders and psychopathologies begin let's take a further look at these phenomena.

STRESS AS AN EVENT

I have in my possession many texts on adjustment psychology, abnormal psychology, and social psychology, some of which do not use the term *stress*, others of which describe and define stress, and still others of which take it for granted that everyone uses the term in the same "under pressure" sense and it, like the terms *hot* and *cold*, needs no placement in a glossary. Stress is sometimes overly defined, sometimes underdescribed, and sometimes just left to the reader to formulate his or her own view. Duty calls for a statement, although there is the danger that once a word had become popularized, refining the terminology through the filter of ongoing theoretical and research efforts will still not remove all the resistance from writer and reader to conceptualize it in current scientific constructs. This is not necessarily a negative statement.

In an early article on stress and coping, Oglivie (1968) related stress levels to positions on the relaxed–tense continuum of Cattell and Scheier's (1963) 16 Personality Factor (16PF) test profile. High scores on tension (tense, frustrated, driven, and overwrought) versus relaxed (tranquil, torpid, unfrustrated). He reported that the physical signs associated with emotional tension and anxiety revealed by the Q4 scale on the 16PF were found represented in clinical work by a broad spectrum of psychosomatic disorders. Psychosomatic disorders—not used at this time diagnostically in the *DSM-III-R* of the APA (1987)—are physical disorders that are attributed to stressful psychological causes largely associated with tension-heightened activity of the autonomic nervous system and that therefore involve anxiety. The diagnostic category psychosomatic disorders (APA, 1952) was changed to the category psychophysiological disorders (APA, 1968). Of this category Kolb (1968) wrote, "The long continued and exaggerated physiological expression of anxiety may eventually lead to structural change in the organ or viscera through which it is expressed" (p. 413).

The problem with the diagnosis, psychosomatic disorder, since the term and concept are still used although the diagnostic category has departed, is that people with certain selected physical complaints are suspected of having psychological causes. Also, many persons with high tension and anxiety levels often do not demonstrate the physical disorders commonly associated with those psychological conditions. Although that is a problem with the psychosomatic diagnosis, it does not obviate the plausibility of physical disorders' having psychological determinants. The problem is really one of discrimination. Oglivie found that the high tension scores provided the most realistic evidence that the psychological stress threshold had been penetrated.

I went to two dictionaries to look at definitions of stress because I felt the common use of the word might be reflected in the dictionary definition and would be indicative of how close the popular usage was to the "scientific" usage. If the comparison of dictionary definitions from the *American College Dictionary* (1956) and the *American Heritage Dictionary* (1985) tells us but one thing, it is that in the early years, stress was related to physics and mechanics, and only later was a mental and emotional definition included. Not that the term was unknown to psychology and psychiatry. Stress reaction disorders are classified and appear in the *DSM* (APA, 1952). Studies of people under stress in catastrophic situations and developmental life stress were well established in the literature by the mid-1950s. The difference between then and now is in the frequent use now of the construct and dynamics of stress not only as the cause of morbid physical and mental disorders but in the general concession that it is a constant event in the lives of people in various levels of vocation and sport. In addition, stress is accepted as a concomitant of serious sport competition and survival, and not just the result of horrible things happening to persons, and may accompany failure to attain realistic or unrealistic goals. It may be part of decision and desire. Perhaps the ubiquitous nature of stress is made no more evident that in sport and no persons may be more susceptible to it than its young competitors.

Hans Selye (1956), probably more than anyone, may be thought of as introducing "stress" into the psychological adjustment literature as a psycho-biological phenomenon to conceptualize an organism's response to noxious stimuli. Although Selye's original work was basically concerned with stress as measured in physiological terms, he could not discard the role of perceptual and learning processes in the stress response. He, like many others, faced the semantic difficulty of that term. Was stress the cause of an organism's adaptive changes or the thing that happened? If stress is only a response then the initiating factor is something else. Selye proposed calling the stimulus *stressor,* while *stress* was defined as the organism's adaptive reaction. No matter what the cause and no matter what the provoking condition, the organism's basic stress reaction was always the same. This reaction to the stressor he called *stress and adaption.* The response to the provoking agent is called the *general adaption syndrome* (GAS).

The GAS is made up of three stages of organismic responses: the alarm reaction, the stage of resistance, and the stage of exhaustion. There is stress at any moment during these three stages although its manifestations change as time goes on. According to Selye, most of the physical or mental exertions, infections, and other stressors that act upon us produce changes corresponding only to the first and second stages. At first they may upset and alarm us but we get used to them. In the course of normal human life everybody goes through these first stages many, many times. Otherwise we could never become adapted to perform all the activities and resist all the injuries that are our lot.

> *Even exhaustion does not always need to be irreversible and complete as long as it affects only part of the body. For instance running produces a stress situation mainly on our muscles and cardiovascular system. To cope with this we have to limber up and get these organs ready for the task at hand. Then for a while we will be at the height of efficiency in running but eventually exhaustion will set in. This could be compared with an alarm reactor as stages of resistance and a stage of exhaustion all limited primarily to the muscular and cardiovascular systems, but such an exhaustion is reversible after a good rest and we'll be back to normal again. (Selye, 1956, p. 64)*

Selye has pointed out that in more traumatic and dynamic situations exhaustion might even be death. The GAS, however, is not synonymous with stress but is rather a component of stress. It is probably apparent at this point that Selye's stress construct is hypothetical and assumed to explain certain human and animal responses after they have occurred.

Selye has said animals low enough on the phylogenetic scale to have no brain and certain nervous system invoke the GAS in stress. To accept the GAS explanation requires a determination to share his view and a willingness to put aside popularized definitions. Selye has spent some effort to clarify his position against a persistent tendency to misunderstand it. Although it is cited in countless modern textbooks, the GAS appears largely academic when it comes to serving the purposes of sports, coaching, and sports psychology. A controversial and highly criticized yet frequently published position, it is has not been the most acceptable notion for the psychologist. Richard Lazarus has a view more amenable to the contemporary psychological view, largely because of its inclusion of the elements of perception in the formation of the stress condition.

In stress study, according to Lazarus (Lazarus & Folkman, 1984), the thrust has moved from dealing with stressors as environmental agents of stress to dealing with the personal perceptions of environmental agents. This is more in line with cognitive and phenomenal positions in psychology and, in one sense radical behaviorism, in which the individuality of reinforcements and punishments is vital to the determination of behavior. The notion that externals are shaped into their meaning by the individual and his or her experiences puts the new emphasis on the individual's perception of things as threatening or otherwise. In other words the creation of stress is an individual and personal event. One person's game is another's terror. Sometimes the acceptance of the event of stress is so established that the image brings on a reactive smile rather than the grimace of horror. (Who would want to enter the ring with heavyweight champion Mike Tyson even for money?) On less of a fantasy level, I was chatting with a colleague about risk sports research, and scuba divers and stress came up. He shook his head. Just the thought of diving brought an anxious look to his face, and I realized that he was in fact in a stress syndrome just from the thought and the power of the image of an activity that he said he would never do (he was virtually phobic about the mask). Well, I thought, I have gone recreational scuba diving, but recreational scuba in clear water off the Caribbean reefs is a pleasurable memory. On the other hand, I have had companions who more enjoy diving down to shipwrecks in the cold, dark, northern Atlantic. The experience and the imagery of that leave me fairly uncomfortable. A good student I know who also happens to be an "elite" athlete dreads being called on, and the cold hand he extends before class may support this. But as a player he is poised, coordinated, and in control no matter what the pressure or the score. He does not, he told me, perceive threat or danger on court.

Selye has said that anything outside of the organism is the stressor and cannot rightfully be called stress, which appears to be a hypothetical construct operating between the stress stimulus and the visible evidence of stress. Selye's view seems more designed for animal research in which stressor stress and visceral response are readily appraised by autopsy or other observable assessment. Lazarus, on the other hand, emphasizes cognitive mediation in stress situations in which the stress-producing stimulus is also considered stress. Lazarus and his associate Susan Folkman (1984), unlike Selye, are concerned mainly with psychological stress, which they define as "as a particular relationship between the person and the environment that is appraised as taxing or exceeding his or her well being" (p. 19).

The view of interpretation as key to stress resembles that of Albert Ellis whose view of psychopathology is basically cognitive. His practice of rational-emotive therapy is based on the assumption that what we label our emotional reactions depends on our conscious and unconscious evaluations. According to Ellis we feel anxious (or depressed) because we strongly convince ourselves that failure at a task or rejection as a significant person is, beyond the ordinary disappointment, "terrible and catastrophic" and he says that hostility is felt because people who behave unfairly absolutely should not act that way and it is utterly insufferable when they do (Ellis, 1973). The implication of this syndrome for highly competitive sport activity and coach–player relationships may be obvious. In Ellis's framework lack of success is accompanied by an irrational feeling of loneliness as "what a worm I am," or in more current wording perhaps "what a wimp I am."

Often both stress and anxiety share billing (Krolme & Laux, 1982; Worchel & Goethals, 1989), sometimes as siblings and sometimes as parent and child. Worchel and Goethals (1989) cautioned us that though stress and anxiety are closely related they are separable phenomena, which could be kept straight by some definition. Stress exists when an environmental demand threatens well being and needs to be dealt with, while anxiety is an emotion that is sometimes felt in facing stress. Anxiety, according to these authors, occurs with uncertainty in how to cope with stress, when we feel that we have not the capacity to deal with it, or when it is felt that it will be overwhelming. Anxiety also may occur with reminders of past threatening or traumatic situations.

ANXIETY AND STRESS

Cameron (1968) called anxiety pathological in adults when it occurs without adequate frustration and is exaggerated or unduly prolonged. Cameron saw the precursor of adult anxiety patterns in the primary anxiety of childhood, which is an irresistible need to discharge tension under any stress that occurs in such activity as crying and generalized hyperactivity. Usually the child is suffering from an unidentifiable stress such as hunger, pain, or discomfort. Early in life, tension from stress cannot be tolerated. Cameron considers that the child in growing to adulthood develops a psychodynamic system that helps him or her to postpone the immediate need for tension relief. However, under certain conditions there may be a pathological regression to the primary mode of anxiety. Such a view falls within a psychoanalytical framework (Freud, 1924). However, descriptions, if not the causes or theories of anxiety, remain largely comparable.

Anxiety is a penetrating feeling of dread and apprehension and impending disaster (Kolb, 1968). Anxiety of higher levels, according to Worchel and Goethals (1989), is something to be experienced. Fear, anger, and feeling in danger; physiological arousal; increased heart and perspiration rate; trembling; and being mentally off balance are components of anxiety. Psychoanalytically, from its sexual origin, it is defined as a reaction to danger (Freud, 1933). Although a number of theorists give varied descriptions, a few common themes run through their accounts of the behavioral consequences of anxiety, which most theorists use as a generic term that includes fear, shame, and guilt (Janis, Mahler, Kagan, & Holt, 1969).

Professional descriptions of anxiety, interestingly enough, seem indistinguishable from popular descriptions. In an informal survey I asked a number of adults what they experience when they have anxiety. Guilt, fear, tension, nervousness, increased heart beat, and worry were frequent signs given. Perhaps anxiety, once a term in the special language of clinicians and researchers, has, like depression and paranoia, entered the psychopathology and language of everyday life (Diamant, 1990). Today most accepted descriptions of anxiety include physiological responses of heightened autonomic nervous system activity. The generally heightened systemic activity generally acknowledged by respondents and theorists alike is of special concern for students of the phenomenon. Other conditions—activation, drive, fear, arousal, motivation, and excitement—demand autonomic nervous system involvement. Schacter's (1964) well-known cognitive theory of emotion developed from emotional–physiological relations addresses and in some ways complicates the problem emanating from the similarity of reactions. Schacter responded to two enduring postulates of emotions proposed by William James (1890). These are (a) that bodily changes follow directly the perception of the exciting fact and (b) that our feelings of the same bodily changes as they occur constitute the emotion. Schacter agreed with the first postulate, saying that a general pattern of visceral reactions followed the arousal of the autonomic nervous system as a characteristic of all states of emotional arousal. However, regarding the second postulate, Schacter said a person's cognitive notion about the situation will steer and influence the person's feelings and emotional behavior and contribute to the label the individual gives that behavior. Schacter took a strong stand that the person tends to evaluate, label, and act on ambiguous body states. He experimentally stimulated the sympathetic nervous system with drugs such as epinephrine. Subjects were then fed true or false information about the expected reactions. Through these experimental manipulations Schacter introduced a wide variety of emotional behavior from the same physiological activity. The application of this to athletic stress, although not yet demonstrated, may offer some promise. Meanwhile the bulk of research dealing with stress and sports emphasizes a number of personality, trait, and mood measurements but relies most heavily, it seems, on the measurement of state and trait anxiety.

Although the notion of state and trait anxiety was described earlier by Cattell (Cattell & Scheier, 1963) its theoretical place in contemporary personality psychology and its application to sports appear to begin seriously with Spielberger (Spielberger, Gorsuch, & Lushene, 1970) and the development of the State–Trait Anxiety Inventory (STAI) and the measurement and conceptual distinction between anxiety as a transitory state versus anxiety as a relatively stable personality trait.

> *Trait anxiety (T-anxiety) refers to relatively stable individual differences between people in the tendency to perceive stressful situations as dangerous or threatening and to respond to such situations with elevations in the intensity of their state anxiety (S-anxiety reactions), and anxiety may also reflect individual difference in frequency and intensity with which state anxiety states have been manifested in the past, and in the probability that S-anxiety will be experienced in the future. The stronger the anxiety trait, the more probable that the individual will experience more intense elevations in S-anxiety in a threatening situation. (Spielberger, 1983, p. 1)*

The STAI, although not the only criterion from which to judge the stressful nature of competitive sports for certain athletes, has become one of those consistently used assessments. The STAI has had wide use as a research instrument in the relation of stress and anxiety to athletic performance. The STAI S-anxiety scales evaluate feelings of apprehension, tension, nervousness, and worry, and in addition to assessing how people feel "right now," the scale may also assess how they felt at a particular time in the recent past or how they may anticipate feeling in a hypothetical situation. The S-anxiety scale has been a valuable indication of transitory anxiety in patients in psychotherapy and behavior modification programs. It may assess anxiety levels induced by a variety of stressors such as surgery or tests. The STAI has been extensively used in medical and psychiatric situations and has played a part in evaluating the outcomes of psychotherapy. The questionnaire is composed of 40 questions (e.g., "I feel content" and "I feel worried") with weighted answers.

The STAI, while having some popularity in its use with athletes, was not specifically designed for sports use. Among other measurements used in researching stress and anxiety in competition are some that have been specifically designed for sports. Martens (1977) has produced an index that is sport specific and is based on the validity and value of athletes' self-reports of what is threatening and anxiety eliciting. The Sport Competition Anxiety Test, which some consider a descendent of the STAI, consists of 15 items relevant to competitive sports. Statements such as "Before I compete I get uptight" are checked on a "hardly ever," "sometimes," and "often" basis. Martens postulated that athletes with higher trait anxiety would be most likely to develop anxiety at the time of competition. Earlier an illustration was given of an outstanding athlete who was not living up to his predictions because he was depressed, not vice versa (fear of success?).

A number of research projects have been confined to the laboratory, whereas others have been field studies. The trend toward field studies may have found inspiration in Martens's (1979) article "From Smocks to Jocks: A New Adventure for Sports Psychologists." Research in the stress of athletic competition has dealt largely with anxiety and mood states. A typical study might use the measures of state and trait anxiety to examine the relation between state anxiety and competency in sports. DeMoja and DeMoja (1986) provided one such example with a nonexperimental correlation study designed to show relation between anxiety and the finishing place in the difficult, complex, and dangerous task of high-level motocross racing. The STAI (Spielberger et al., 1970) was administered to 32 riders 30 min before the beginning of a race. The experimenters found a negative correlation between state anxiety and position of finish—the lower the state anxiety, the higher the order of finish. However, the riders higher in trait anxiety performed better information processing. DeMoja and DeMoja attributed this to these riders' being accustomed to processing information under high arousal conditions (the track was uncommonly sandy). The authors' observation of the unfamiliar characteristics of the track as an anxiety-arousing factor finds support from the Fenz and Jones (1972) case study on the effect of uncertainty on anxiety. Fenz and Jones tested arousal reaction as judged by heartbeat and respiration on an expert parachutist and found uncertainty to produce a disruption of the orderly pattern of physiological responding. An early investigation of the relation of precompetitive anxiety to performance (Fenz, 1975) found marked differences in anxiety between experienced and inexperienced parachutists as well as between poor and good performers. Experience has a prominent role in knowing what to expect and in dealing with the unexpected (i.e., uncertainty).

DeMoja and DeMoja (1986) suggested further research on the role of state–trait anxiety as well as the employment of relaxation and mental preparation. Weinberg, Seabourne, and Jackson (1982) wished to study whether visual motor behavior rehearsal (VMBR) over an extended period would be efficacious in reducing state anxiety and therefore improve performance (somewhat suggested by the DeMoja and DeMoja research). They gave the STAI to members of a university karate club and compared the performance of a single-exposure group with that of an extended-exposure group and found reduction in state–trait anxiety with the exposure to VMBR. However, a continuous practice group of VMBR with a significant drop of state anxiety did not show karate improvement when compared with the no VMBR practice group, "despite physiological evidence that the practice of relaxation increases alertness and develops less anxiety and greater stability" (Weinberg et al., p. 151).

The study by Weinberg et al. does not clarify the issue. They found that although steps could be taken to reduce state anxiety, the reduction need not be followed by improved performance. Highlen and Bennett (1979) examined anxiety patterns and concluded that wrestlers who qualified for berths on the Canadian World Wrestling Team had lower scores in competitive and precompetitive anxiety. Gould, Weiss, and Weinberg (1981) found no differences in anxiety patterns in wrestlers with winning and losing records in Big Ten wrestling. Later Gould, Horn, and Spreeman (1983) reacted to Heyman's (1982) comment that there might be some unexamined variables such as age and experience that need to be examined in order to gauge more accurately the role of anxiety and athletic success. Gould et al. (1983) extended Gould et al.'s (1981) study by examining age and trait anxiety as well as competitive state anxiety as variables in wrestling success. They found, as did others (Mortens & Gill, 1976; Scanlan & Passer, 1978, 1979), that trait anxiety played a part in the levels of competitive state anxiety, but their work could not support previous findings that athletic success, at least in wrestlers, was negatively related to competitive state anxiety. They suggested as an explanation for the difference in studies that multitudinal factors of anxiety be considered (i.e., cognitive, performance, and behavioral); of course this reopens the total question of arousal and cognitive pairing. The researchers did not find that age and experience were related to the wrestlers' anxiety levels, although these variables interrelated with other variables such as confidence and placing. This seems, after a fashion, to have been demonstrated by the Weinberg and Genuchi (1980) field study. Here the authors employed Oxendine's (1970) concept of optimal arousal or anxiety levels for different skill, practice, and stress levels used in various sports. State anxiety scores would thus be much lower for optimum performance in golf and archery and could be much higher in weight lifting and football blocking where arousal is often sought by the participant. Weinberg and Genuchi in essence found anxiety not at higher or even moderate levels, but rather at the lowest levels, was promotive of successful competition in golf. They explained this as relating to the precision required by golfing compared with the blending of strength and complexity required by some other sports, in which arousal might be more related to successful outcomes. Cook et al. (1983) noted that golfing ability per se could be related to state anxiety.

It would appear from a sampling of the literature that the final inning of the anxiety–performance game has not been played. One would think that Morgan's (1978) longitudinal study of athletes from freshman to seniors might have answered most questions concerning an inverse relation between sports success and anxiety. From beginning to end there were enough significant relations between personality factors based heavily on what could be determined as anxiety and competitive success—enough for Morgan to believe that success might be predicted on the basis of tests. However, understanding the prediction problem of these assessments, he did not recommend them for definitive selection purposes. Morgan extended this theme to his now classic descriptive label of successful athletes, "the iceberg profile" (Morgan, 1980). The profile is made up of tension, vigor, fatigue, depression, anger, and confusion scales. Not specifically anxiety, these may easily be thought of as components of anxiety (or stress). A person with cool is not commonly or clinically thought of as one who is anxiety ridden. Of course a word of caution is now needed for those examining stress and competition. Inferences may be drawn from Morgan's work that personalities reflecting the stress of life may be more likely to carry it into athletic endeavor, or that the never-ending competition for a place on the team is an exacerbating force, or perhaps that persons of certain life-styles and experiences develop a confident and cool personality that wears well in competition. Perhaps a myriad of intellectual, social, and genetic factors affecting these questions should be scrutinized. Currently gender as a (genetic?) (social?) variable in sport anxiety is getting some of that scrutiny.

Rainey and Cunningham (1988) investigated issues related to competitive trait anxiety (CTA) among 64 male and 64 female varsity athletes. It appeared from the study that because women's sports was given less attention than men's sports, expectations or criticism had less relation to CTA. However, the more female athletes placed importance on sports, the higher was their CTA. Werk (1979) investigated the relation between sex roles and CTA in undergraduate male and female psychology students. The males chosen for the study chose masculine sex roles and the females chose feminine roles as measured by the BEM Sex Role Inventory. Masculine males had lower CTA related to sport competition than did feminine females, thus demonstrating relations between CTA and sex role orientation.

Comparisons between the studies (Rainy & Cunningham, 1988; Werk, 1979) are limited by the differences in study samples, one comprising basically psychology classes and the other comprising varsity athletes. In addition, as cautioned by Rainy and Cunningham their National Collegiate Athletics Association (NCAA) III athletes present different variables than, for example, would NCAA I athletes, on whom pressure to succeed is greater. Segal and Weinberg (1984) explained gender and anxiety as a relation in competitive sports and concluded that it is a consistent finding that females exhibit higher levels of CTA than males, with CTA being defined as "the tendency to perceive competitive sports situation as threatening and to respond to these with feelings of apprehension and tension" (p. 153). They found sex rather than sex role orientation related to the higher female scores, recommending emotional support and equal opportunity to girls engaging in sports as a "step in the right direction in reducing anxiety and negative consequences that have long been associated with participation in sport" (p. 158).

CONCLUSION

Although this chapter began with a dramatic illustration of the possibility of psychological damage to athletes as a result of the demands of athletic survival and victory, it seems the focus on anxiety in sports is more on the psychological malfunctioning behind losing than on the preservation or improvement of an athlete's mental health. However, this is not entirely so. Stability, at least as measured in low levels of anxiety and tension, was found to be the hallmark of the successful athlete compared with the nonsuccessful athlete.

Morgan (1978) noted that the winning athlete compared with the nonwinning athlete was generally lower on state and trait anxiety and tension. In *Psychology Today* Morgan's (1980) article "Test of Champions: The Iceberg Profile" carved that concept in ice, if not stone. He stated that the profile of successful Olympic contenders for wrestling indicated that the winners scored significantly lower on tension, depression, anger, fatigue, and confusion and higher on vigor on the Profile of Mood States (McNair, Lorr, & Droppleman, 1971). Tension and confusion are popularly accepted correlates of anxiety and certainly of stress. These are also mental health variables, and Morgan suggested the regular monitoring of mood swings "that could impair performance and might require some form of counseling or psychotherapy" (p. 102).

In this chapter I have shuffled a small stack of terms that mean stress, that are equated with stress, or that are signs of stress. We find *stress* and *anxiety* used interchangeably and separately. For example, Singer's (1975) *Myths and Truths in Sport Psychology* has in its index "stress, pp. 103–108" and "anxiety, pp. 103–108." On top of that, *drive, activity, arousal,* and even *motivation* may be synonymized. In an attempt to contribute to clarification, some theoretical elaboration on semantics and nomenclature has been made, and even if there may not be a noticeable difference from other definitional attempts, it does at least keep before the reader the importance of terminology and theoretical concepts.

A number of researchers suggest at least that, especially in athletic skills of higher complexity, anxiety levels may interfere with performance—that competitive state anxiety may be related to trait anxiety or even gender. There are suggestions in the literature for extensive and diverse measures of resolving sports-inhibiting anxiety (e.g., Nideffer, 1985).

Elsewhere in this book the idea that exercise, especially of the aerobic type, may have mental health value by way of reducing stress, anxiety, tension, and depression is introduced. Might athletes, especially those engaged in sports requiring marked cardiovascular effort, have lower anxiety levels than nonathletic peers? Simono (1968) found, when comparing the scores on the Taylor Manifest Anxiety Scale, that among male college students varsity athletes produced statistically higher anxiety scores than did nonathletes (who may or may not have been physically active). This could raise questions about a chronicity of stress in athletes except perhaps among the "elite" athletes (Morgan, 1980). Simono suggested an "emotional reactivity and excitability" (p. 111) as factors in athletic competition. Certainly far from understood, the relation of athletics and stress needs continued investigation. When I raised the question to one coach, he said he could understand the stress that some players go through even just waiting on the bench—but he added quickly that this never happened to him (a superstar, he probably had the "iceberg profile"). A second coach responding to the same line of questioning said that the players didn't have any stress—it was the coaches. I shelved his answer, but a few days later the following Associated Press release appeared in the Charlotte Observer: "Saturday, July 29, 1989, [Joe] Morrison's widow says stress caused coach's heart attack. Je Vena Morrison, widow of South Carolina's football coach Joe Morrison, reportedly has filed a claim with the state workers compensation commission claiming her husband's fatal heart attack was caused by job stress" (p. 1A). Friedman, Werner, Brown, Breall, and Dixon's (1986) major 4 1/2-year study of 1,013 myocardial infarction patients supported relations among stress, personality, and coronary heart disease as well as the positive effect of counseling in the reduction of heart attack deaths. Shouldn't we consider that if "the child is father to the man," might not the player be parent to the coach?

REFERENCES

American college dictionary. (1956). New York: Random House.

American heritage dictionary. (1985). New York: Houghton-Mifflin.

American Psychiatric Association. (1952). *Diagnostic and statistical manual of mental disorders.* Washington, DC: Author.

American Psychiatric Association. (1968). *Diagnostic and statistical manual of mental disorders* (2nd ed.). Washington, DC: Author.

American Psychiatric Association. (1987). *Diagnostic and statistical manual of mental disorders* (3rd ed., rev.). Washington, DC: Author.

Barker, J. P., Dembo, T., & Lewin, K. (1941). Frustration and regression: An experiment with young children. *University of Iowa Studies of Child Welfare, 18*(1), 1–314.

Bugelski, B. R. (1956). *The Psychology of Learnings.* Buffalo, NY: Holt, Rinehart, and Winston.

Cameron, N. (1963). *Personality Development and Psychopathology; A Dynamic Approach.* Boston: Houghton Mifflin Company.

Cattell, R. B., & Scheier, L. H. (1963). *Handbook for the IPAT Anxiety Scale questionnaire.* Champaign, IL: Institute for Personality and Ability Testing.

Cook, D., Gansnedes, B., Rotella, R., Malone, C., Bunker, L., & Owens, D.

(1983). Relationship among competitive state anxiety, ability, and golf performance. *Journal of Sport Psychology, 5,* 460–465.

Cratty, C. J. (1989). *Psychology in contemporary sport.* Englewood Cliffs, NJ: Prentice-Hall.

DeMoja, C. A., & DeMoja, G. (1986). State-trait anxiety and motocross performance. *Perceptual and Motor Skills, 62,* 107–110.

Diamant, L. (1971). The function of choice in the psychotherapy of a stutterer. In L. Diamant (Ed.), *Case studies in psychopathology* (pp. 260–265). Columbus, OH: Charles E. Merrill.

Diamant, L. (1977). Clinical contributions to dwarf symbolism. *Psychoanalytic Review, 6,* 611–619.

Diamant, L. (1990). A note on the possibility of a paranoia of everyday life. *Psychoanalytic Review, 77,* 201–218.

Dollard, J., Doob, L. W., Miller, N. E., Mower, O. H., & Sears, R. R. (1939). *Frustration and aggression.* New Haven, CT: Yale University Press.

Ellis, A. (1973). *Humanistic psychotherapy: The rational–emotive approach.* New York: McGraw-Hill.

Fenichel, O. (1945). *The psychoanalytic theory of neurosis.* New York: W. W. Norton.

Fenz, W. D. (1975). Coping mechanisms and performance under stress. In D. M. Landers (Ed.), *Psychology of sport and motor behavior II* (pp. 3–24). University Park, PA: Pennsylvania State University.

Fenz, W. D., & Jones, G. B. (1972). The effect of uncertainty on mastery of stress. *Psychophysiology, 9,* 615–619.

Fine, R. (1986). *Narcissism, the self, and society.* New York: Columbia University Press.

Freud, S. (1924). A connection between a symbol and a symptom. In *Collected Papers of Sigmund Freud.* London: Institute of Psychoanalysis and Hogarth Press.

Freud, S. (1933). New introductory lectures on psychoanalysis: Anxiety and instintual life. *Abstracts of the standard edition of the complete psychological works of Sigmund Freud,* (Lecture XXXI, p. 502). New York: International Universities Press.

Friedman, M., Werner, D., Brown, B., Breall, S. B., & Dixon, T. (1986). A behavior and its effect on cardiac recurrences in post myocardial infarction patients: Summary of the recurrent coronary prevention project. *American Heart Journal, 112,* 2.

Gould, D., Horn, T., & Spreeman, J. (1983). Competitive anxiety in junior elite wrestlers. *Journal of Sport Psychology, 5,* 58–71.

Gould, D., Weiss, M., & Weinberg, R. (1981). Psychological characteristics of successful and non-successful Big Ten wrestlers. *Journal of Sport Psychology, 3,* 69–81.

Heyman, S. R. (1982). Comparisons of successful and unsuccessful competitors: A reconsideration of methodological questions and data. *Journal of Sport Psychology, 4,* 295–300.

Highlen, P. S., & Bennett, B. B. (1979). Psychological characteristics of successful and unsuccessful competitors: An exploratory study. *Journal of Sport Psychology, 1,* 123–137.

Horner, M. S. (1972). Toward an understanding of achievement related conflicts in women. *Journal of Social Issues, 28,* 157–175.

James, W. (1890). *The principles of psychology.* New York: Henry Holt.

Janis, I. L., Mahler, G. F., Kagan, J., & Holt, R. R. (1969). *Personality: Dynamic development and assessment.* New York: Harcourt, Brace and World.

Kolb, L. C. (1968). *Noye's modern clinical psychiatry.* Philadelphia: W. B. Saunders.

Krohne, H. W., & Laux, L. (1982). *Achievement stress anxiety.* New York: Hemisphere Publishing.

Lazarus, R. S., & Folkman, S. (1984). *Stress appraisal and coping.* New York: Springer.

Martens, R. (1977). *Sport Competition Anxiety Test.* Champaign, IL: Human Kinetics.

Martens, R., & Gill, D. L. (1976). State anxiety among successful and unsuccessful competitors who differ in competitive trait anxiety. *Research Quarterly, 16,* 29–37.

McNair, D. M., Lorr, M., & Droppleman, L. F. (1971). *Profile of Mood States manual.* San Diego: Educational and Industrial Testing Service.

Meichenbaum, D. (1977). *Cognitive behavior modification: An integrative approach.* New York: Plenum Press.

Miller, N. E. (1944). Experimental study of conflict. In J. N. V. Hunt (Ed.), *Personality and the behavior disorders* (Vol. 1, pp. 431–465). New York: Ronald Press.

Morgan, W. P. (1978). Characteristics of successful and unsuccessful oarsmen. *International Journal of Sport Psychology, 9,* 119–133.

Morgan, W. P. (1980, April). The test of champions: The iceberg profile. *Psychology Today,* pp. 92–102.

Nideffer, R. M. (1985). *Athletes' guide to mental training.* Champaign, IL: Human Kinetics.

Ogilvie, B. C. (1968). Psychological consistencies with the personality of high level competitors. *Journal of the American Medical Association, 205,* 156–162.

Oxendine, J. B. (1970). Emotional arousal and motor performance. *Quest, 13,* 23–32.

Rainey, D. W., & Cunningham, H. (1988). Competitive trait anxiety in male and female college students. *Research Quarterly for Exercise and Sport,* *59*(3), 244–247.

Scanlan, T. K., & Passer, M. W. (1978). Factors related to competitive stress among male youth sports participants. *Medicine and Science in Sports, 10,* 103–108.

Scanlan, T. K., & Passer, M. W. (1979). Sources of competitive stress in young female athletes. *Journal of Sport Psychology, 1,* 160–169.

Schacter, S. S. (1964). The interaction of cognitive and physiological determinants of emotional state. In L. Berkowitz (Ed.), *Advances in experimental social psychology* (Vol. 1, pp. 49–81). New York: Academic Press.

Segal, J. D., & Weinberg, R. S. (1984). Sex, sex role orientation and competitive trait anxieties. *Journal of Sport Behavior, 7*(4), 153–159.

Selye, H. (1956). *The stress of life.* New York: McGraw-Hill.

Simono, R. B. (1968, March). Personality characteristics of athletes. *Journal of College Personnel,* pp. 109–111.

Singer, R. N. (1975). *Myths and truths in sport psychology.* New York: Harper & Row.

Spielberger, C. D. (1983). *Manual for the State–Trait Anxiety Inventory.* Palo Alto, CA: Consulting Psychologists Press.

Spielberger, C. D., Gorsuch, R. L., & Lushene, R. E. (1970). *Manual for the State–Trait Anxiety Index.* Palo Alto, CA: Consulting Psychologists Press.

Wark, K. A., & Willig, A. F. (1979). Sex role and sport competition anxiety. *Journal of Sport Psychology, 1,* 248–250.

Weinberg, R. S., & Genuchi, H. (1980). Relationship between competitive trait anxiety, state anxiety and golf performance: A field study. *Journal of Sport Psychology, 2,* 148–154.

Weinberg, R. S., Seabourne, T. G., & Jackson, A. (1982). Effects of visuomotor behavior rehearsal on state–trait anxiety and performance: Is practice important? *Journal of Sport Behavior, 5*(4), 219–220.

Worchel, S., & Goethals, G. R. (1989). *Adjustment: Pathways to personal growth.* Englewood Cliffs, NJ: Prentice-Hall.

7

SPORTS, EXERCISE, AND EATING DISORDERS

Julie A. Pruitt and Ruth V. Kappius

University of North Carolina at Charlotte

Pamela S. Imm

Medical University of South Carolina

If you watched the 1988 Olympics, the Pan Am Games, or the World Games you may have noticed a number of women athletes who were emaciated, with elbows, knees, and collar bones protruding. Cheeks and eyes often appeared sunken, and yet they were able to perform amazing physical feats. If you looked at the bodies of those athletes, especially the women who competed in gymnastics and long distance running, it would have been difficult to distinguish their physical forms from those of anorexic women. Their body weights and percentage of body fat were so low that these women athletes resembled prepubescent girls rather than adult women. To even the casual observer, it may have seemed possible that at least some of these athletes were suffering from an eating disorder, such as anorexia and/or bulimia.

Anorexic individuals are those who (a) refuse to maintain a normal body weight (15% below expected weight for their height, build, and age), (b) have an intense fear of getting fat, even when emaciated, (c) have a distorted body image (i.e., they see themselves as fat when they are objectively quite thin), and (d) in females, have missed at least three consecutive menstrual cycles (American Psychiatric Association [APA], 1987). The diagnostic criteria for bulimia are engaging in episodes of binge eating (rapid consumption of a large amount of food in a short period of time) a minimum of two times per week, followed by some form of purging behavior, such as self-induced vomiting, laxative abuse, strict dieting, fasting, or vigorous exercise. To meet these criteria the bingeing must have been present for at least 3 months, the individual must feel out of control during binges, and there must be persistent overconcern with body shape and weight (APA, 1987).

The concern that some long distance runners may be very similar to anorexic individuals was expressed by a group of physicians in the *New England Journal of Medicine* in 1983. Yates, Leehey, and Shisslak (1983) proposed that running may be an analogue of anorexia. The authors suggested that a subgroup of runners becomes so obsessed with running and with body perfection that this focus becomes self-destructive. This type of detrimental pattern occurs with anorexic individuals who become so obsessed with thinness that they place themselves in medical danger. In addition, the desire for thinness is valued over every aspect of their lives. Yates et al. (1983) maintained that runners, in a similar fashion, place tremendous value on success in running and will continue to run despite physical injury or medical danger. As would be expected, this article sparked a heated debate. A number of other authors wrote virulent articles protesting this hypothesis. Responses to the article included the following criticism excerpted from a letter to the editor of the *New England Journal of Medicine*: "There is a need for medical information about running so that physicians can advise the 31 million Americans who run, but *there is no need for articles like this*. I hope that in the future the *Journal* will apply the same criteria to articles about running that it applies to articles on other topics" (italics added, excerpted from material originally appearing in Wells, "Letter to the editor," *New England Journal of Medicine*, p. 47, 1983).

The debate about the relationship between excessive exercise and anorexia was complicated by the research findings from three areas. First, excessive exercise is a common symptom seen in both anorexia and bulimia. Second, researchers have found significant rates of eating disorders in athletes. Third, in a very different area of research, Epling, Pierce, and Stefan (1983) proposed an elegant animal model in which they suggested that exercise, in conjunction with food deprivation, actually induces anorexia in laboratory rats.

In this chapter we first present the literature surrounding this debate and the evidence that excessive exercise is a common feature of both anorexia and bulimia. Then the animal model for exercise-induced anorexia is presented. In the final sections we review the data on the incidence of eating disorder in athletes and the data that suggest that athletes and patients with anorexia and bulimia may be quite dissimilar.

RUNNING AS AN ANALOGUE OF ANOREXIA

Yates et al. (1983) interviewed approximately 60 male runners who ran more than 50 miles per week. They reported that the personality characteristics of these men are similar to those of women with anorexia. They referred to these men as "obligatory runners." The central feature that appears to differentiate these men from other runners is that for them "running becomes a consuming goal that preempts all other interests in life" (Yates et al., 1983, p. 252).

Yates et al. (1983) presented seven major comparisons between anorexics and obligatory runners. First, difficulty with the expression of anger and the lack of ability to cope with conflict are often common problems for anorexic patients (Garner & Garfinkel, 1985). Yates et al. reported that this same pattern of avoidance of anger and conflict occurred in the runners they studied. Second, both groups have extremely high self-expectations. They continually set higher and higher goals that remain unreachable. Yates et al. referred to this as "a single minded quest for an elusive ideal" (1983, p. 253). For anorexic patients this means seeking ever lower weights (Garner & Garfinkel, 1985), while runners seek ever faster times and longer distances. Third, both groups exhibit an extremely high tolerance for pain. Anorexic patients exercise and refuse food despite emaciation and fatigue (Crisp, 1967). Obligatory runners run despite painful injury or illness. Fourth, both groups easily become depressed when they are prevented from engaging in their chosen patterns of behavior and may use these behaviors to cope with depression. Anorexic individuals often appear depressed as they gain weight (Garner & Garfinkel, 1985), as do the obligatory runners when they are unable or not permitted to run. Fifth, anorexic individuals and obligatory runners tend to be fairly socially isolated and lack close relationships (Bemis, 1978). Sixth, both groups appear to use these behaviors to help establish a sense of identity. The self-statement that "I am a runner" or "I am thin" becomes the primary means of self-definition. Sixth, these obsessive behaviors frequently begin during a time of stress and identity confusion. For the anorexic individuals this often occurs during the confusing time of adolescence (Bemis, 1978). Obligatory runners may also experience a similar identity confusion during midlife or midcareer crisis. In addition, these behaviors serve to differentiate both groups from other "less dedicated people" (Yates et al., 1983, p. 254). The seventh issue for both groups is one of control. The extremely restricted diet or the extreme dedication to exercise makes them feel in control of themselves and their environment (Garner & Garfinkel, 1985). A major part of this control, for both groups, revolves around food and weight. The anorexic individual's obsession with weight is a cardinal symptom of the disorder, while for obligatory runners low body weight is seen as necessary for successful performance. In summary, these two groups differ from normal runners and dieters in that "their behavior became pathological as a result of an extreme degree of constriction, inflexibility, repetitive thoughts, adherence to rituals and need to control themselves and their environment" (Yates et al., 1983, p. 254).

In presenting these data, Yates et al. (1983) discussed three case studies but relied extensively on clinical impressions without presenting specific data. The lack of scientific evaluation of their hypothesis may mean that it is partially or entirely inaccurate.

EXCESSIVE EXERCISE IN ANOREXIA

The cardinal feature of anorexia is "refusal to maintain body weight over a minimal normal weight for age and height" (APA, 1987, p. 65). Anorexic patients maintain this low body weight through a variety of behaviors including severe food restriction, self-induced vomiting, laxative abuse, diuretic abuse, and vigorous exercise. There is a clear consensus that a substantial percentage of anorexic patients use exercise as one of their primary means of losing weight. In fact, hyperactivity was included in an early set of diagnostic criteria used in conducting research with anorexia nervosa patients (Feighner et al., 1972).

In 1874, Sir William Gull wrote what is considered to be one of the earliest descriptions of an anorexic patient, "The patient complained of no pain, but was restless and active. This was in fact a striking expression of the nervous state for it seemed hardly possible that a body so wasted could undergo the exercise which seemed so agreeable" (Gull, 1874). In a similar vein, A. H. Crisp stated, "These patients often walk great distances, rarely settle, have a sense of inner intense restlessness, spend their time doing vigorous physical exercises and can be heard by their parents pacing up and down in their bedrooms at night" (Crisp, 1967, p. 121). Further descriptions of the nature of this behavior come from Hilde Bruch. Bruch stated that although some patients' overactivity was directed toward "athletics and sports, more often, these activities appear to be aimless, e.g. walking by the mile, chinning and bending exercises, or just refusing to sit down or literally running in circles" (Bruch, 1962, p. 190). This overactivity continues despite emaciation: "The actual amount of exercise may not be large but appears remarkable, in view of the state of starvation" (Bruch, 1962, p. 190). This activity clearly has an obsessive flavor to it and may include very ritualized exercise programs (Casper & Davis, 1977; Garner, Garfinkel, & Bemis, 1982). Garner et al. (1982), for example, reported that one patient's exercise routine required that "passing street lamps and mail boxes had to be followed by jogging for one block. Initial reduction in her exercise program could only be accomplished by mapping safe exercise routes that were poorly lit with inadequate postal service" (p. 18).

Estimates of the number of anorexic patients who engage in excessive exercise range from 14% (Halmi, 1974) to 65% (Crisp, 1967). However, specifying how much exercise is "acceptable" and healthy and how much is too much is extremely difficult. Only one study has directly compared the activity level of anorexic patients with that of other women. Blinder, Freeman, and Stunkard (1970) found that anorexic inpatients with free access to passes walked an average of 6.8 miles per day compared with an average of 4.9 miles per day found in women of normal weight living in the community.

Many researchers have reported that anorexic patients were very active and interested in sports before they became anorexic. They often come from families that place a high emphasis on sports and athletics (Bruch, 1966; Crisp & Burns, 1983; Crisp, Hsu, Harding, & Hartshorn, 1980; Kron, Katz, Gorzynski, & Weiner, 1978). As the disorder progresses and weight loss increases, it appears that this goal-directed activity (e.g., sports, dance, or gymnastics) becomes more and more frantic and disorganized. Vandereycken, Depreitere, and Probst (1987) stated that "anorexics become prey to a kind of impersonal, ego-dystonic urge to move" (p. 253). They are described as exhibiting "a generalized rushing around" (Crisp & Burns, 1983, p. 8).

This overactivity appears to serve a number of functions. Naturally, overactivity results in burning calories and thus increasing weight loss. The resulting exhaustion also serves to suppress hunger (Casper & Davis, 1977). Reports of similar "restless" behavior frequently occur in studies of starvation in humans, where it seems to be due to efforts to find food (see Casper & Davis, 1977, for a discussion of the literature on human starvation). In starvation studies, however, subjects generally try to conserve energy, which is clearly not the case in anorexia. Some anorexic patients do eventually reach a state in which they complain of exhaustion and fatigue. Crisp (1967) reports that this is the period in which they are most likely to appear depressed.

Excessive, ritualized exercise may also serve a number of psychological functions. It may play a part in magical or superstitious thinking about weight maintenance (e.g., "I'll gain weight if I don't run at least 5 miles and do 150 sit-ups"). Excessive exercise may also serve as a defense against paralyzing depression, a means of self-punishment, or a means of coping with negative feelings such as anxiety, anger, or depression (Garner et al., 1982; Johnson & Conners, 1987).

EXCESSIVE EXERCISE IN BULIMIA

Bulimia is a psychiatric disorder characterized by engaging in binge eating, that is, eating a large amount of food in a discrete period of time, followed by some form of purging (APA, 1987). As is true in anorexia, this purging behavior can include any of the following: self-induced vomiting, abuse of laxatives or diuretics, strict dieting or fasting, or vigorous exercise. Prior to 1987, excessive exercise had not been specifically included in the diagnostic criteria as a means of purging. Thus, it is not surprising that little has been written about this phenomenon. Pyle, Mitchell, and Eckert (1981) reported that 76% of bulimic patients studied reported exercising daily as a means of weight control. More recently, Powers, Schulman, Gleghorn, and Prange (1987) also reported that 76% of the bulimic patients they studied used excessive exercise to counteract the effects of binge eating.

Further research in this area is clearly warranted. There are at least three possible reasons for the relative lack of information on exercise in bulimia compared with that found in the research on anorexia. First, this symptom has only recently been specifically included in the official diagnostic criteria. Second, defining the phrase "excessive exercise" is clearly difficult and subjective. Finally, this phenomenon is much less striking in bulimic patients than it is in anorexic patients because of the difference in their body weights. Seeing an emaciated woman exercising for hours at a time is more notable than seeing a woman of normal weight engaging in exactly the same behavior.

AN ANIMAL MODEL
OF EXERCISE-INDUCED ANOREXIA

Epling et al. (1983), in a comprehensive review of the literature, found evidence of a relation between physical activity and self-starvation in animals when food is restricted. Falk (1977) reported that animals whose weight was reduced 20% and who were given limited amounts of food only at scheduled times quickly developed "excessive and persistent behaviors" (p. 325). These behaviors included excessive wheel running, excessive licking, polydipsia (excessive drinking), and other unusual behaviors.

Epling et al. (1983) found that in most of the animal studies that included a restricted diet, in which food was presented only at scheduled intervals and the animals had access to a running wheel, the animals spontaneously increased their activity level. At the same time the animals decreased their food intake and often literally starved to death. This behavior is often described as "schedule induced" and seems to occur when there is a combination of restricted diet and a scheduling of food delivery (Falk, 1977).

Although it may be a quantum leap from schedule induced behavior in animals such as polydipsia and wheel running (Falk, 1977) to the development of anorexia in athletes, there is evidence of the development of similar schedule induced behaviors in humans. Wallace, Sanson, and Singer (1978) demonstrated that when humans are placed on a strict food delivery schedule they show an increase in strange behavior, for example, fidgeting, tapping, and pacing, much like the schedule induced behaviors found in the animal studies. This theory suggests that anorexia may not "cause" excessive exercise, but rather excessive exercise may "cause" anorexia.

RATES OF EATING DISORDERS IN ATHLETES

Athletes who participate in sports in which size and bulk are considered to be an asset, such as football and basketball, appear to be in little danger of developing an eating disorder. However, athletes who participate in sports in which thinness is considered an asset or a necessity, such as gymnasts, distance runners, light-weight crews (sculling), dancers, or jockeys, or in sports in which it is necessary to maintain a particular weight, such as wrestling, the picture changes. These athletes may be at risk for developing an eating disorder because of the measures used to obtain and maintain an "ideal" body weight for the sport. Although little research has been done in this area, two studies have looked at the weight loss practices of college athletes.

Rosen, McKeag, Hough, and Curley (1986) surveyed approximately 200 female collegiate athletes to determine which weight loss practices they use. Rosen et al. found that 32% of these athletes reported that they used at least one method of weight control that might be considered pathological (i.e., self-induced vomiting or laxative abuse, diet pill use, and/or diuretic abuse). Black and Burckes-Miller (1988) expanded on the work done by Rosen et al. In addition to asking about self-induced vomiting and the use of laxatives, diet pills, and diuretics, Black and Burckes-Miller included questions about excessive exercise, fad diets, fasting, self-starvation, and enemas in their measure concerning weight control methods. The questionnaire was completed by approximately 700 male and female college athletes. Not surprisingly, a majority (59%) of athletes reported that they engaged in excessive exercise as a means of controlling weight. In addition, Black and Burckes-Miller found that approximately 25% of athletes in their study restricted their caloric intake to near starvation levels (600 calories or less)! This is truly remarkable considering the caloric output necessary for training and competition. Fasting was another popular method of weight control, with 12% reporting that they fasted two to three times per month. Fad diets (10%), self-induced vomiting (6%), laxative abuse (4%), and diuretic abuse (1%) were all methods of weight control reported by athletes (Black & Burckes-Miller, 1988).

Reports suggest that it is common practice for collegiate and high school wrestlers to intentionally lose 3–20% of their preseason weight prior to weight certification (Boe, 1985; Hansen, 1978). In theory, qualifying to wrestle in the lowest possible weight class gives the wrestler an advantage. Thus, the most drastic weight loss occurs in the few days before an official "weigh-in." Prior to weigh-in, wrestlers often restrict both food and fluid intake and often spend time in sweat boxes or rubber suits to increase the loss of body fluid. In the time between weigh-in and the match, the athlete attempts to regain as much of the lost weight as possible (Hansen, 1978). The issue of the relationship between these pathological efforts to induce weight loss and the clinical syndromes of anorexia and bulimia shall be discussed shortly.

Dancers have also been found to engage in pathological weight loss programs at an alarming rate. Hamilton, Brooks-Gunn, and Warren (1985) and Garner and Garfinkel (1980) found that 33–43% of female ballet dancers have high scores on a measure of anorexic symptoms. During follow-up interviews with those dancers scoring in the clinical range, 7% were found to have anorexia. Other estimates of the prevalence of anorexia in professional dancers range from 3.5% (Garner & Garfinkel, 1980) to 15% (Hamilton et al., 1985).

The estimates of the rates of bulimia in dancers have been as high as 19% (Hamilton et al., 1985).

Exhibiting anorexic and/or bulimic behaviors is not the same as having the disorder. The question that this research raises is, Are all of these athletes in as much psychological trouble as individuals with eating disorders?

ARE ATHLETES DIFFERENT?

The controversy sparked by Yates et al. (1983) led to the publication of a number of studies that contradicted the hypothesis that running is an analogue of anorexia. Goldfarb and Plante (1984) found that only a small percentage (14.5%) of the competitors in a 10-km road race exhibited high scores on a measure of fear of fat. The runners' overall mean scores indicated a lower than normal fear of fat. Thus, the majority of this sample of runners failed to show one of the cardinal symptoms of anorexia, a fear of fat. Blumenthal, O'Toole, and Chang (1984) compared the scores of anorexic patients with those of "obligatory runners" on the Minnesota Multiphasic Personality Inventory (MMPI; Hathaway & McKinley, 1948), an instrument widely used in personality assessment. The anorexic patients scored much higher than the runners on eight of the nine clinical subscales of this test. (This figure omits Scale 5, which is a measure of masculine/feminine orientation and is not commonly considered to be of clinical significance.) The anorexic patients clearly exhibited significantly more psychopathology than did the athletes. Using the Jackson Personality Inventory (Jackson, 1976), Wheeler, Wall, Belcastro, Conger, and Cumming (1986) found no evidence of psychopathology in a sample of high-mileage (40 or more miles per week) runners or low-mileage (20–29 miles per week) runners. In another study of the difference between anorexic patients and women runners, Owens and Slade (1987) administered the Setting Conditions for Anorexia Nervosa Scale (SCANS; Slade & Dewey, 1986), which provides a measure of perfectionism and satisfaction, to a group of anorexic patients and a group of women marathon runners. They found that although the runners and the anorexic patients scored equally high on the measure Perfectionism, the runners were more like normal, nonrunning women on the measure Dissatisfaction with Self. In fact, the runners scored significantly lower than the anorexic patients on this measure. This indicates that although the runners were very perfectionistic they were clearly not dissatisfied with themselves. Anorexic patients, unfortunately, scored very high on this measure of self-dissatisfaction.

Two additional studies focused on female high school athletes. Johnson, Lewis, Love, Lewis, and Stuckey (1984) found no relation between bulimic behaviors and frequency of exercise in this population. Mallick, Whipple, and Huerta (1987, in a comparison of female high school athletes, a group of other high school girls, and a group of eating-disordered patients, the athletes received the highest scores on a measure of self-esteem (the Offer Self Image Questionnaire for Adolescents; Offer & Howard, 1972). The eating-disordered patients' scores indicated significant problems on the Psychopathology, Body and Self Image, Emotional Tone, and Social Relationships scales. Both the athletes and the high school group scored within the normal range on all sub-scales of this measure. However, Mallick, et al. (1987) failed to conduct a statistical comparison of the three groups.

One final study of the relation between eating disorders and athletecism should be mentioned. Joseph, Wood, and Goldberg (1982) examined the rates of anorexia by college major. They found a significantly higher prevalence of anorexia in women majoring in dance and drama than in women majoring in English and physical education. They interpreted these findings as indicating that "individuals at risk for developing anorexia nervosa will gravitate toward areas of culture where there is increased focus on *body* image but *not* on *physical exercise*" (Joseph et al., 1982, p. 53, italics added). Women who were "athletic" were no more likely to be anorexic than other women, with the exception of those women athletes for whom success in their field required thinness.

In evaluating these studies, it is of some interest to note that four of the studies reported findings suggesting that the athletes evaluated were not exactly prime examples of good mental health. The runners whom Goldfarb and Plante (1984) described as exhibiting the "greatest zealousness" had scores on a personality inventory that indicated that they were "assertive, obsessive, perfectionistic and anxious" (p. 296). With the exception of assertiveness, these characteristics are also commonly seen in both bulimic and anorexic patients (Bemis, 1978; Schlesier-Stropp, 1984). In addition, it is of interest that 15% of Goldfarb and Plante's sample did have a high score on a measure of fear of fat, one of the cardinal symptoms of both anorexia and bulimia. Blumenthal et al. (1984) found that 21% of the runners they studied exhibited a significant elevation on at least one of the clinical subscales of the MMPI, indicating that these runners were experiencing difficulty in one or more areas. Finally, Wheeler et al. (1986) found that 20% of runners had high scores on a measure which assessed symptoms of anorexia. They scored more than 2 standard deviations above the mean for nonrunners. The high-mileage runners studied also significantly overestimated the width of their waists in comparison with control subjects. Thus these individuals endorsed many of the symptoms of anorexia, including a distorted body image.

SUMMARY

In summary, a substantial number of athletes exhibit distorted and destructive eating behaviors and engage in dangerous weight control practices. These include severely reducing caloric intake, fasting, self-induced vomiting, laxative or diuretic abuse, and other means of inducing dehydration. However, only a small percentage exhibit both the disordered eating patterns and the psychological symptoms of eating disorders. Of the groups of athletes discussed, it would appear that the wrestlers are the most likely to engage in very destructive purging behaviors. Although empirical studies have not been completed, it appears that these destructive behaviors disappear at the end of the wrestling season. The long-term effect of these behaviors has yet to be assessed. The American College of Sports Medicine (1976) suggested that even the short-term effects of these behaviors may negatively affect performance. They maintain that of two wrestlers in the same weight class, the one whose body weight has not been drastically cut for competition may be stronger and more effective than one who lost weight in order to compete in a lower weight class.

For women athletes the distinction between exhibiting destructive eating patterns and having anorexia nervosa or bulimia nervosa is more difficult. We hypothesize that the central difference between extremely committed athletes who do destructive things to their bodies and anorexic and bulimic individuals who engage in the same destructive behaviors is self-esteem. Anorexic and bulimic individuals do not like themselves; they do not feel good about themselves even in the light of success. They have a difficult time saying "I won" or "I succeeded," often feeling that they are still not good enough. Athletes who exhibit these dangerous patterns but feel good about themselves are not likely to be anorexic or bulimic. This is not to say that bingeing, severely restricting food intake, or performing any form of purging is ever a safe or reasonable means of achieving athletic goals.

To be highly successful, an athlete must make the sport a high priority in his or her life; in fact it may need to be the highest priority at times. However, it cannot be the *only* priority. We have seen many anorexic and bulimic individuals who see food as their best friend, because it is always there, always working to diminish psychological pain or helping them to cope with other feelings. Having only one point of focus, one means of coping, one goal, or only one "friend" may be potentially pathological and destructive. Although athletic success is a worthy goal, young athletes should be encouraged to develop a balance in their lives including academics and an active social life. They should be encouraged to perform in their sport at the level that is consistent with the normal growth and development of their bodies. Parents and coaches should become aware of the potentially dangerous weight loss practices in which athletes sometimes engage and actively discourage their use.

REFERENCES

American College of Sports Medicine. (1976). *Medicine and Science in Sports, 8,* xi–xii.

American Psychiatric Association. (1987). *Diagnostic and statistical manual of mental disorders* (3rd ed., rev.). Washington, DC: Author.

Bemis, K. M. (1978). Current approaches to the etiology and treatment of anorexia nervosa. *Psychological Bulletin, 85,* 593–617.

Black, D. R., & Burckes-Miller, M. E. (1988). Male and female college athletes: Use of anorexia nervosa and bulimia nervosa weight loss methods. *Research Quarterly for Exercise and Sport, 59,* 252–256.

Blinder, B. J., Freeman, D. M. A., & Stunkard, A. J. (1970). Behavior therapy of anorexia nervosa: Effectiveness of activity as a reinforcer of weight gain. *American Journal of Psychiatry, 126,* 77–82.

Blumenthal, J. A., O'Toole, L. C., & Chang, J. L. (1984). Is running an analogue of anorexia nervosa? An empirical study of obligatory running and anorexia nervosa. *Journal of the American Medical Association, 252,* 520–523.

Boe, E. E. (1985). The physiological and psychological consequences of excessive weight loss in athletics. *Journal of the National Athletic Trainers Association, 20,* 233–242.

Bruch, H. (1962). Perceptual and conceptual disturbances in anorexia nervosa. *Psychosomatic Medicine, 24,* 187–194.

Bruch, H. (1966). Anorexia nervosa and its differential diagnosis. *Journal of Nervous and Mental Disease, 141,* 555–566.

Casper, R. C., & Davis, J. M. (1977). On the course of anorexia nervosa. *American Journal of Psychiatry, 134,* 974–978.

Crisp, A. H. (1967). The possible significance of some behavioral correlates of weight and carbohydrate intake. *Journal of Psychosomatic Research, 11,* 117–131.

Crisp, A. H., & Burns, T. (1983). The clinical presentation of anorexia nervosa in males. *International Journal of Eating Disorders, 2,* 5–10.

Crisp, A. H., Hus, L. K. G., Harding, B., & Hartshorn. (1980). Clinical features of anorexia nervosa. *Journal of Psychosomatic Research, 24,* 179–191.

Epling, W. F., Pierce, W. D., & Stefan, L. (1983). A theory of activity-based anorexia. *International Journal of Eating Disorders, 3,* 27–46.

Falk, J. L. (1977). The origin and functions of adjunctive behavior. *Animal Learning and Behavior, 5,* 325–335.

Feighner, J. P., Robins, E., Guze, S. B., Woodruff, R. A., Winocur, G., & Munoz, R. (1972). Diagnostic criteria for use in psychiatric research. *Archives of General Psychiatry, 26,* 57–63.

Garner, D. M., & Garfinkel, P. E. (1980). Socio-cultural factors in the development of anorexia nervosa. *Psychological Medicine, 10,* 647–656.

Garner, D. M., & Garfinkel, P. E. (1985). *Handbook of psychotherapy for anorexia nervosa and bulimia.* New York: Guilford Press.

Garner, D. M., Garfinkel, P. E., & Bemis, K. M. (1982). A multidimensional psychotherapy for anorexia nervosa. *International Journal of Eating Disorders, 1,* 3–46.

Goldfarb, L. A., & Plante, T. G. (1984). Fear of fat in runners: An examination of the connection between anorexia nervosa and distance running. *Psychological Reports, 55,* 296.

Gull, W. W. (1874). Anorexia nervosa. *Transactions of the Clinical Society of London, 7,* 22–28.

Halmi, K. A. (1974). Anorexia nervosa: Demographic and clinical features in 94 cases. *Psychosomatic Medicine, 36,* 18–26.

Hamilton, L. H., Brooks-Gunn, J., & Warren, M. P. (1985). Sociocultural influences on eating disorders in professional female ballet dancers. *International Journal of Eating Disorders, 4,* 465–477.

Hansen, N. C. (1978). Wrestling with "making weight." *Physician and Sportsmedicine, 6,* 107–110.

Hathaway, S. R., & McKinley, J. C. (1948). *Minnesota Multiphasic Personality Inventory.* New York: Psychological Corporation.

Jackson, D. N. (1976). *Jackson Personality Inventory manual.* Port Huron, MI: Research Psychologists Press.

Johnson, C., & Connors, M. E. (1987). *The etiology and treatment of bulimia nervosa.* New York: Basic Books.

Johnson, C., Lewis, C., Love, S., Lewis, L., & Stuckey, M. (1984). Incidence and correlates of bulimic behavior in a female high school population. *Journal of Youth and Adolescence, 13,* 15–26.

Joseph, A., Wood, I. K., & Goldberg, S. C. (1982). Determining populations at risk for developing anorexia nervosa based on selection of college major. *Psychiatry Research, 7,* 53–58.

Kron, L., Katz, J. L., Gorzynski, G., & Weiner, H. (1978). Hyperactivity in anorexia nervosa: A fundamental clinical feature. *Comprehensive Psychiatry, 19,* 433–439.

Mallick, M. J., Whipple, T. W., & Huerta, E. (1987). Behavioral and psychological traits of weight-conscious teenagers: A comparison of eating-disordered patients and high- and low-risk groups. *Adolescence, 22,* 157–168.

Offer, D., & Howard, K. I. (1972). An empirical analysis of the Offer Self-Image Questionnaire for Adolescents. *Archives of General Psychiatry, 27,* 529–533.

Owens, R. G., & Slade, P. D. (1987). Running and anorexia nervosa: An empirical study. *International Journal of Eating Disorders, 6,* 771–775.

Powers, P. S., Schulman, R. G., Gleghorn, A. A., & Prange, M. E. (1987). Perceptual and cognitive abnormalities in bulimia. *American Journal of Psychiatry, 144,* 1456–1460.

Pyle, R. L., Mitchell, J. E., & Eckert, E. D. (1981). Bulimia: A report of 34 cases. *Journal of Clinical Psychiatry, 42,* 60–64.

Rosen, L. W., McKeag, D. B., Hough, D. O., & Curley, V. (1986). Pathogenic weight-control behavior in female athletes. *Physician and Sportsmedicine, 14,* 79–86.

Schlesier-Stropp, B. (1984). Bulimia: A review of the literature. *Psychological Bulletin, 95,* 247–257.

Slade, P. D. & Dewey, M. E. (1986). Development and preliminary validation of SCANS: A screening instrument for identifying individuals at risk for developing anorexia and bulimia nervosa. *International Journal of Eating Disorders, 5,* 517–538.

Vandereycken, W., Depreitere, L., & Probst, M. (1987). Body-oriented therapy for anorexia nervosa patients. *American Journal of Psychotherapy, 41,* 252–259.

Wallace, M., Sanson, A., & Singer, G. (1978). Adjunctive behavior in humans on a food delivery schedule. *Physiology and Behavior, 20,* 203–204.

Wells, R. J. (1983). Letter to the editor. *New England Journal of Medicine, 309,* 47.

Wheeler, G. D., Wall, S. R., Belcastro, A. N., Conger, P., & Cumming, D. C. (1986). Are anorexic tendencies prevalent in the habitual runner? *British Journal of Sports Medicine, 20,* 77–81.

Yates, A., Leehey, K., & Shisslak, C. M. (1983). Running—An analogue of anorexia? *New England Journal of Medicine, 308,* 251–255.

8

THE RIGHT PLACE IS HERE, THE RIGHT TIME IS NOW: TAIJI AS MENTAL AND PHYSICAL THERAPY

Jeffrey F. Meyer

University of North Carolina at Charlotte

> *I was born seven years after the start of the century in the wrong time, the wrong place, and into the wrong family. I am not insensible of the paradox: It is this which made me. (Loren Eiseley, in Heuer, 1987, p. 117)*

I once met an unusual woman, a sort of hermit who lived alone among the pines, rocks, and rhododendrons of the North Carolina mountains. She built a house that fit perfectly into a wooded hollow in the high country, and she was as happy there as a badger in her den. She planted a garden, cut wood, and lived in quiet and perfect contentment, without electricity and without plumbing. Most people, she told me, do not know what perfect silence is, or perfect peace, because even their "silence" is marred by the humming of a refrigerator or the ticking of a clock. She blended into her environment like a shy but clever animal.

But she did not "fit" into her body. She was not fat but big and square like a large man, except for her very large breasts. It was the breasts, I think, that especially bothered her. She did not say it in so many words, but as I got to know her better, I understood that she imagined them as huge weights which impeded the freedom of her spirit. Like a latter-day Gnostic or Cathar, she felt trapped in her frame of flesh. And although she denied being religious, I knew that she looked toward a future when she would be free of what she imagined as her incongruous corporal form.

I know a man, too, who once confided to me that he did not like his body.

It was soft, fleshy, unathletic, and faintly girlish. "Ever since high school I can remember the feeling of revulsion toward my own body," he said.

These two accounts of physical discontent remind me of the blessing and curse of the West, which is to feel the more universal dimension of being in the wrong body, in the wrong place at the wrong time. From the tripartite "chariot" of Plato, to the distinction between body and soul by Aristotle, to the split sensibility of Descartes, Western man (not woman perhaps) has felt the painful gap between the body and the perception of what he "really" is.

This particular *corporal* discontent connects with another: the *local* discontent that led to the quest, the search, the pilgrimage, the journey to a better land, to the garden of the Hesperides, to Ilium, to Jerusalem, to Rome, to Mecca, to Heaven, to the place where the true and the real were to be found. Throughout the great works of our literature the homeless wanderer searches for a true home: Abraham, Gilgamesh, Ulysses, Aeneas, Dante, Bunyan, Milton. All suffer from "ectopia," the disease of being "in the wrong place." Chanting of their distress in the world, the chorus in T. S. Eliot's *Murder in the Cathedral* sing: "Here is no continuing city, here is no abiding stay. Ill the wind, ill the time . . . " Framed in more homely sentiments, there is the Irish saying: "There are green hills, far away."

There is no parallel to this in the Chinese tradition, which is one of fixity, stability, and harmonizing into the landscape, the home given to the Chinese by their ancestors. In the Confucian cemetary near Qufu in Shandong, one can find the grave of Confucius and graves of his descendants for nearly 2,500 years. I saw a tombstone that said that the deceased was of the 77th generation of the family of Confucius, a continuity that can be duplicated nowhere else in the world.

Nor is there a strong sentiment for individual transcendence. More typically, the Taoist sage or Confucian scholar sought "long life," or immortality through posterity. Valery contrasted the European and non-European worlds of thought as follows: "One, occupying the greater part of the globe, remained as though immobile. . . . The other was a prey to perpetual restlessness and search. . . . Europe burst out of its borders, went out to conquer other lands" (Valery, 1962, p. 313).

Olympic-type athletics, epitomized by the marathon run, characterize the physical/athletic expression of Western restlessness. Today jogging, cycling, pumping iron, and various other oxygen-burning, painful activities are their successors. The fox gnaws at the bosom of the West. Spartan hardness, scaling mountains, traversing deserts, fording streams, and the vein-popping and turgid muscles of the bodybuilding magazines are all expressions of this same spirit. These are not always pleasant prospects, but they have made us, paradoxically, what we are.

Taiji (also written *T'ai chi*), a form of exercise native to China, represents the opposite in nearly every way. It is the physical expression of oriental fixity, harmony, at-oneness with the body and locality, the feeling of being at home in the world. Although it is said to be popular now in the United States, there are few who have mastered it. Perhaps this is because it goes against nearly every tendency and habit of the West. It is slow, it is pointless, it "gets nowhere," it is "soft," it takes too much time out of the day. If my limited experience as a teacher is any indication, approximately 1 out of 10 who begin practicing Taiji learn the complete form, and only one-tenth of those who do learn it continue to practice it.

AGAINST THE WESTERN GRAIN

So let us be clear about Taiji. It should not be advertised as the latest "fix," the New Age way of achieving the same goals we have sought all along. It is better conceived as a bitter or at least strange-tasting medicine, an "antidote" to pervasive Western tendencies such as competition, efficiency, goal oriented-ness, and practicality. Only those who feel a kind of discontent with the cultural norm will want to master and maintain this practice.

There are two basic aspects of Taiji, which are seen by the Chinese as complementary. One is the martial art (*wu shu*) or the method of self-defense. The other is "breath work" (*qigong*) by which an individual learns to regulate the passage of an element in the body called *qi* (pronounced "chee"). Both of these aspects require comment.

Taiji is the oldest form of martial art known to China and, in the eyes of its proponents, the best and most effective. There are the stories of skinny little men who can repel the attacks of 250-pound monsters. But I have always had my doubts about Taiji's martial efficacy, feeling that for most people other forms such as gongfu, karate, judo, or aikido are probably quicker and more practical ways to self-defense. Perhaps with the right teacher and unremitting practice alone and with partners, an individual could achieve a level of compe-tence that would allow Taiji to be used effectively for self-defense. But most Chinese, from my observation, are older persons who practice it for reasons of health and mental strength.

If you watch the flow of movement in a Taiji form (there are several main schools or "family" styles of form such as Yang, Wu, and Chen, together with innumerable variations within each—in fact there are almost as many forms of Taiji as there are masters who teach it), you will see the martial movements, the punches, kicks, blocks, and so forth. But all in slow motion. Somehow what the practitioner learns in the school of slow movements, he or she must apply in the event of an actual attack. Yet the practice of Taiji is more mental than physical. As my teacher often admonished, "Use your mind, not your muscles!"

I once taught Taiji to a woman in her 70s. She had no illusions about using it for self-defense. But when the course was completed, she wrote me a letter saying how Taiji had raised the level of her self-esteem and self-confidence. Her daughter was in politics, so she had felt duty-bound to help her campaigns by canvassing, but was terrified every time she walked up to the door of a stranger's home. After learning Taiji, she wrote that "the fear completely disappeared."

My own experience tells me that the use of Taiji for self-defense is not a matter of learning a bag of physical tricks to repel an aggressor. Somehow, as it did in the case of my elderly friend, it creates an egoless calmness and confidence that take away the conditions or need for real battle. It is like the sword of Chuang Tzu. "Thrust forward [it] meets nothing before it; raised, it encounters nothing above; pressed down, it encounters nothing beneath it," but "it brings harmony to the wills of the people and peace to the four directions" (Tzu, 1970, p. 342). Of the mental state sought in Taiji, it is said that "at the time of practice, though there is no one present, it seems as if there were; when in a fight, though the opponent is there, it seems as if he were not" (Shi, 1958, p. 34).

The "breath work," or *qigong,* that is an essential part of Taiji presents another problem. It is at the heart of Chinese ideas about the nature of the human body and health and medicine. Simply put, the theory of *qi* says that the body is laced with meridians or veins through which flows the element called *qi,* and if one is to be strong and healthy this *qi* must circulate through the body unobstructed. Disease is caused by blockages. Taiji is a regimen that promotes the generation of and circulation of this element. The problem for us Westerners is that this element is not measurable on scientific instruments, and the meridians are not revealed by anatomical dissection or x-ray photography. Yet they are the very basis of acupuncture, acupressure, and all other forms of traditional Chinese medicine. Using paradigms of Western religion, we find we must have faith in the existence and functioning of *qi* and the meridians. Yet the term "faith" is not an appropriate concept to match the way the Chinese feel about *qi.* They simply take it for granted.

Qi is usually translated as "breath," or perhaps better, "energy" or "vitality." It is not the same as the breath that goes in and out of our lungs, or the greater air that flows through the universe, but at the same time it is not entirely different. Needless to say, no breathalizer will discover its presence. Perhaps the best way to describe it in accord with Chinese ideas is as a "universal element," a fundamental constituent of which the energy of our bodies and the air we breathe are manifestations. In any case, unless we accept the reality of *qi,* much of Taiji will not make sense. And this is very hard for a non-Chinese person to do.

REST LIKE A MOUNTAIN, MOVE LIKE A RIVER

What do we see when we watch a person practicing Taiji? I use the term "practicing" instead of the usual term "playing," which comes from the fact that the Chinese word *da,* the word used for most sports, is also used for Taiji. You *da* baseball, basketball, Ping-Pong, and so on, and you *da* Taiji. While I like the word "playing" because it conveys the idea of purposeless activity, I use "practice" instead to divorce it from competitive athletics and to suggest the deeper purposes not found in ordinary sports. For the vast majority of Chinese who practice it, Taiji is in no way competitive. When you watch a person practicing Taiji, you see a person with her feet planted together, who stands erect but not ramrod straight, who looks forward at nothing in particular, and is relaxed but not slack. She sinks slightly into a mildly flexed position as her feet move to shoulder width apart.

Then the form begins. "All motion begins with rest; when at rest be like an immoveable mountain, when moving, be like the great and ever flowing rivers" (Shi, 1958, p. 3). In performing these simple initial moves the practitioner is imitating the cosmogony, which begins in transcendent unity, divides, multiples, and becomes the "ten thousand things" (a Chinese cliché meaning all that exists). As the *Tao Te Ching* says, "The Tao begets one; one begets two; two begets three; three begets the ten thousand things" (Lau, 1963, p. 103). In the long Yang style that I practice, there follows a sequence of 108 movements or "forms," many of them with very colorful names, such as "grasping the sparrow's tail," "the white crane beats it wings," "embrace the tiger, return to the mountain," and "cloud hands." In all of these movements there is a continuous alternation between gestures of attack and retreat, aggression and passivity, expansion and contraction, forward and reverse.

The movements are expressive of what the Chinese call *yin* and *yang,* maintaining that all that exists is a combination of these two complementary opposites, whose unceasing movement produces the continuous change that marks existence as we know it. There is no stopping, but a continuous flow from one movement to the next. The motions continue like spirals of endless circles, fluctuations in the rhythms of nature. The energy of the body imitates, or really is a part of, the energy that flows through all of nature. "The way of life is never to stop, but to fluctuate, to ebb and flow, expand and contract, in recurring cycles, like the seasons" (Shi, 1958, p. 20). When finally the form concludes, the feet come together again and the practitioner has "returned to the source." Here, in true Chinese spirit, the journey has been an inward one, and the questor finds the goal to be in the same place where the journey had begun.

Again, contrary to Western thinking (and perhaps to most human thought patterns generally), Taiji teaches that the control center of the body is not brain but belly. More accurately, all movement is said to originate from the *dantian* (field of cinnabar), a center in the lower abdomen, below the navel and near the base of the spinal cord. The *dantian* is the pivot of the body, the source of *qi.* The upper body must be held straight above this foundation, with no leaning or wobbling. The waist turns there, and when the upper body does bend low, it bends from this point. Of course the *dantian* does not show up on x-ray photographs, but even as a symbol, imagining this lower center of gravity as my physical center produces a sense of stability and balance.

Finally, the sort of strength developed in Taiji is not physical in the normal sense. Faithful practice, year after year, does not produce muscular development, except in the legs. The muscles of the back, chest, neck, and arms remain undeveloped. They are to be relaxed and loose. All the movements promote fluidity in the motions of the arms. Tension, which is thought to block the flow of *qi*, is the enemy of health and strength. Furthermore, there appears to be little or no aerobic advantage to the practice of Taiji (Mucci, 1989).

The legs, on the other hand, do become conditioned and muscular, because Taiji is done, from beginning to end, in a sort of "horse riding" stance, with knees slightly bent. This position is what dancers call "pelvic tilt." In this sense, Taiji is similar to jogging, in that it promotes the development of leg strength but not arm strength (unless one runs with weights). In Taiji, however, the true source of power is not even the legs, but the earth beneath. A classic text on Taiji says "The feet are planted on the ground as if they were growing roots," and "the center of support is *under* the feet" (Shi, 1958, p. 45, italics added). "When at rest, be like an immoveable mountain, when moving, be like the great and ever flowing rivers." This is the source of the supposed rocklike solidity of the Taiji practitioner.

Taken together, the ideas mentioned above describe a form of physical exercise based on a "mystic" physiology that is scientifically unverifiable and uses practices alien to Western patterns of thought and behavior. Yet it undeniably has attracted a following, myself included. There are Taiji training centers and teachers in all major cities in the United States, regional associations, countless books on the subject, magazines, and newsletters whose circulation continues to grow. Let me offer some conjectures to account for the popularity of Taiji.

There are, of course many New Age types who will try anything: Taiji, Yoga, transcendental meditation, EST, and so forth. I'm not sure this is a bad thing, because it shows at least openness to change and a willingness to experiment. But those whose cup of tea is the new and different will soon quit Taiji, because it becomes "old" and tedious very rapidly, if you are looking for a quick fix. In the following discussion, I focus instead on more enduring reasons for practicing this form of martial art, which is often called "meditation in motion."

For the very same reasons that it "goes against the grain," Taiji is useful in treating some of the maladies that infect us in modern Western culture. For those whose lives have fallen into patterns of ceaseless activity, it teaches the lesson of slowing down. For those whose minds are crammed with anxieties and distractions, it says stop the mindless chatter, tether the monkey, calm down. You can achieve a lightness and clarity by which you can be at one with yourself and your surroundings. For those whose lives are best described by metaphors of struggle and battle, it says that true strength is quiet and reserved, possessing the sort of power than never need be exerted. Save your energy for when it is really needed. Be like the cat, the image of languid relaxation, until the moment it springs on its prey. For those who are afraid, it teaches self-confidence. For those who are too busy to slow down, it offers the paradoxical advice to accomplish more by knowing when to stop. "Better stop short than fill to the brim/Oversharpen the blade, and the edge will soon blunt/When the storeroom fills with gold and jade, no one can guard it" (Lau, 1963, p. 65).Therefore, the *Tao Te Ching* advises, "When you've accomplished something, hide! That is the Way of Heaven" (Lau, 1963, p. 65). Such advice no doubt speaks to the condition of many in our affluent society.

Taiji teaches the continuities between the human world and the world of nature. Like Oriental thought generally, it perceives humans as part of nature, and a fairly humble part at that, not the "lords of creation." Nature is the *Tao*, the Great Way, the great teacher. Much of Taiji literature shows a deep sensitivity to the patterns of nature, seeing in them models for imitation if one wants to live a more successful human life. According to the mythology of Taiji, its founder watched a fight between a crane and a snake, and from the motions of these animals began to develop the forms of Taiji.

Most generally, like all life, Taiji follows the patterns of *yin* and *yang*, naturally flowing from one to the other, from advance to retreat, aggression to defense, from exposure to protection just as in nature there is the passage of the seasons, the alternation of day and night, heat and cold, darkness and light. "The way of life is never to stop, but to fluctuate, to ebb and flow, expand and contract, in recurring cycles, like the seasons" (Shi, 1958, p. 20). But, more specifically, individual motions of the forms are said to be imitations of nature. The adept practitioner of Taiji is said to be so sensitive that "his touch is like the touch of a dragon fly on the surface of the water." No bird can escape from his palm, for to fly away the bird must find some resistance, but when the adept practitioner feels the first hint of thrust he yields and the bird cannot take off. With that finely developed sensitivity to aggression, no one can lay a hand on him.

Leg movements are supposed to be catlike, sure-footed and unerring. One should watch with the relaxed vigilance of a gliding bird of prey, and move like the inchworm which retreats only to move forward. Even the world of vegetation is sought out for instruction. The arms and hands should follow the body as branches of the willow follow the trunk in a breeze or as seaweeds undulate to the motions of the waves and tides.

Although recognizing the difference between human and nonhuman nature, Oriental thought has chosen to emphasize the continuities rather than the split between the two worlds. Western thought has done the opposite and mourned the divergence between humans and their animal cousins and the loss of innocence that is implied. In Taiji one is supposed to revert to the original state, not only through the imitation of patterns in nature, but in the very emptying of the mind which suggests a return to the unself-conscious state of the animal or the innocence of the child.

WHAT TAIJI CAN AND CANNOT DO

Leaving aside the question of its efficacy as a martial art, what can a person expect to gain from the faithful practice of Taiji over a long period of time? As mentioned earlier, it does not accomplish bodybuilding, it has no aerobic advantage, and I seriously doubt that it would help anyone trim inches off the waistline, though it certainly would firm up the legs. In the estimation of all Chinese who practice it, it is useful in treating sicknesses and diseases, such as heart disease, high blood pressure, arthritis, and many others (Liu, 1986). One would probably have to accept the theory of *qi* circulation and the meridians in order to believe that these claims are true. And yet I cannot doubt the sincerity of the people who have told me how Taiji helped them to cure a sickness or overcome some physical problem that had resisted conventional medical treatment.

Recent scientific experiments indicate that Taiji has many of the same good effects as accomplished meditation, in particular a 33% slower rate of breathing, and an 11% improvement in breathing efficiency. Hirai (1975) and others have shown the value of meditation in lowering the brain waves, increasing heart rate, lowering blood pressure, increasing galvanic skin response, and generally increasing the activity of the autonomic nervous system and the dissipation of lactic acid, thus producing the same restorative effects as periods of sound sleep.

Assuming the physiological and mental (or psychic) values of meditation, I would like to propose a particular value in the practice of Taiji that surpasses that of other meditational forms. One of the great difficulties faced by people who practice meditation is how to translate the values of meditation into daily life. Too often the feeling of calmness and centeredness of the time of meditation is lost when an individual leaves the privacy of the room, the woods, or the temple, and is thrown once again into the pressured situations of ordinary living. Unlike seated mediation, Taiji's calmness is already projected into patterns of motion and behavior, and is therefore more easily translated into the world of activity where we spend most of our waking hours.

I recall that when I first learned Taiji I became much more conscious of my body—its sensations, processes, and movements. I found this fascinating, like a child discovering a new toy. I would stand in a certain way, move in a certain way, and occasionally attract the stares of bystanders by my behavior. The strangeness has gone away, but I still become periodically aware of the "miracle" of movement, and can sometimes gain a certain balanced state of mind as I walk down a hill, climb stairs, balance on a ladder, and so forth, simply by recalling the original rediscovery of my body. A friend of mine who is a professional masseur has developed a method of Taiji and massage that enables him not only to give a better massage in a physical sense, but to achieve an important state of mind while he works. My suggestion is that Taiji, as meditation in motion, could infuse or inform any sort of physical activity.

Perhaps *harmony* and *balance* are the two words that best capture the essence of Taiji. I like these words because they have definite physical manifestations, yet represent an ideal state of mind—one of health, energy, and composure. Success in human life requires harmony with nature and with other human beings, and this often has to be achieved in the midst of potentially distressing situations. This is what Shi (1958) refers to when he speaks of "the mysterious knack of 'preserving your center' while responding to the changes which go on about you" (p. 21). Balance is poise, and a balanced person is one who is not at the mercy of fear, anger, ego, or addictions. It represents perhaps the highest ideal of Taiji as a mental discipline, and also its limitations. I have already described the ideal. From a Western perspective Taiji seems at this limit to be too cautious, with the full power of motion and feeling always held in check:

> *watchful, like someone crossing a winter stream.*
>
> *alert, like those aware of danger.*
>
> *courteous, like visiting guests.*
>
> *yielding, like ice about to melt. (Lau, 1963, p. 71)*

As Delza (1985) put it, Taiji counsels us never to throw ourselves into a position that we cannot get back out of, "never allowing one to expend oneself in a gesture of finality" (p. 15). "Better stop short than fill to the brim/Oversharpen the blade, and the edge will soon blunt," says the *Tao Te Ching* (Lau, 1963, p. 65). The phrase "gesture of finality" could hardly be improved upon to express what it is that Taiji warns us against. And if as a method of self-protection these are good pieces of advice, one must ask if certain life situations might not require that we push beyond such limitations.

In this respect, one thinks of the opposite spirit expressed in such phrases as "throwing oneself into the breech" and "leap of faith" from Western culture. They may reflect the Western penchant for risk taking, which at its best is courageous and selfless, but at its worst is reckless and destructive. Certainly we have seen plenty of both in the story of Western civilization. On the other hand, the Taiji attitude (and by extension, the Chinese mentality) at its best bespeaks humility, peace, and harmony, but at its worst an overcautious craving for mere self-preservation. Rather than compare the two, it would be wiser to measure each by success within its own context.

REFERENCES

Delza, S. (1985). *T'ai chi ch'uan: Body and mind in harmony.* New York: SUNY Press.

Heuer, K. (Ed.). (1987). *The lost notebooks of Loren Eiseley.* Boston: Little, Brown.

Hirai, T. (1977). *Zen meditation therapy.* Tokyo: Japan Publications.

Lau, D. C. (trans.) (1963). *Lao Tzu: Tao Te Ching.* Baltimore: Pengiun Books.

Liu, D. (1986). *T'ai chi ch'uan and meditation.* New York: Schocken.

Mucci, G. (1989). Scientific study clarifies t'ai chi ch'uan benefits. *T'ai Chi, 13,* 2–6.

Shi, T. (1958). *Taijichuan pu niewaigong yenjilu [Taijichuan illustrated: A brief examination of interior and exterior forms].* Taipei: Huawen.

Watson, B. (trans.) (1970). *The complete works of Chuang Tzu.* New York: Columbia University Press.

Valery, P. (1962). The European. In *The collected works of Paul Valery: Volume 10. History and politics.* New York: Bollingen Pantheon Books.

III

SOCIETY AND THE INDIVIDUAL PERFORMER

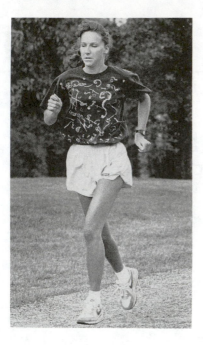

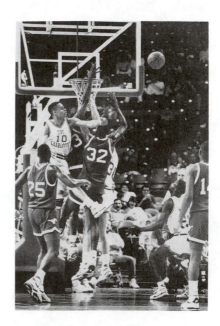

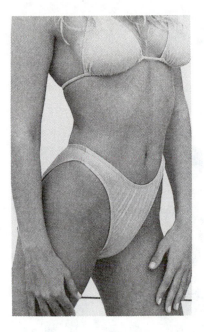

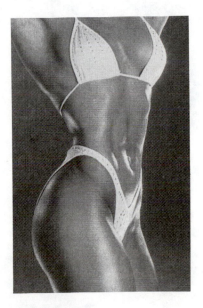

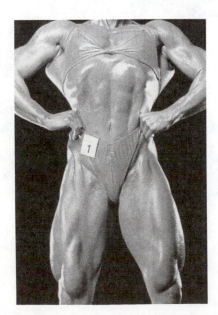

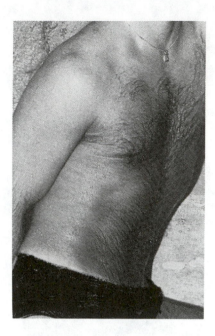

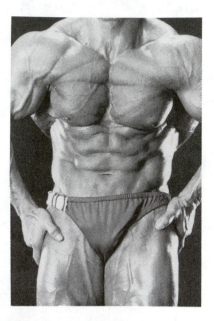

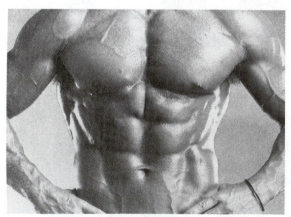

9

SPORTS IN THE WORKPLACE: DO THEY PAY?

Jo Ann Lee

University of North Carolina at Charlotte

The research described in this chapter was conducted with the intent of answering two questions. First, do sports programs benefit the organization/employer in terms of a more productive, more efficient organization? For example, might employees' participation in sports programs improve communications among participants, build trust, and enhance working relationships? Second, does sports participation pay off for the individual participant? For example, do certain participants in sports activities get special treatment or benefits from the employer or immediate supervisor because of the player's sports prowess? My investigation of these two questions suggests affirmative answers to both questions.

The topic of discussion in this chapter is sports programs that include employees of one organization playing together. There are differences across the organizations described in terms of (a) whether the employees play against each other or play against other organizations and (b) the amount of support extended by the organization. Some sports activities among employees are formed haphazardly by the employees themselves with no sponsorship or intervention by the employer, whereas other organizations provide varying amounts of monies, equipment, or facilities for the programs.

The fact that many employers have invested much time, effort, and money in the development and implementation of employee exercise and fitness programs (Falkenberg, 1987) indicates their belief in the effectiveness of these programs. However, many employers appear to have overlooked the value of sports programs and have not identified characteristics of successful sports programs. Falkenberg (1987) mentioned in her critique of the research related to the impact of employee fitness programs on work-related variables that approximately 50,000 business firms promote physical activity. In contrast, my literature review found no articles or books directly focusing on sports in the workplace.

I believe that employers would benefit from developing and implementing organized sports programs for their work force. My opinion is based on the research on informal groups in the workplace, interviews I held with a number of participants of sports programs, and the latest research on socialization and corporate culture. For instance, an employer-sponsored sports program for employees may serve to socialize the new employees by subtly communicating aspects of the corporate culture to them in a relaxed atmosphere. A result of organized sports programs could be increased overlap of the formal and informal work groups.

The majority of the information in this chapter refers to how organizations/employers could use sports to increase the productivity of the organization as a whole because (a) the literature on organizational behavior includes several critical phenomena (e.g., informal groups, socialization, and corporate culture) related to this issue and (b) the persons I interviewed spoke more about this issue than about how individual employees may benefit in their professional pursuits because of their athletic prowess. In the first two sections of this chapter, I briefly describe and discuss the relevant organizational phenomena that I believe are related to sports in the workplace. Next, I discuss the comments made by my interviewees. I then discuss how sports are related to the organizational phenomena discussed in the first two sections. Finally, I focus on a few situations in which individual employees have benefited from their sports prowess.

As Diamant mentions in Chapter 1, there are distinctions among sports, exercise, and fitness. Specifically, sports uniquely includes both competition and recreation. These distinctions of sports must be kept in mind while reading this chapter.

INFORMAL GROUPS

There are two types of groups in organizations: formal and informal. Formal groups are those that are formed by the employer. There are two types of formal groups: command and task. Command groups are those that one would find on an organizational chart, which shows the different levels and different units in the organization. Task groups are more temporary and are formed to accomplish a specific task or objective.

In contrast, informal groups are those that are formed by the employees. These groups are not planned, as are formal groups, and are not explicit. In fact, the constituents of the informal groups may change several times while the formal groups stay intact, or vice versa. There are two types of informal groups: friendship and interests. Friendship groups are constituted of persons who have a nonwork relationship. Persons in these groups are likely to socialize together away from the workplace. Interest groups are constituted of persons who share a common goal or objective, for example, restricting smoking in the workplace. Usually, the greater the overlap between formal and informal groups, the more productive the organization will be. This occurs because members of informal groups tend to exert more effort than members of formal groups in assisting each other in accomplishing the work goals.

The impact of informal groups on organizational productivity is a well-researched, well-known phenomenon. Study of informal groups dates back to the classic Hawthorne studies of the 1930s (Roethlisberger, 1980) and the Tavistock study of coal mining (Trist & Bamforth, 1980). The Hawthorne studies were originally designed to study the effects of illumination on productivity. However, the investigators in both the Hawthorne studies and the Tavistock study discovered that the social environment as well as the physical environment affected organizational productivity. In the Bank Wiring Observation Room Study, which was part of the Hawthorne studies, it was found that co-workers often disregarded the boundaries of formal groups and worked according to the boundaries of informal groups. Consequently, members of friendship groups who were members of different command groups assisted each other with their respective jobs.

Closely related to the concept of informal groups are the concepts of corporate culture and the process of socialization.

CORPORATE CULTURE AND SOCIALIZATION

These two concepts are discussed together because socialization refers to the *process* of teaching the corporate culture (Pascale, 1984). Corporate culture is "the pattern of basic assumptions, values, norms, and artifacts shared by organization members" (Cummings & Huse, 1989, p. 421). "Socialization is the process by which organizations shape the attitudes, thoughts, and behavior of employees" (Davis & Newstrom, 1985, p. 54). Socialization refers to the process of assimilating employees by

1. helping them develop work skills and abilities,
2. helping them acquire appropriate role behaviors,
3. helping them adjust to the work group and its norms, and
4. teaching them the organizational values (Feldman, 1980).

The topic of corporate culture has been of prime interest in the business world for the past decade since competition from Japan has become extremely fierce and threatening to the U.S. economy. The success of the Japanese companies has led many to study and write about their corporate culture and culture characteristics that would benefit companies in the United States. Some of the best known books are *Theory Z: How American Business Can Meet the Japanese Challenge* (Ouchi, 1979), *The Art of Japanese Management* (Pascale & Athos, 1981), *In Search of Excellence* (Peters & Waterman, 1982), and *A Passion for Excellence* (Peters & Austin, 1985). What these books seem to have in common is their focus on corporate *values* as critical to success. The acceptance of others' values is partly dependent on the amount of trust there is between the concerned parties. Many of the characteristics of the informal groups already discussed appear to be also characteristic of the successful corporate culture. More specifically, members share a sense of trust and respect for each other, share common attitudes and values, and assist each other as needed. It is noteworthy that Ouchi (1979) emphasized the importance of "subtleties" to the successful corporate culture in the evaluation and understanding of co-workers and subordinates. He stated, "A foreman who knows his workers well can pinpoint personalities, decide who works well with whom, and thus put together work teams of maximal effectiveness. These subtleties can never be captured explicitly, and any bureaucratic management will do violence to them" (p. 7). Sports provides an opportunity to observe the subtleties of the individual employees.

Admittedly, employer-sponsored sports programs alone will not be sufficient to teach the corporate culture to the employees. However, they represent one strategy for this purpose.

INTERVIEWS WITH PARTICIPANTS
OF ORGANIZATION'S/EMPLOYER'S SPORTS PROGRAMS

This research was not designed as a survey study and admittedly does not include a representative sample of all the types of organizations. Rather, this study serves as an exploratory investigation of the effects of organized sports in the workplace. I interviewed employees of organizations that have or have had sports programs. Their comments are summarized below, with a focus on what they perceived as the advantages and disadvantages of having such activities. In general, the interviewees endorsed organized sports programs in the workplace under certain conditions. In addition, I found that the interviewees described the benefits of the programs using the same terminology also used to describe the benefits of informal work groups and of having an appropriate corporate culture.

I do not use the names of individuals or organizations, in order to protect their privacy. I chose to include public and private sector organizations because they often have very different organizational cultures. The organizations include a city and a federal government agency, a university, two service organizations, and an industrial manufacturer. Please note that, although my employer is located in Charlotte, North Carolina, the organizations of the interviewees are not necessarily located in Charlotte. To provide the reader with a framework, I present the organizations in terms of the amount of employer involvement in the sports program, starting with the organization with the least employer involvement. However, the reader will learn that this dimension may not be the most important determinant of the success of the sports program.

A City Police Department

The interviewee is the current training director for the police department, which employs approximately 400 employees. Cliques for various sports, such as golf, martial arts, hunting, softball, scuba diving, and tennis, have formed informally. According to the interviewee, the advantages of having sports activities among co-workers include (a) the development of trust among them, (b) their learning cooperation, (c) their meeting people not normally encountered during the regular work day, and (d) the use of one scale (ability in the sport) to evaluate all persons. However, in his opinion, whether or not these advantages are realized depends on the amount of communication involved with the sport, the amount of danger involved with the sport, and whether or not the skills needed for the sport are the same skills needed for the job. For example, I may trust you with confidential information concerning the workplace if I have already trusted you with my life in sports (e.g., in scuba diving). As might be expected, the interviewee believes there is a big difference between individual sports and team sports in terms of their respective contributions toward achieving the listed advantages. When people play as a team, some of the social distance that has been established at the workplace disappears.

Interestingly, many of the employees have failed to take advantage of the agency's fitness program. This could be because the jobs involved are physically demanding. However, the employees seem willing to and do get together to participate in a sport when they feel it is not required and when there is more social discourse. According to the interviewee, persons at different occupational levels tend to join different types of sports. For example, most of the members of the golf clique are civilians or sworn officers not assigned to street duty. They are, in the interviewee's opinion, slightly more intelligent than the average employee in the department. According to him, "the golfers" have developed a network among themselves. Using their network, they are able to bypass channels and are able to accomplish some tasks in a few hours that might take those who are not members of the clique several days. As a result, the golfers have gained power that is not explicitly written anywhere. For example, both the person in charge of handling supplies and the person in charge of budget are golfers. When the budget person needs some supplies, he calls the supply person. Usually the supply person responds immediately and does not require the budget person to complete the paperwork immediately. However, according to the interviewee, the supply person requires him (a non-golfer) to complete the specified paperwork and go through the specified channels according to the rules. Consequently, it takes the interviewee much more time to obtain supplies.

The interviewee believes that the contacts he has made through sports activities have benefited him, both professionally and socially. He said that he has made good friends through sports, because sports serves as a common interest. He added that sports helps to break down barriers based on race and gender. With sports, the only thing that is judged is one's ability. He told of his joining some of the officers on the firing range when he was a new hiree and how it helped his socialization into the department. His experience could also be generalized to minorities and female employees. That is, getting the job is only part of the employment process. One's acceptance by one's co-workers and supervisor is another part of the process toward professional success. For example, some black employees may feel isolated when no effort is made by the current employees to socialize with them outside of the workplace. The interviewee mentioned that sports were the only commonality between him and a certain black employee. They differed along other dimensions, such as politics and religion.

On the other hand, employee morale and organizational commitment may decline if some employees perceive that certain star athletes on the company team receive special treatment. This is reflected in the comments of my next interviewee.

A National Transportation Company

The interviewee was an employee in one of the offices that at the time of her employment had about 100 employees. According to her, she witnessed several examples of favoritism given to two employees who were star softball players on the company team. One of the players was the pitcher and the other was the leading scorer. The league in which the team played was citywide and was very competitive. As one might guess, only a few employees (13–14) were chosen to play on the team. The team was all male; women could participate by attending the games. The company had worked hard to get into the league. The company played against other companies with a similar type of work force (i.e., blue collar). The supervisor of the two star players served as the team coach and no supervisors were on the team.

Before the sports program was started, according to the interviewee, there was a great deal of cohesion among the employees and most of them supported the new program. Most of the employees had tried to work together, which made the job more enjoyable. However, that unity started to crumble as inequities and injustices in terms of the supervisors' differential treatment of the employees became conspicuous. The company had good intentions when it started the softball team. The softball games were a big deal. The interviewee said that the team was viewed by the company as "a way of establishing [the company] as a visible company in the area because a lot of people came to the games. It was a source of prestige and a valued activity for the employees. It was thought of as a social event for the employees."

Where did the company go wrong? To begin with, friction developed between two groups: those who played and those who did not play. The two star players did anything they wanted to do, even things that went against company policy. Moreover, they were very blatant about violations. For example, the two would blatantly take 30-min breaks instead of the allotted 15 min. The violations were very obvious to the other employees. Although the co-workers did not complain to the supervisor about the long breaks, resentment developed among the other employees. Eventually, others tried to get away with taking longer breaks. Elaborate schemes were devised to trick the system for clocking out for breaks. Other persons who took breaks longer than 15 min were reprimanded. The co-workers did not report the two for break violations because of the previously established cohesion in the group.

Another example of favoritism toward the two star players was the supervisor's allowing the two to leave early (e.g., at lunch time) every time there was a game. The other employees were not granted this privilege. In fact, if other employees did leave work early, they were reprimanded. The interviewee did not notice any violations or special treatment for the other team members at first. Later, the perceived inequities led many of the other employees to try to get away with the same violations. This resulted in a decrease in performances. When people started slacking off, a domino effect occurred. The unity that was there in the work group started to crumble. The other employees said, "If they don't have to work then I am not going to work."

In addition, the supervisor at times ignored complaints made about the star players by customers and the supervisor gave the two players prime work assignments. If complaints were made about other employees, punitive action was taken, such as time off without pay. The prime work assignments were supposed to be made on the basis of superior job performance. Giving the two players these assignments was not justified, according to the interviewee, because they were not pulling their weight. In fact, the two often would talk to each other on the job rather than doing their work. The supervisor would ignore their negligence.

The one other sports activity sponsored by the company was a tennis tournament. It was open to all employees, but mostly men played. The employees played against each other instead of against other companies. The tennis activity was short-lived compared with the softball games. The interviewee did not observe any favoritism toward any of the tennis players.

A Federal Government Agency

In contrast to the situation at the previous organization, the sports program at this government agency seemed to help build trust and a sense of teamwork among the employees, according to the interviewee from the agency. The two offices are about the same size, 100 employees each; the participation rate was about the same, about 10%; the degree of involvement by management seems to have been about the same, a low to moderate degree of involvement. The difference between the two organizations seems to be how the supervisors in the respective organizations treated the players versus the nonplayers. The different behaviors of the two supervisors toward their respective players and the non-players seem to reflect different values and attitudes of the two organizations.

The government agency's sports program included a women's softball team and a men's basketball team. The softball team was limited to female government employees. All levels of government (i.e., local, state, and federal) were included. The basketball team was open to all employees of the agency, but no women joined. Both leagues were initiated by the city personnel department. The interviewee served as the coach of the women's softball team and he played on the basketball team. He worked at the agency while the sports program was active and continues to work there today when there is no sports program; therefore, he was able to provide a comparison of the work environment between the two eras. According to him, there is a noticeable difference in the organizational climate between the two eras. In his opinion, there seemed to be "a sense of identity and a sense of camaraderie" when the agency was active in the sports program. He also said that the sports activities broke down barriers of authority, race, gender, educational level, and occupational level, and a sense of teamwork developed. Both the softball and basketball activities taught the people how to "work together toward a common goal." One possible reason for the deterioration of the barriers was that the activities gave the employees something that everyone could talk about and it put everyone "on the same level." Although no supervisors played, the professionals in the office played with those in clerical positions.

Whereas the women's softball team was composed of members of other government agencies in addition to those employees of the interviewee's agency, the basketball team was limited to the agency's employees. The basketball team was initiated because some men in the office wanted some exercise and fun. However, the agency did not have a coordinator for the sports program. This may be one reason why the sports activities ceased.

The interviewee's explanation of how the sports activities benefited the organization concerned how people got a chance to get to know each other. He explained that an employee could get a sense of whom he or she could depend on both in the sports activity and at the workplace. If a player did not show for the game, the players were disappointed in that person. He believed that such unreliability indicated disrespect and/or lack of concern for the coach and the teammates. This led to distrust in that person. He added that the business world looks for many characteristics that are displayed in sports, for example, ability to cooperate and dependability. He also noticed that the people who played in the various sports usually were the same people who submitted their names for promotion and took more risks in the workplace. According to the interviewee, sports participation is valuable information for the supervisor. He said that if in doubt about a person's effort at work, go watch the person play a team sport and you will detect laziness, not giving full effort, level of commitment to getting the job done, and how well the person gets along with others. He saw consistency in behaviors at work and on the field.

In his opinion, his participation in the sports activities benefited him personally. He said that his participation affected his attitude toward his job. He had had some dissatisfaction with certain aspects of the job. The sports provided a distraction from the unpleasant aspects. It was one way of coping for him. One advantage of his coaching was that it gave him a feeling of what it was like to manage, to make decisions and live with them. It taught him a lot about how to deal with people. It helped him in the performance of his job by teaching him the importance of having a strategy in order to accomplish his job. He also learned the importance of maintaining control over his emotions. He admitted that he learned much about himself, for example, that he is competent to make good decisions about people. Sports gave him a feeling that he always had a chance to succeed and this philosophy carried over to the workplace. When the agency's team won he felt the agency was great. The down side was that when they lost he felt bad about everyone.

I inquired about any differential treatment at the workplace for players versus nonplayers and good players versus poor players. He admitted to some difference in treatment and he said that it was "subtle and effective." The difference that he explained appeared actually to be more beneficial than destructive. According to him, the women who played softball developed a sense of confidence that spilled over to their work performance. They seemed to develop a sense of self-assurance. Those with less education than others may have felt they were equal to those with better education and better positions. The office is 50% men and 50% women, with most women at lower level positions. When the men watched the women play softball, that showed the men's interest and support. That contributed to the respect the women had for themselves and the respect the men had for the women.

Interestingly, the interviewee said there were differences among the different basketball teams in terms of how they played and the differences were consistent with the differences among their types of occupations. Professions seem to take their mode of operation to the playing court. For example, the team composed of lawyers tended to have planned a strategy. According to the interviewee, the players on that team were generally aggressive, very technical, very conservative, and very intelligent. They passed the ball around and they understood teamwork. They played like lawyers; for example, they disputed calls. In contrast, blue-collar workers were more "laid back," did not dispute calls, were more physical, and did not have a plan. Teams representing private companies that had a lot of stress on the job aimed their stress at their opponents. These teams showed a lot of anxiety and hostility. There was much rivalry among such teams, and the players were easy to arouse and upset. It made the interviewee wonder how the companies kept their respective teams together. According to him, the government league was more relaxed.

A Utility Company

This company has offices in several locations. Some of the offices have taken advantage of the company-sponsored sports program whereas others have not. Approximately 50% of the workers participate in the program. The interviewee, the business office supervisor, is currently in an office that does not participate in the sports program. However, a year ago she worked in one of the offices that did participate in the sports program. Consequently, she was able to offer her perspective of the work environment with and without the sports participation. Her earlier office, with more than 1,000 employees, was much larger than her current office, which has about 100 employees. She feels the benefits of the sports activities are so great that she continues to play with her former co-workers. She has been involved in the sports program for 2 years.

The company provides financial support for various sports, such as softball, basketball, volleyball, and bowling, and has published guidelines for the formation of teams. One of the rules requires that an equal number of men and women compose the team. The interviewee is a member of the volleyball team. According to her, the employees' participation in the sports activities enhanced the communications among the employees and provided an opportunity for the employees to get to know each other. She gave the following example of how the sports program has benefited the organization. Before the sports program, there was friction among the three departments on her floor. The departments competed against each other and did not talk to each other. There was a desire to eliminate the friction because of concern for some recent hirees. They did not want the recent hirees to experience the friction that existed. The "floor" organized a sports team, including all three departments, to participate in the sports activities. The sports activities gave the three different departments something to talk about; it gave them a common interest. This led to better work relationships and communications. The co-workers felt like the other workers were more like friends. In the interviewee's opinion, "The better you know someone individually and personally, the better you can work with them and all that spills over into the workplace." According to her, the company fosters a family feeling and the sports activities enhanced the family concept and commitment. With the interviewee's group of teammates, there is more to the sports than the actual playing. After the game, the team usually socializes over drinks. The social aspect of corporate sports has helped to lead to other types of social activities, such as weekend socializing.

The interviewee added that she enjoys playing against other teams from within the company more than playing against other companies, because she has an opportunity to see and to become familiar with other employees of the company whom she does not usually see. I asked if friction and destructive competition ever developed among opposing teams. She said that the players are never mad at each other. She added that the fact that the employees must volunteer to coordinate the sports program shows that the employees are very interested in the program. (The company used to have a sports coordinator, but this position no longer exists.)

Her participation in the program has helped her specifically as a supervisor, the interviewee said, because it improved her relationship with her subordinates. It put her on the same level with her subordinates, some of whom could play better than she. They saw her in a different light and she saw them in a different light. They had to depend on each other to win. She wants to develop a sports program at her current office. She added that her participation has facilitated her working relationships with male workers. The men seem to respect her more professionally because of her athletic skills, and their compliments about her athletic skills boost her self-confidence. The men seem to respect all the female players because they at least try.

The only disadvantage of sports in the workplace that my interviewee mentioned was that feelings and egos could be damaged if an "arrogant supervisor" played on the team. According to her, if the supervisor feels that he or she must call the shots on the playing field then he or she may feel emasculated when that is not allowed. Similarly, if the team consists of timid subordinates who feel they must follow the orders of the supervisor, then the goal of better relationships and camaraderie will not be achieved. It is important for the supervisor to know the goal of the sports program. Apparently, the players on her team have the right perspective. The department supervisors on her floor as well as the manager over the entire floor play, and the workers appreciate it. The manager's playing has not caused a chill over the team and their playing relationships. In her words, "It is good when supervisors and the subordinates are at the same level. The big advantage of sports is that the subordinates can call the shots and give the supervisor orders during the game because they cannot do this on the job."

An Industrial Manufacturer

This company, like the preceding one, has several locations and the employer is very involved with the company sports program. Some form of a sports program has been around about 50 years. According to one of my interviewees, the company is very interested in the employees as individuals and their health. The particular office of the two interviewees has approximately 2,600 employees. About 15% of the employees participate in the sports program. The company provides most of the finances needed for the sports. There are a golf course and tennis courts on the grounds, and volleyball, basketball, and bowling facilities are provided. In addition, the company finances and organizes an awards banquet each year. The program involves only employees of the company, and no games involve other companies.

The first interviewee was a general foreman of a department who has been with the company for 10 years at various locations and in different positions. He has been at this office for 4 1/2 years. He has three shift foremen under him and 150 hourly people in his department. He is involved with all of the sports activities except basketball. I asked him if he felt that having the sports program made a difference in the working relationships among his subordinates and between himself and his subordinates. He said it definitely does make a difference and he believes that if there were no sports the relationships would be different. In fact, when he first moved to this office he formed a three-team softball league within his department for the purpose of getting to know the people in his department. With an office of 2,600 people, he felt he would not be able to get to know the people in his department through the regular company softball league, because the company teams would include only a few people from his department. The three teams in his department league played each other and he would rotate among the teams. The result was a very strong relationship between himself and the hourly employees. He felt that when he had to reprimand his employees for some work-related issue they took it better, because they considered him a friend. He may have talked to them about softball just an hour before he had reprimanded them.

Among the benefits of playing with subordinates, he included the fact that sports allow one to see a different side of others. He also added that employees appear more motivated on the job because of the strong relationships that develop. Similarly, the employees get to know people from other departments. The plant is so big, making it difficult to become acquainted with many employees during the regular workday. The employees are able to develop connections and build networks. As the interviewee said, "You remember people in other departments who can help you accomplish some work task."

The company seems to involve the family members of the employees. For example, the company holds "baseball night," to which the employees' families are invited and the interviewee invites his teammates over to his house. The company does seem to be very family oriented. In fact, second and third generations of families are currently employed with the company and multiple members of families are working there. In addition, retirees from the company are invited to baseball night.

The company policy that requires each team to have at least one woman seems to help integrate women into the workplace. The job requires close working relationships among co-workers and the sports seem to engender a mode of cooperation between men and women. For example, the interviewee mentioned that he noticed than when a female employee needs help with a machine her male co-worker tends to run to help. Sports provides a more enjoyable atmosphere within which to learn how to cooperate. I asked how the company assimilates people who do not play. He said that the company has other activities for them to develop the teamwork concept, for example, quality productivity improvement teams. These teams travel together out of town to visit customers. In other words, although all employees may not participate in the company sports program, this does not have to pose a problem. The sports activities may be a very effective way of assimilating employees into the workplace and building teamwork, but it does not have to be the only means.

The interviewee mentioned only one disadvantage of having the sports activities: Some of the employees may vent ill feelings toward those players perceived as representing management (i.e., the salaried people from the main office).

The second interviewee from this company was a woman in the public relations department. She serves as coordinator of the sports program even though it is not officially part of her job description. Apparently, her duties related to the sports program evolved as the employees became more interested in the activities. Most of the activities are organized by volunteers, which reflects the employees' commitment to the program. Her main comment about her participation on the volleyball team was that it allows her to meet and become acquainted with employees from other parts of the plant whom she would not meet otherwise. According to her, the complex is so big that the relationships that have developed with the sports program probably would not have developed without it because the people probably would not have met. She said that the sports activities serve as a good assimilation device for employees. In her opinion, the development of a close relationship via volleyball is very obvious because the games include salaried and hourly employees.

This interviewee could not think of any disadvantages. She said that the sports activities are geared to the work schedule. Consequently, employees cannot use their participation in the sports activities as an excuse to get out of work.

A University

I chose to include a university in this research for two reasons: (a) to find out how athletic prowess may help college graduates locate and succeed in jobs and (b) to learn more about the foreign professional sports teams owned by companies. This section does not include any reference to the involvement in sports of the faculty or administrators of the university.

First, I talked with the assistant director in marketing and public relations. According to him, many businesses wish to hire college athletes for management trainee positions because they believe that athletes are well-rounded individuals. The assistant director agreed with this assumption. He remarked that athletes usually have characteristics that are helpful in business: motivation, aggressiveness, interpersonal skills necessary to work well with other people on a team, and ability to handle many different duties concurrently. Specifically, for the past 3 years a certain company has asked the interviewee for the names of one or two of the university's best athletes for the company's management trainee program. The interviewee also mentioned that some companies may seriously consider an applicant's sports prowess if the company has an intermural sports team (e.g., softball or basketball) in which they compete against other companies in the same business.

The assistant director also talked about the overseas professional sports teams owned by nonsports companies and the companies' hiring of American athletes. According to the interviewee, the companies use sports to enhance their image and to advertise their company. The overseas companies are benefiting from sports in a slightly different way than mentioned earlier. That is, the players on their teams are employed to play the sports and are not employed to work in a capacity related to the company's primary function. However, the sports programs may still engender a feeling of commonality and identity with the company among the regular employees of the company.

I also talked with a former college basketball player who had played for an overseas professional team. He said that he knows of companies that seek to hire athletes and coaches because they feel these two groups of people have certain personality characteristics important for success in business. They are attractive to companies for another reason: name recognition. Their names are so well known by the general public that they enhance the image of the company and enhance the value of the company's product. He told me of another situation in which an athlete was hired by a large company in a given city just so the person could play for the semiprofessional softball team in that city. According to my interviewee, there are numerous cases involving star athletes who retire from the sports industry and find it easy to secure jobs in business or politics.

Summary of Interviewees' Comments

Some common themes appear to run through the interviewees' comments and opinions. Except for the interviewee from the national transportation company, the interviewees seem to agree that sports in the workplace tended to produce many positive outcomes. I believe the primary positive outcomes that were repeatedly mentioned were the building of trust and improved communications among the employees. The other positive outcomes that they repeatedly mentioned, including enhanced cooperation among the employees, enhanced commitment to the job and the organization, increased self-respect and self-confidence, and the development of networks among the employees, probably sprang from the two primary outcomes. In addition, an organized sports program was seen as an opportunity for employees to meet co-workers and as a vehicle for assimilating and socializing new employees into the work force. More than one of the interviewees expressed the belief that the above benefits were achieved by sports activities because all the players were judged by the same standards. That is, all employees from various organizational units and at different occupational levels were judged according to their sports abilities. As a result, preconceived stereotypes (e.g., those based on race, gender, educational level, and occupational level) were weakened.

The interviewee from the national transportation company was the one interviewee who focused on the negative outcomes of having a sports program. However, other interviewees alluded to possible problems that could emerge. The negative outcomes mentioned include differential treatment by supervisors toward players versus nonplayers, offended supervisors who wanted to give all the orders on the playing field, and hostile behavior during the sports activities by employees who vented ill feelings about their employer or management.

THE RELEVANCE OF SPORTS TO INFORMAL GROUPS, SOCIALIZATION, AND CORPORATE CULTURE

The phenomena of informal groups, corporate culture, and socialization are intricately interrelated. For example, informal groups can serve as a valuable vehicle by which to socialize new employees and teach them the corporate culture. Although the term "corporate culture" has caught on, there are few prescriptions regarding how to socialize the employees into the culture (Brief, 1982; Pascale, 1984; Schein, 1984). This is where organized corporate sports programs can play a role. Sports programs offer one way that the socialization process can be accomplished. I believe they can contribute tremendously, albeit subtly, to the socialization process (see Pierce, Stillner, & Popkin, 1982). For example, including new employees in the sports activities may lead to the development of informal groups. In turn, within these informal groups, information concerning the corporate culture may be effectively disseminated. Moreover, participation in sports activities may also benefit current employees. Their participation in sports activities may lead to the development and maintenance of informal groups among them. Their observations during sports activities may improve or reinforce their understanding of the corporate culture. As mentioned by the federal government agent, playing together allows the employees the opportunity to witness how their co-workers and supervisors react to events and to each other.

The benefits to the organization of having informal groups can be great. Compared with members of formal groups, members of the informal groups tend to work harder to assist each other in the accomplishment of the work goals, resulting in increased productivity. The reader must note, however, that informal groups can work to the disadvantage of the organization, if the informal groups do not accept the philosophy, values, and/or rules of the organization. The peer pressure to conform to the group's values and attitudes is very powerful and difficult for the individual members to resist (Davis & Newstrom, 1985), and the group members may conform to the group's rules instead of the organization's when there is a conflict between the two (Roethlisberger, 1980). In fact, many of the benefits of the informal groups could turn into problems for the organization. For example, the network that developed among the golfers at the police department excluded the interviewee. He could eventually become unbearably frustrated and leave the department.

Also, the sports activities that may have facilitated the development of the informal groups may create some problems. Important information is often exchanged on the playing court or field, and work-related contacts are made. The employees not included in the sports activities may not be privy to this information, leading to suspicion among co-workers and/or confusion about the information. There are other possible disadvantages to having corporate sports programs. Some people may feel left out or inferior in athletic ability, thus defeating the purpose of the program. This may happen if the company's work force includes a mixture of men and women, age groups, and/or racial groups. The company should include something for everyone, either different sports and/or different levels of participation in the different sports. For example, all employees could be invited to attend as spectators, as is done by the industrial manufacturer. The purpose of the program will also be defeated if, as the interviewee from the utility company mentioned, the players maintain the company hierarchy on the playing field or court, with the supervisors continuing to call the shots.

Within any organization there will be differences of opinions regarding the desirability of having an organized sports program. This point is not evident from the accounts of the interviewees, because only one perspective is offered. If more persons within each organization had been interviewed, it is very likely that conflicting opinions would have surfaced. These differences of opinions may derive from differences in levels of participation and/or differences in occupational levels. For example, the reader probably noticed the dramatic difference of opinions between the interviewee from the transportation company and the interviewee from the federal government agency. The different perceptions of these two could reflect the different perceptions of a nonparticipant versus a participant and/or a subordinate versus a supervisor.

The organization should, of course, use a sports program to its advantage, not to its detriment. Certain safeguards for the success of the program may be implemented, although there will never be a guarantee of a problem-free program. To begin with, the attitudes and values of the company (i.e., the corporate culture) should be understood by management before the implementation of a sports program. In addition, the treatment of the players and nonplayers as well as all other behaviors emanating from the sports program should reflect those values and attitudes. The sports activities should serve as a vehicle by which the values are communicated. Finally, the organization should develop and promulgate guidelines for the implementation of the sports program. In the next section I list some guidelines that organizations may find helpful.

SUGGESTED GUIDELINES FOR EFFECTIVE CORPORATE SPORTS PROGRAMS

The goals of any corporate sports program will have a low probability of being realized if the program is left to materialize haphazardly. Below is a list of suggested guidelines that may be helpful in the development and implementation of a program. I formed this list on the basis of the comments of the interviewees.

1. The sports program should be voluntary. If employees are pressured to play, the purpose of the program will be defeated. The sports activities will become another work task that they must complete. However, all who wish to join should be included. Those who do not wish to actively play should be invited and/or encouraged to attend as a spectator. Make it a family affair in which spouses and children are invited.
2. There should be guidelines regarding the composition of the teams, ensuring that persons of all races, ages, and occupational levels and both genders are included. This may facilitate the deterioration of stereotypes and barriers.
3. It should be made explicit to all employees that work roles (e.g., supervisor and subordinate) are left at the office and do not count on the playing court or field.
4. Team sports (e.g., volleyball) are better than individual sports or sports

which involve few players (e.g., tennis). Select sports that require much social discourse, interaction, and cooperation.

5. Hold games regularly, perhaps once a week, and throughout the year.
6. Neither star athletes nor any players (versus nonplayers) should be given preferential treatment in the workplace. Such differential treatment could cause group cohesion to crumble and lead to a decrease in productivity, as happened with the transportation company.

HOW SPORTS IN THE WORKPLACE MAY BENEFIT THE INDIVIDUAL EMPLOYEE

The present research was started with the intent of addressing two issues: how sports in the workplace may benefit the organization and how sports in the workplace may benefit the individual employee. The majority of the chapter has been devoted to the first issue because most of the collected information addressed it. However, the interviews revealed two specific situations in which the individual benefited because of his or her athletic prowess: (a) when companies wanted to hire people with certain characteristics and (b) when the company supervisor gave preferential treatment to the star players.

The first situation was mentioned by the university interviewees. Both stated that they knew of some companies that have specifically sought athletes and/or coaches because of the personality characteristics that they were assumed to have. The second situation was discussed earlier as a negative outcome for the organization in which the performance levels declined. The star players in the transportation company gained certain privileges in the workplace because of the sports abilities, but the company as a whole suffered in the long term. One should also notice that other benefits that were mentioned as positive outcomes for the organization could be construed as benefits for individual employees. For example, the network of golfers in the police department benefited individuals because they were able to accomplish some tasks much quicker than individuals not in their network. The important point to be grasped is that what is good for the individual is not necessarily good for the organization.

REFERENCES

Brief, A. P. (1982). Undoing the educational process of the newly-hired professional. *Personnel Administrator, 27,* 55–58.

Cummings, T. G., & Huse, E. F. (1989). *Organizational development and change* (4th ed.). New York: West.

Davis, K., & Newstrom, J. W. (1985). *Human behavior at work: Organizational behavior* (7th ed.). New York: McGraw-Hill.

Falkenberg, L. E. (1987). Employee fitness programs: Their impact on the employee and the organization. *Academy of Management Review, 12,* 511–522.

Feldman, D. C. (1980). A socialization process that helps new recruits succeed. *Personnel, 57,* 11–23.

Ouchi, W. (1979). *Theory Z: How American business can meet the Japanese challenge.* Reading, MA: Addison-Wesley.

Pascale, R. (1984, May). Fitting new employees into the company culture. *Fortune,* pp. 28ff.

Pascale, R., & Athos, A. (1981). *The art of Japanese management.* New York: Simon and Schuster.

Peters, T., & Austin, N. (1985). *A passion for excellence.* New York: Random House.

Peters, T. J., & Waterman, R. H., Jr. (1982). *In search of excellence.* New York: Harper & Row.

Pierce, C. M., Stillner, V., & Popkin, M. (1982). On the meaning of sports: Cross cultural observations of super stress. *Culture, Medicine, and Psychiatry, 6,* 11–28.

Roethlisberger, F. J. (1980). The Hawthorne experiments. In D. Mankin, R. E. Ames, Jr., & M. A. Grodsky (Eds.), *Classics of industrial and organizational psychology* (pp. 29–39). Oak Park, IL: Moore.

Shein, E. H. (1984). Organizational socialization and the profession of management. In D. A. Kolb, I. M. Rubin, & J. M. McIntyre (Eds.), *Organizational psychology: Readings on human behavior in organizations* (pp. 7–21). Englewood Cliffs, NJ: Prentice-Hall.

Trist, E. L., & Bamforth, K. W. (1980). Some social and psychological consequences of the longwall method of coal-getting. In D. Mankin, R. E. Ames, Jr., & M. A. Grodsky (Eds.), *Classics of industrial and organizational psychology* (pp. 316–344). Oak Park, IL: Moore.

10

GENDER EXPECTATIONS AND SPORTS PARTICIPATION

Arnie Cann

University of North Carolina at Charlotte

Few people would challenge the claim that athletics have been a traditionally male domain. Only recently have females entered this domain in sufficient numbers to attract the attention of social scientists. As women and girls have crossed the barriers to their participation in athletics, the role of gender in sports has become an active research focus. Many fine summaries of the broad issues related to gender already exist (e.g., Boutilier & SanGiovanni, 1983; Mangan & Park, 1987). The purpose of this chapter is to draw on this literature in order to examine how expectations based on gender affect the access of females to sports, the reception of females as athletes, and the personal adjustment of females to the role of athlete. A model based on recent developments in social cognition (see Fiske & Taylor, 1984, for a detailed review) is developed that relates gender stereotypes to the social interactions that encourage or discourage females' participation in athletics.

WOMEN, SPORTS, AND THE SOCIAL CONTEXT

A Brief History

The evolution of sports and physical fitness activities in American society involves two quite separate histories, divided according to the gender of the participants. No consideration of the current status of women in sports and fitness activities or of the importance of gender in sports can be undertaken without an appreciation for the differences in these histories.

The controlling social systems and changing attitudes toward women have dramatically influenced the acceptance and involvement of women in sports. Although the social forces that influenced women's participation in sports activities are the same ones that affected women's lives in general over the past 150 years, the impact of these forces on participation in athletics was probably more extreme. Certainly in this instance, as in many others, sports represents an intriguing microcosm of the larger social system. A comprehensive history of gender and athletics is not attempted here; many excellent reviews exist (e.g., Gerber, 1974; Park, 1987; Struna, 1987). However, a brief overview is provided to establish a context within which the importance of gender can be understood.

In the 19th century sports and other physical fitness activities were of little concern when life-styles required regular strenuous physical activity to ensure survival. Although some athletic competitions were staged, these usually amounted to comparisons of physical skills developed in the pursuit of other, nonrecreational activities. It was only when leisure time became available, and life-styles were not so physically demanding, that sports, and the relation of gender to sports, became an issue requiring "social" guidelines. An inexact but reasonable date for beginning the examination of sports participation and fitness activities as events separable from daily requirements is the mid-1800s. During this Victorian era, the upper class, a segment of the population with ample leisure time to fill, developed recreational activities and established the salience of gender in decisions about participation in sports.

The Victorian concept of the ideal woman was a concept appropriate only for the upper class, and it was established as much to justify excluding women from many endeavors as it was to honor them (O'Neill, 1971). Women were granted protected status within society and were expected to insulate themselves from the supposed dangers of the world outside the home. The qualities that were advanced as desirable for the ideal woman were in direct contradiction to those suited to athletic participation. An ideal woman was delicate, soft, and gentle. A pale appearance and a lack of muscular development were features of attractiveness. Strenuous activities would alter this appearance and were considered possible hazards that might endanger the woman's valued ability to have children. Furthermore, athletic involvement would most likely draw the woman from the safety of the home.

The sports and recreational activities that were acceptable for women encouraged relatively passive participation and were designed to facilitate social interactions, not fitness. Upper class women engaged in sports like tennis and golf in the safe environment of private clubs. Some exceptions to this rule gradually began to appear in the special environments created by the women's colleges that were becoming more common. Although athletic activities at women's colleges were often carried out away from the public view, the women were being encouraged to participate in team sports and to use sports as a means to achieve physical fitness. Eventually, departments of physical education were established at these colleges, and as a result of these changes women gained minimal acceptance for participation in a variety of true sports activities.

By the beginning of the 1900s, social forces were creating additional important changes that broadened opportunities for women. At the international level, sports were becoming more visible. The establishment of the Olympic Games made athletic success a goal tied to national prestige. In America, the women's movement, with its push for voting rights, changed the image of women. World War I, and the pressures it placed on the social system, brought women out of the home and into the workplace. All of these factors conspired to remove constraints that had limited the choices of women. As a result, the years between 1920 and 1936 represent a period of rapid growth for women's athletics. Many new events were added to the Olympics for women, and women began participating openly in most of the popular team and individual sports. The changes, dramatic as they appeared to be, in no way meant that women and men were accepted as equals on the athletic fields. In subsequent years, there was a certain amount of backlash, with occasional attempts to limit the involvement of women in the Olympics and other organized sports activities.

Sports Participation by Girls and Women: The Current Situation

Today, traditional barriers to females' participation in most sports have been removed or seriously weakened (Acosta & Carpenter, 1985). Title IX of the Higher Education Act of 1972 has forced many educational institutions to reassess their procedures and work more seriously toward achieving a degree of equity between men's and women's opportunities. However, equality clearly has not been achieved. Only quite recently has it become possible for women to seriously consider careers in athletics (Brodie, 1989). What has been achieved is that women can participate in athletics and fitness activities if they choose. The social implications of their choices to take advantage of these opportunities remain to be investigated.

With formal barriers to participation in athletic activities reduced, has there been a move toward more active involvement by girls and women? According to the results of a recent national survey, changes are evident. The Wilson

Report (1988) described a survey of parents and daughters concerning reported encouragement of and actual participation in sports or fitness activities. The survey, conducted in cooperation with the Women's Sports Foundation, assessed the involvement of girls ages 7–18 years in sports. Although the data are all self-reports, and therefore subject to many sources of bias, they should reflect the current relevance of sports as perceived by girls and their families.

The results indicated that almost 90% of parents believed sports to be just as important for girls as for boys, and 97% of the parents felt fitness activities were important and beneficial for girls. There was little evidence of a rigid dual system in which sports were perceived as a male-only domain. Of the girls surveyed, most (82%) were currently involved in some form of sports or related fitness activity. An even larger proportion (89%) expected to be active in such activities as adults. A trend that cannot be clearly interpreted because longitudinal data were not collected indicated that the rate of participation was highest for the youngest girls and lowest for the oldest. This might mean that older girls tend to drop out of activities or that younger girls are now receiving even more encouragement to participate. In choosing between these two possibilities, it must be noted that there are, without question, fewer opportunities for girls to participate in organized sports activities after they leave the school system, so a stronger personal commitment may be required for girls to continue their participation. Older girls also reported that competing interests drew them away from sports. A large proportion of those quitting indicated that they were now "more interested in boys" (47%), suggesting that boys were perceived as a "competing" interest.

The factor that most influenced girls' interest in sports was parental participation in athletic activities. If their parents were engaged in sports, girls were much more likely to be involved as well. Evidently, as both parents become more active in athletics they send a clear message of acceptance and encouragement to their daughters.

Although acceptance and encouragement of women and girls in sports may be growing to the point that gender differences in involvement are minimal, the social implications of participation are not the same for both genders. Some questions remain to be answers. Are girls and boys encouraged equally to participate in athletics without restrictions, or do different rules and opportunities for participation apply? When girls or boys decide to discontinue sports, are equivalent attempts made to persuade them otherwise? Will girls' participation, compared with boys' participation, be met with the same reactions by others, or is the girl's decision to discontinue one that results from actual or perceived social pressures? The remainder of this chapter examines the role of gender stereotypes in influencing the acceptance and evaluations of women in sports and fitness activities.

GENDER STEREOTYPES

Overview of Function and Content

Gender stereotypes are cognitive structures that contain the organized set of beliefs an individual holds concerning the supposedly reliable differences between males and females. Stereotyped beliefs often play a crucial role in directing interpersonal interactions. Like other stereotypes, one obvious benefit of the gender stereotype is that it can minimize the cognitive effort required to form impressions or make predictions about others. A richness of information can quickly be assumed about individuals because they belong to a stereotyped group (female or male). Expectations can be formed to facilitate initial interactions with group members. Because much of the information contained in the stereotype is based on observed behavioral differences, correct decisions may sometimes result. If expectations are adjusted following contradictions, the stereotype remains potentially useful.

The content of the gender stereotype can be traced back to Victorian views of the ideal woman. Research has consistently identified clusters of qualities perceived by the majority of individuals, both male and female, to represent typical masculine and feminine styles and preferences. The clusters have been described using a variety of terms designed to capture the stylistic differences represented, but the essence of the distinction has remained relatively constant. Broverman, Vogel, Broverman, Clarkson, and Rosenkrantz (1972) found clusters associated with masculinity and femininity that they labeled "competency" and "warmth/expressiveness." Spence and Helmreich (1978) described the clusters that emerged in their research as "instrumental" (masculine) and "expressive" (feminine). Others have resorted to the obvious descriptors of "masculine" and "feminine" (Bem, 1974; Williams & Best, 1982). The prevailing preference is to avoid the sexual associations inherent in the terms masculine and feminine by employing terms originally proposed by Bakan (1966). Masculine qualities, those reflecting assertion and a desire to master, are characterized as "agentic," whereas the feminine qualities, which reflect a concern for others and a desire to avoid conflict, are termed "communal."

The descriptive terms that usually are associated with the agentic category are "aggressiveness," "independence," "dominance," "activity," "adventurousness," and "competitiveness." The communal category includes the descriptive terms "gentle," "emotional," "understanding," "tactful," "quiet," and "dependent." These descriptions have been shown to be relatively consistent in a cross-cultural examination of 30 nations (Williams & Best, 1982), indicating a very general acceptance of the major differences between the two categories. Similarly, the stability of gender stereotypes across time also has been assessed, and the results indicate little change in perceptions, at least within the United States, from 1957 through 1978 (Werner & LaRussa, 1985).

Despite the consistency and the stability of the perceptions of gender-based differences, the actual behavioral differences as a function of gender appear to be minimal. Maccoby and Jacklin (1974) reviewed more than 1,000 research reports in which gender differences were assessed. They found clear support for only four areas of gender difference in behaviors or abilities. Males did score higher on mathematics and visual–spatial abilities and were typically more aggressive in their behaviors. Females were superior in verbal skills. For the other potential areas of difference, no consistent pattern of differences was apparent. Recent reviews of the literature employing meta-analyses have confirmed there are few reliable differences between the genders, and the differences that are reliable are often quite small (Hyde & Linn, 1986).

Comparisons of observed behaviors provide further confirmation of the very limited utility of gender stereotypes for predicting a specific individual's behaviors. In an examination of children's play behavior, Lott (1978) found little evidence of actual behavioral differences consistent with the gender stereotype. Similarly, Brown (1979), in a review of leadership studies, reported that in leadership situations there were few differences between males and females in the styles of influence used. Thus, it is obvious that even though gender stereotypes are quite firmly entrenched, they are likely to be a source of considerable error when used to predict an individual's behaviors.

Recent research has provided a mechanism for understanding the stability of gender stereotypes despite their lack of validity. Eagly and Steffen (1984) proposed that the continued categorization of males and females as communal or agentic is primarily the result of the apparently stable distribution of the sexes into identifiable social roles. According to Eagly and Steffen, "If perceivers often observe a particular group of people engaging in a particular activity, they are likely to believe that the abilities and personality attributes required to carry out that activity are typical of that group of people" (p. 735). Apparently, observers give little attention to the reasons for sexual segregation of roles or to the possibilities that individuals within roles have abilities that extend beyond the limits of the role.

In our society and in most others, women are more often seen in caregiver roles: mothers, nurses, and child-care workers. Because these roles would seem to require behaviors that are communal in order to be successful, the occupants are assumed to be high in communal qualities. The fact that men are most often seen in roles perceived as achievement oriented or requiring strength or activity leads observers to conclude that men must be higher on these dimensions. Thus, observations made on a daily basis could serve to support highly stereotyped assumptions when they indicate a high degree of role segregation by gender.

Data are available to support such conclusions. For example, one recent survey of more than 400 organizations found that 59% of the companies had work forces that were completely segregated by gender; women exclusively filled certain jobs, and men exclusively filled others (Bielby & Baron, 1984). Moreover, despite the increase in two-income families, child-care responsibilities and housekeeping tasks are still carried out primarily by women (Gilbert, 1985). As long as there is this significant separation of the typical roles filled by men and women, it is unlikely the general assumptions made about gender-differentiated traits and abilities will change.

What would be the effect of disrupting the current patterns and redistributing individuals into varying roles? Apparently, if the information that roles are no longer segregated by gender was made salient enough, indicating no necessary connection between gender and social roles, significant changes in our assumptions about gender stereotypes could result. To test this proposal, Eagly and Steffen (1984) presented instances of specific men or women performing in communal or agentic roles (homemakers vs. employees). They found that the traits assigned to the individuals varied more as a function of the role than the sex of the person. Those portrayed in communal roles were judged as communal, and those in agentic roles were imagined to be highly agentic. In fact, they found that women in agentic roles were actually perceived to be more agentic than men in the same role. Eagly and Steffen suggested that participants assumed women in these roles were in them by choice, and therefore these women must be especially high in agentic qualities. Perhaps some recognition is given because these women are assumed to be functioning counter to the expected role. It follows that as more examples of individuals in nontraditional roles appear, the usual assumptions about gender-based differences may gradually diminish. Of course, there may be costs to bear if possessing agentic qualities also implies a deficit in communal qualities. The implications of assumptions that the categories (agentic and communal) may be mutually exclusive deserves further examination before Eagly and Steffen's results can be considered a basis for optimism.

The Gender Stereotype as Schema:
A Process Approach

Recent research on stereotypes has shifted from an emphasis on identifying content to a consideration of the processes by which stereotypes impact on social decision making (Hamilton, 1981; McCauley, Stitt, & Segal, 1980). Stereotypes are now proposed to be one of the types of cognitive schemata (Fiske & Taylor, 1984) that influence social perception processes. Cognitive schemata are organized systems of information concerning an object or concept. They include the individual's knowledge about specific qualities associated with the object and assumptions about relations among the qualities. The information is stored as abstractions, representing a generalized image of the target not tied to idiosyncratic characteristics. A schema would be "activated" when the object or concept is made salient to the person, most often because of an actual or anticipated interaction. The gender schema, containing the gender-stereotyped beliefs about males and females, would be activated in any interactions in which gender is a salient factor.

The presence of a schema implies a top-down cognitive processing model (Abelson, 1981). Reality construction is seen as an active process. The observer's assumptions play an active role in determining how data are interpreted during interactions. The top-down view is in contrast to a bottom-up, or passive process, in which any data presented during interactions are assumed to guide the observer's processing. The gender stereotype would be considered a *role* schema, because it contains information about characteristics and appropriate behaviors for a broad social category of individuals. Role schemata would exist for any common roles we encounter in social interactions.

The impact of a schema can be seen in three main areas of cognition: perception, memory, and inferences. An individual, guided by a schema, would be more likely to (a) attend to schema-appropriate rather than schema-inappropriate stimuli; (b) store schema-consistent information in memory more easily; and (c) draw inferences that were logically consistent with the relations specified in the schema. This strategy facilities processing when the specific situation matches the schema, but disrupts accurate processing when schema-inconsistent information is encountered. For example, a police officer would be seen as a safe individual to encounter on a dark street late at night because the police officer role includes protecting people from dangers. For this reason, a criminal dressed as a police officer would be able to take advantage of unsuspecting citizens. The citizens would not expect or be prepared for criminal behavior from the police officer.

The existence of a role schema based on the gender stereotype provides a mechanism for understanding the continuing difficulties faced by women and girls in gaining acceptance for their sports-related interests and activities. The gender schema establishes expectations about behavioral and interest characteristics of females that will guide the inferences and actions of those with whom the girl or woman interacts. These expectations are probably not consistent with athletics, so interactions will be directed into other areas. The gender schema may, in fact, influence many females as they make personal choices about their athletic involvement, leading them to see such interactions as inappropriate and therefore leading them to avoid participation. Just as others may judge females according to gender-schematic beliefs, females may judge themselves by reference to this commonly accepted standard.

One especially noteworthy outgrowth of research on schematic processing is the identification of an expectancy confirmation process (Darley & Fazio, 1980) whereby there is a tendency to confirm one's expectations by selective attention to certain stimuli or by unintentionally eliciting schema-consistent behaviors from others. This expectancy confirmation process reveals why significant changes in stereotyped assumptions are difficult to achieve. Darley and Fazio (1980) have described the sequence of actions and decisions that characterize the process and have demonstrated the almost inevitable confirmation of expectations. Initially, the perceiver approaches an interpersonal interaction with a set of schema-based expectancies about the person with whom they will interact (the schema might be a gender schema, for example). The perceiver's expectations determine whether an interaction may be avoided or limited in its scope. An interaction would be pursued only if the other party is expected to respond positively to the content of the desired interaction. In a discussion with another person, for example, a topic will be selected on the basis of assumed common interests. If an interaction does occur, either by choice or because it cannot be avoided, the perceiver selects an initial behavior based on the expectations derived from the schema. The behavior most likely constrains the options of the other person because it requires a response; it does not grant the other person complete freedom to choose a behavior.

The target, the person with whom the interaction is taking place, must then interpret the other's behavior and decide on an appropriate response. The target could interpret the perceiver's action as due to the qualities of the perceiver (a reflection of the perceiver's abilities or interests), due to some situational forces (a behavior forced by external pressures and not due to the perceiver's characteristics), or as due to the target's own qualities (a behavior somehow elicited from the perceiver by some quality of the target). The interpretation made by the target could affect the target's impression of the perceiver or the target's self-image. Regardless of the interpretation, the target must decide whether to respond with a behavior that will support or contradict the perceiver's apparent expectations. Behaviors that contradict the expectations may be avoided because they are likely to disrupt the interaction.

No matter what the target's interpretation, the perceiver still will have to make a separate interpretation once the target selects a response. The perceiver will tend to ignore or discount instances that contradict the expectancy and will readily accept those that confirm it. The top-down processing characteristic of the schema leads to highly selective processing. Seldom would an expectancy change simply because of an isolated disconfirmation. In the end, the perceiver and the target are likely to leave the interaction with the expectations contained in the schema even more rigidly held. Contradictory information has been avoided or ignored and many schema-consistent responses have resulted from external pressures caused by trying to avoid a disruption of the interaction. Little has been done to force a significant change in beliefs. Whenever strong expectations control interpersonal interactions, this expectancy confirmation process can suppress any possibilities for significant changes in beliefs.

GENDER AND ATHLETICS

The social research on gender and athletics has emphasized three general issues: the socialization of girls into athletics, the perceptions of girls and women as athletes, and the role conflicts experienced by girls and women involved in athletics. In the following sections, each issue is considered separately. Representative research is reviewed and followed by a final section describing the application of a gender schema model to these issues. By integrating recent insights from the social cognition literature with the descriptive results from sports psychology, a useful process model for understanding gender issues in sports should be evident.

Socialization of Girls into Athletics

The interest in sports socialization has focused on identifying the general factors that influence children's choices about involvement in sports or other athletic activities. Researchers recognized that athletic ability alone was not likely to predict participation. The social system must provide support and opportunity for participation before that talent can be translated into active sports involvement (McPherson, 1978). Using social learning theory (Bandura, 1977) as a theoretical foundation, researchers initially searched for the role models who might consistently guide children's sports decisions. However, when this notion was tested and evaluated, it was rejected as inadequate. A broader based social role–social system approach was proposed by Loy, McPherson, and Kenyon (1978) that assumed that the important influences on children's sports involvement encompassed multiple social systems (family, peers, and school) within which individual role models served special functions. The underlying processes and sources of influence were assumed to be common for boys and girls. Unfortunately, the evidence on which the model was based came almost exclusively from an examination of male athletes, so the generality of the model could not be proven.

Greendorfer and her colleagues (Greendorfer, 1977, 1979, 1987; Greendorfer & Ewing, 1981; Greendorfer & Lewko, 1978) subsequently provided extensive evidence indicating that there are important gender differences in decisions about sports participation. In fact, Greendorfer (1987) found that the general social role–social system model actually predicts sports participation for female nonathletes more effectively than it predicts participation for female athletes. One consistent finding is that for boys and for girls the family plays a crucial role in determining sports participation (Greendorfer, 1979; Snyder & Spreitzer, 1973, 1976, 1978). In families in which parents are actively involved in athletics, girls and boys are likely to develop sports interests that will continue even into adulthood.

Greendorfer (1979, 1983; Greendorfer & Lewko, 1978) suggested that major difference affecting the socialization of girls and boys into sports is the consistency of the process. Boys' interests in sports are likely to be supported in any family situation, regardless of parental involvement in sports. The influence would be stronger if parents were serving as role models, but even without these models the encouragement would probably occur. Beyond the family, boys will be quite naturally exposed to peer role models or alternative adult role models. At every age level, boys are more likely to be active in sports than are girls (Lewko & Ewing, 1980). The boys also will have many readily available opportunities to participate in sports through school or other organized sports institutions (e.g., Little League Baseball and Pee Wee Football).

Girls, however, will find little encouragement outside of the family. The family must provide the environment within which the encouragement and rewards for athletics can be obtained. When both parents model and encourage sports activities, the girls will likely interpret involvement as a normal and natural choice. Having established a positive view of sports activities in the family, a young girl may carry this interest beyond the confines of the home. If the family fails to set the tone for sports activities, the girl will find very few models, peer or adult, outside the family to emulate, and other institutions will do little to cultivate or support the female's interests. For example, whereas peers and the schools are influential in determining boys' choices about sports, neither is as strong a factor in influencing girls' decisions (Greendorfer, 1977; Greendorfer & Lewko, 1978). In fact, for girls, the number of role models appears to be decreasing, at least within the ranks of women coaches and athletic administrators (Acosta & Carpenter, 1985). Given the lack of traditional social systems to support an interest in sports, female socialization into sports must be seen as the exception, rather than the rule.

Perceptions of the Female Athlete

The girl or woman who emerges from this socialization experience having successfully established herself as a competent or active athlete may now have to endure social suspicion as the result of her accomplishment. The stereotypic successful athlete is believed to have the qualities of drive, aggressiveness, and self-confidence (Tutko, Ogilvie, & Lyon, 1969). These are characteristics that overlap dramatically with those of a "typical male." Thus, many observers may assume that the female athlete must possess qualities that contradict one of the relevant social categories she appears to occupy (female or athlete). She cannot be both masculine and feminine. The likely implications of this perceived contradiction are either a devaluing of the woman's accomplishments because she is believed to possess predominantly feminine qualities (i.e, she must not be a very good athlete), or a perception of the woman as masculine (or less feminine), to achieve consistency with the expected "masculine" qualities of the athlete. In either case, there would be a corresponding social rejection for failing to meet social expectations.

Both of these effects seem evident to social scientists examining the sports social system. Concerns have routinely been expressed about the general public's tendency to perceive successful female athletes as "masculine" and therefore failures in the female role (Eitzen & Sage, 1978; Felshin, 1974; Harris, 1980; Mrozek, 1987; Rohrbaugh, 1979). Similarly, the devaluing of the female athlete is apparent, with the prestige of being a female athlete often being challenged. Women have had to endure claims that their activities are less worthy of financial or public support. They also have suffered as a result of the lower prize monies available as rewards for success in women's professional events, and the incredibly limited media coverage of women's athletics (Boutilier & SanGiovanni, 1983).

Given the social realities of the difficulties faced by female athletes, research assessing perceptions of female athletes has provided little information to aid in understanding the reported problems. Early analyses portrayed the female athlete as an aggressive, frustrated, and unfeminine woman (Malumphy, 1971), suggesting for the female athlete both a break from the feminine role and a personal dissatisfaction. Unfortunately, subsequent research efforts have not assessed commonly held perceptions of woman athletes in a way that allows for a clear interpretation of the implications of occupying potentially contradictory roles. Many studies require respondents to simply rate the social category "woman athlete," with occasional comparisons of male and female reactions to the category. Interpreting any results obtained using these methods is difficult because it is unclear whether the respondents are truly considering the dual categories of woman and athlete when they respond. If respondents are reacting to only one or the other category, without confronting the integration of roles implied by the combination, they are not truly judging the female who is an athlete.

In research requiring separate identification of the qualities associated with various roles women might take, it is clear that there is little overlap between the qualities assigned to the traditional images of women and those assigned to the female athlete. For example, the "female athlete" is expected to be active, aggressive, confident, and adventurous; these qualities are more commonly attributed to males. The "housewife," however, is characterized as communal: faithful, gentle, sensitive, sympathetic, and kind (Clifton, McGrath, & Wick, 1976). Moreover, the "female athlete" is judged as quite distinct from images of the "ideal woman." "Girlfriend" and "mother" are the roles rated as similar to the "ideal woman" (Griffin, 1973). Despite this clear separation of roles, there is little evidence in this literature indicating negative assessments of or a rejection of the female athlete. She is simply seen as agentic, an expectation perfectly consistent with the athlete role. Although the athlete role also is recognized to be distinct from the traditional female roles, ratings reveal little about how respondents are resolving the obvious inconsistency they recognize.

Comparisons of males' and females' attitudes toward females' participation in sports reveal a tendency for males to be less accepting of the females (Nixon, Maresca, & Silverman, 1979). The gender differences are quite general, appearing in response to questions about likely talent, interests, and appropriateness of participation, but the males' attitudes are most often found to be less positive than the females' attitudes rather than truly negative. Males' biases also lead them to see individual sports, those typically judged as more feminine, rather than team sports, as most appropriate for women (DeBacy, Spaeth, & Busch, 1970), but the basis for this distinction is not clear. The gender bias is apparently one that develops early, because it is present even among young (Grades 3–6) children (Selby & Lewko, 1976). Especially discouraging was the finding that among the older boys surveyed, active participation in sports actually lowered their acceptance of girls in sports.

A difficulty in determining whether these results indicate a general, although somewhat gender-biased, acceptance of the female athlete is that almost all studies have requested responses to the nonspecific cases of a "female athlete" or women/girls in athletics. The respondents are judging a category, not a person. The difficulties reported by female athletes and noted by social scientists observing actual athletes were responses experienced by particular individuals. Obviously there are potentially important differences between these two situations. What would happen if respondents in these research situations were presented with a person who was a female athlete: Would the responses be the same or would the conflict between the two stereotypes now cause a serious dilemma? The probable differences in social perception processes when judging a category versus a person are considered later in this chapter as a way of understanding these contradictions. After all, if the impressions of female athletes are relatively positive, as the research suggests, why have women experienced such difficulty gaining acceptance for their sports activities?

Role Conflict

The female athlete combines two roles, that of female and that of athlete. She must establish a style that allows her to function comfortably in both roles. Because the female athlete is attempting to present two apparently opposing social images, the communal style of the typical female and the agentic qualities of the athlete, she may experience role conflict. The problems created are really twofold. First, the woman or girl must deal with her own learned expectations about appropriate behaviors for the two conflicting roles. If she holds traditional views about women and about athletes, she must sort out her image of self in reference to the contradictions. Second, she must deal with the external pressures created by others' reactions to her attempts to occupy two contradictory roles. According to Sage and Loudermilk (1979), "One of the oldest and most persistent folk myths, and one of the main deterrents to female sports participation, has been the notion that vigorous physical activity tends to masculinize girls and women. . . . Thus, consciously or unconsciously, athletic achievement has been equated with a loss of femininity" (p. 89).

Sage and Loudermilk (1979), in one of the first attempts to assess role conflict, examined both perceived and experienced role conflict. In a sample of female collegiate athletes they found nearly half (44%) perceived little or no role conflict, and more than half (56%) had experienced little or no role conflict. They did report, however, that women involved in sports judged to be the least feminine did experience a significantly greater amount of role conflict. A similar survey of female high school athletes provided comparable results. Many (37%) perceived role conflict to be little or no problem, and half had little or no problem with experienced role conflict (Anthrop & Allison, 1983). For the high school sample, the differences between those participating in traditionally feminine sports as opposed to traditionally masculine sports did not emerge.

Although both of these studies indicate that role conflict for female athletes is not a serious problem, a more likely possibility is that the data do not portray the true impact of role conflict. One weakness of these initial studies is their failure to provide any meaningful comparisons in order to determine the level of role conflict present in comparable groups. Recent studies have shed some light on this issue by comparing female athletes with female nonathletes. Results indicate that although there are differences between the female athletes and the female nonathletes, with athletes perceiving and experiencing more role conflict, the overall level of role conflict for athletes remains low (Desertrain & Weiss, 1988).

A potentially critical comparison of female athletes' experiences to those of male athletes and male nonathletes has not been made. Less conflict would be expected for these two groups of males, because the roles are not clearly contradictory, but little is known about existing levels of conflict among males. It has been suggested that such role conflicts do exist for male athletes (Stein & Hoffman, 1978), but no studies have directly compared either male athletes with nonathletes or female athletes with their male counterparts. Without that information, it is difficult to truly assess whether role conflict experienced by female athletes is high or low, relative to males' experiences.

The existing research also fails to assess the impact role conflict may have in determining persistence in athletics. The low levels of role conflict in high school and college athletes may reflect the outcome of a selection process. Only those females who avoided or survived serious role conflict may be represented in these groups. Many females who might otherwise have pursued an interest in athletics may have dropped their interest in athletics because of the role conflict they experienced. An assessment of role conflict at the time a decision is made to discontinue participation in athletics might be the most useful way to measure the impact role conflict has on females engaged in athletic pursuits.

Although existing results suggest fairly low levels of role conflict, Butt (1987) has identified a variety of strategies or presentation styles she believes female athletes have adopted to deal with the conflict inherent in their multiple roles. The strategies include (a) adopting clearly separate roles; (b) becoming "the athlete" while performing but presenting a "feminine self" when not (see also Harris, 1975); (c) presenting superficial femininity by providing instances of feminine behavior just for public appearances, while being guided by the athlete role in establishing a self-identity; (d) adopting a consistently agentic role by forsaking the female role; (e) becoming the chameleon (image maker type) who adopts whatever appearance is needed to please the currently salient powers; or (f) adopting a stereotype-free approach by behaving and feeling unconstrained by any role expectations. Only in the last case has role conflict truly been avoided, and Butt offers no basis for estimating how many female athletes have been able to adopt this, or any, of the proposed strategies.

Many women apparently survive whatever amount of role conflict is created without significant psychological damage. For these female athletes, there may be a support system that helps to prevent them from major conflict and allows them to pursue athletic interests. Snyder and Spreitzer (1983) suggested that the family often serves to shelter the female athlete from role conflict by supporting variations from traditional roles. If the young girl does not rigidly accept the traditional definitions of gender roles, the identification with the athlete role should cause less conflict. Because the family plays a major part in transmitting gender roles, it also could encourage more flexible views.

Summary

Overall, the research indicates that the social climate for females in athletics is not supportive. Girls receive much less encouragement to enter into sports activities, and the social system is poorly designed to facilitate their possible interests in sports. Females who do manage to establish an identity as athletes must then deal with the gender-biased perceptions of others who may question their competence or their femininity. Each female athlete must confront her own beliefs, and decide how she will handle the implied conflicts between the two roles she has adopted. At the core of these problems lie the stereotypic beliefs about the typical qualities of males and females and the processes through which the stereotyped beliefs affect social decision making.

A GENDER SCHEMA APPROACH
TO GENDER AND ATHLETICS

The top-down information-processing strategy characteristic of a gender schema means that reality construction will be guided, for most individuals, by the traditional beliefs of the gender stereotype. The gender schema has the potential to influence the expectations that set the stage for many interactions, the information that is processed during the interactions, and the conclusions that are drawn following these interactions. In addition, because schematic processing applies to judgments about the self as well as assessments of others, the implications extend to self-examinations relevant to gender identity. A gender schema model helps to explain why females encounter difficulties establishing themselves in sports activities. The implications of a gender schema model for each of the issues reviewed are considered below.

Impact on Socialization Processes

What prevents girls from being socialized into sports? Obviously, one major factor concerns the contrasting beliefs about females and athletes. Stereotypic beliefs about females are in direct contrast to those associated with successful athletic performance. More important, however, is the process through which these beliefs, in the form of the gender schema, influence the interactions that take place with girls. The beliefs determine the expectations people bring with them to interactions with girls. The expectations play a major role in determining their choice of behaviors in social situations. Stereotyped expectations have often been found to influence even initial perceptions of an individual (Brigham, 1971; Klatzky, Martin, & Kane, 1982; Taylor, Fiske, Etcoff, & Ruderman, 1978). Thus most people, guided by the traditional expectations of the gender schema, would not assume athletics are relevant in interactions with girls. Interactions involving athletic activities or discussions about sports would be very unlikely to occur. The effect is that the gender expectations terminate interactions even before they can begin. The woman or girl will have few opportunities to develop or to provide evidence of her athletic interests or abilities. At the same time, those who hold stereotyped views will effectively avoid exposing themselves to contradictory information. The expectations will be safely preserved.

When sports do enter into interactions with girls, the gender schema will filter the information and create a reality consistent with the expectations. The top-down processing will ensure that schema-consistent information has a priority in determining the outcome of the interaction. For example, gender expectations of parents begin to influence the perception of a child almost from the moment of birth. Children less than a day old have been described by parents in gender-typed terms (Rubin, Provenzano, & Luria, 1974). Girls were described as softer, smaller, and cuter than were boys. This occurred despite a lack of real differences in physical size or responsiveness as recorded by the attending physicians. Lott (1978) also reported that parents and teachers claimed to have observed gender-typed behaviors in a group of kindergarten children even though the actual observed behaviors were far less gender-typed than claimed. Despite a lack of real behavioral or physical differences, a lack of differences that was noted earlier in reference to the content of the gender stereotype, the expectations resulting from the gender stereotype lead the perceiver to find much evidence consistent with gender-biased beliefs.

One might ask whether the children are actually attending to the suggestions that gender stereotypes define the acceptable social roles. Are the children adopting self-defining schemata based on gender stereotypes? The evidence indicating that children are well informed about gender expectations is compelling and abundant. Just as parents see behavioral differences in infants, other children will report seeing clear instances of gender-appropriate behavior in other children. Three- and 5-year-old children who watched a videotape of two infants who had been randomly labeled as a boy or a girl, reported that the "girl" was smaller, weaker, quieter, and softer than the "boy." At 18 months of age, children already have developed gender-typed preferences for toys used during free play (Fagot, 1974). As they get older, children's requests for new toys are clearly gender stereotyped. By the time the child is 3 years old, most expressed preferences are gender consistent, with boys requests being especially gender stereotyped. Although toys selected by parents were more likely to be gender-neutral educational toys, very few cross-gendered toys were ever requested or given (Robinson & Morris, 1986). The child is being submerged in a gender-typed social world.

Children also seem to recognize the gender-segregated characteristics of the adult world. Children show extensive knowledge of adult occupational roles (Gettys & Cann, 1981) and expected behavioral styles (Connor, Serbin, & Ender, 1978; Goldman & Goldman, 1983; Leahy & Shirk, 1984). They know which gender fills the various roles in society, and they recognize the distinction between agentic and communal styles. Their evaluations and expectations also are gender biased. They expect gender-stereotype-consistent performers to be more competent and desirable in their careers or related activities (Cann & Garnett, 1984; Cann & Haight, 1983), and they judge behaviors that are inconsistent with expectations as inappropriate (Sandidge & Friedland, 1975).

The gender schema clearly represents an important force in socialization of girls and boys into sports. The gender schema would usually guide interactions with girls away from sports or athletics and, by implication, probably convince girls that these activities must be inappropriate. Because most adults and children share the views represented in the gender schema, the cumulative effect across a variety of interactions would be to discourage any attempts by a girl to become involved in sports. It would take salient role models and a supportive environment to motivate an individual female to persist in seeking involvement in sports. The claims by Greendorfer (1977, 1979) and Snyder and Spreitzer (1978) that parental involvement in sports is one of the best predictors of sports participation by girls is consistent with a gender schema view. Parents who participate in athletics are less likely to see athletics as a gender-specific activity, so their female children are not going to experience constant subtle discouragement. Such girls are also less likely to develop a self-image that precludes sports.

Impact on Perceptions of the Female Athlete

Once a girl or woman has established herself in the athlete role, despite the social pressures opposing her, she faces a new dilemma. The top-down processing caused by the gender schema should lead most people to expect her to possess qualities inconsistent with the athlete's role, creating a potentially biased view of the female athlete. Although research using nonspecific instances of female athletes, requiring respondents to judge social categories, not individuals, has found no significant bias against the female athlete, self-reports by women athletes and observations of the social climate suggest a less optimistic conclusion. The issue to be considered is, What happens when respondents encounter a specific woman athlete, rather than the nonspecific social label "female athlete"?

In the case of an actual female athlete, the perceiver most likely sees and begins reacting to a female, not an athlete. Regardless of the context, the information immediately available to the perceiver is more likely to activate the gender schema than the schema associated with the role of athlete. Thus, it is the content of the gender stereotype that initially affects the perceptions of the female athlete, determines storage and retrieval of specific information about her, and influences the inferences drawn about her. With judgments made about a nonspecific social category (female athlete) presented without a particular referent, it is less likely that the schema activated would be the schema for a female. There may even be a tendency to focus on the more specific descriptor "athlete," because it more narrowly defines the task for the perceiver. The category "female athlete" is noteworthy not because it requests a judgment about a woman, but because one must evaluate an athlete. Thus, the respondent might be able to focus on the athlete role without truly attending to the additional information that the athlete is a female. On the other hand, when judging an identifiable woman who also is an athlete, the contrasts between the two roles are probably much more salient and troublesome to the respondent.

The process predicted using a gender schema model would be as follows. When the gender schema is activated by the presence of a female, the expectations about communal or "feminine" qualities are salient to the perceiver. The introduction of the athlete role now forces a consideration of highly contrasting qualities. The conflict for the perceiver becomes real. The simple solution is to deny one of the woman's roles. This could result in a perception of either an unqualified athlete or an unfeminine woman. Even if the perceiver does admit the specific woman is an exception to the general case, cognitive effort expended in thinking about exceptions to schema expectations often strengthens the original stereotyped beliefs (O'Sullivan & Durso, 1984). The perceiver retrieves readily available information, the schema-consistent information, while considering the exception. This effort makes the consistent information more salient and provides an opportunity for its rehearsal.

Information about the female athlete presented after the initial perceptions also will be affected by the gender schema. Observers will likely remember those elements that are consistent with the activated schema and, unless forced to consider them, will forget or distort those inconsistent with it (Cohen, 1981; Rothbart, Evans, & Fulero, 1979; Snyder & Uranowitz, 1978). When information about the woman is recalled, it will be interpreted to deny stable influences, attributing the deviation from expectations to some transient, unstable cause (McHugh, Duquin, & Frieze, 1978). Similarly, when inferences must be drawn about future behaviors, another's success at a counterstereotypic activity is less likely to be used to predict success at related activities (Cann & Palmer, 1986). This strategy allows the observer to dismiss the event as irrelevant to expected future behaviors, further protecting existing beliefs and expectations. An impressive athletic performance by a female need not imply a stable underlying ability, so biases about female athletes can endure.

The extent of the difficulties people encounter when dealing with counterstereotypic information, information that challenges expectations, can be seen even on simple picture memory tasks, when the social implications of the information are less obvious. Children presented with pictures depicting males and females performing either traditional or counterstereotypic events have much more difficulty remembering the counterstereotypic images (Cann & Newbern, 1984; Liben & Signorella, 1980; Martin & Halverson, 1983). The memory deficit occurs despite the usually impressive performance of children on picture memory tasks. Other recent evidence suggests that an evaluative bias based on gender expectations exists even in these simple memory tasks. Adult participants asked to memorize phrases of the form "Jane is a good doctor" were influenced by the evaluative information as well as by the stereotype consistency of the person–job pairings. Recall was greater for the stereotype-inconsistent information when the evaluative information was negative (Jane was a bad doctor) rather than positive, with the reverse pattern evident for stereotype-consistent pairings (Cann, 1986). Obviously, the information that is available about proper role behaviors is not merely descriptive. Variations are coded in evaluative terms.

The female athlete faces an imposing challenge in establishing a social identity. She will likely be judged by the expectations most salient to those with whom she interacts. She is a female attempting to present agentic, or masculine, qualities along with communal qualities. The gender schema that guides social information processing draws attention away from her athletic talents; they may not even be noticed. Her athletic accomplishments that are evident will be devalued, attributed to transient causes, whereas her failures will be more easily remembered by observers. The expectancy confirmation process that characterizes our dealings with exceptions to social expectations interferes with the interpretation and retention of any evidence that might reduce our biased views. The notion of a female athlete is "wrong" within the context of the gender schema, so there must be something wrong with the information suggesting she exists or with her.

Impact on Role Conflict

The gender schema and the athlete schema contain expectations that are a potential conflict for the female in developing her self-image. These two roles, when defined in traditional terms, require qualities often perceived as stylistic opposites. To understand the personal conflict a female athlete would experience, however, a third schema must be introduced. Each individual has a self schema (Markus, 1977), that is, "general information about one's own psychology [that] makes up a complex, easily accessible verbal self-concept that guides information processing about the self" (Fiske & Taylor, 1984, p. 149). The self schema contains those self-conceptions and personality dimensions that are most important to individuals and those in which they see themselves as extreme or distinct. These dimensions become especially salient for the individual and will attract the individual's attention in decisions about the self and in evaluations of others (Cacioppo, Petty, & Sidera, 1982). The self schema operates as do other schemata to guide perceptions, memory processes, and inferences. When thinking about the self, the self schema is more likely than general role schemata (e.g., gender or athlete schema) to be salient to an individual and to guide his or her information processing (Kuiper & Rogers, 1979; Rogers, 1981).

When a woman's self schema mimics the communal qualities from the traditional gender schema, indicating a self-definition in traditional gender-typed terms, she will face a clear conflict when adopting the athlete role. Her self-analyses and self-evaluations well reflect the same difficulties described earlier in the discussion of perceptions of the female athlete. She must confront the implied challenges to her "femininity" or to her competence as an "agentic" athlete as she judges herself relative to each role. Her attempts to integrate the two roles will likely be a persistent source of frustration that may force a choice between the competing self-images.

Women who recognize the assumptions of the traditional gender schema, but do not adopt those qualities in defining themselves, may avoid much of the expected role conflict as they engage in sports activities. Development of a self schema that does not contradict involvement in sports or success as a female would eliminate the comparisons that fuel role conflict. One alternative to traditional gender-typed views that has been suggested as a positive self-definition for female athletes is characterized as psychological androgyny (Bem, 1974; Duquin, 1978). An androgynous self schema incorporates both agentic and communal qualities, with choices among behavioral styles dictated more by situational demands than by gender role definitions. The person who is androgynous is not constrained by the limits implied by gender stereotypes. Female athletes who have a more androgynous self-conception should experience less role conflict when their self schema is integrated with either the gender schema or the athlete schema.

If role conflict discourages many females from continuing in athletics, then females who have a more androgynous self schema, and thus less conflict, should be more likely to survive as athletes. Evidence supporting this proposal can be found in a number of recent investigations. Salisbury and Passer (1982) found that women who participated in sports considered less "feminine" (e.g., soccer, basketball, and long-distance running) were much more likely to have liberal gender stereotypes. These women saw fewer restrictions as applicable to women's behavioral options. Having broadly defined the acceptable behaviors for women, these athletes were able to pursue less traditional activities without role conflict. More directly relevant are the results reported by Butt and Schroeder (1980) and Myers and Lipps (1978). They found that successful athletes from a variety of sports not judged as "feminine" were more likely to score high on agentic qualities, but that they did not reject communal qualities. They simply accepted agentic qualities without a perceived contradiction; they were androgynous. These women do not survive role conflict; they simply avoid its impact.

An androgynous self schema affects more than just self-assessments. Because the qualities in the self schema are considered especially important, they will often be used in judging others. Thus, those individuals with androgynous self schemata are less likely to be concerned about the gender appropriateness of their decisions concerning athletics and are less inclined to use gender consistency as a criterion in judging others' choices (Matteo, 1988). Perhaps a requirement for clarifying the findings on role conflict among athletes will be a careful assessment of gender-stereotyped beliefs *and* beliefs about the self. An awareness of the self schema's importance provides a possible mediating factor in determining when role conflict should exist for the individual.

CONCLUSIONS

Gender stereotypes have often been implicated in the failure of girls and women to gain reasonable access to athletics. Without question, the presence of stereotyped beliefs that validate male participation in athletics as consistent with the male role, while challenging female involvement as inconsistent, and therefore inappropriate, make females' attempts to participate more difficult. Unfortunately, the processes by which gender stereotypes produce social barriers to females have never been clearly specified. As an initial step in this direction, a gender schema model has been proposed. Operating as a schema, the gender stereotype will influence interactions with females at multiple levels. Expectations derived from the gender schema will lead most people to avoid athletics or sports as a focus of interactions with females. In addition, the gender schema will distort information about female athletes or females' athletic accomplishments, justifying a conclusion that their efforts reveal failure, either as an athlete or as a female.

Participation in athletics by females will be generally accepted only by changing the traditional notions about gender differences or by protecting girls from these beliefs so that their self-images will not reflect the implied restrictions on behavioral styles. The family environment must play a dominant role in creating the needed changes. Girls who receive encouragement from their families, and who see appropriate role models in the family, will be less inclined to classify themselves using traditional gender stereotypes. As a result, these girls will avoid judging either themselves or others according to gender-typed standards. A second important factor in breaking the cycle of gender expectations may be the media. Through the media, we might see both the communal side of the successful male athlete, and the agentic potential of females. A broader definition of the successful athlete could emerge that is less gender biased. As a starting point, if more females are presented in the media successfully engaging in athletic activities, the perceived contradiction between being female and being athletic will be weakened. It is the limited availability of role models for girls and women that allows the traditional views to be sustained. As Eagly and Steffen (1984) demonstrated, the segregation of roles by gender supports the continuation of stereotyped beliefs. Recent trends in physical fitness participation by girls suggests a movement in the right direction. More girls and women are actively involved, but if gender-biased expectations are not seriously challenged, this trend may not continue.

REFERENCES

Abelson, R. P. (1981). The psychological status of the script concept. *American Psychologist, 36,* 715–729.

Acosta, R. V., & Carpenter, L. J. (1985, August). Women in athletics: A status report. *Journal of Physical Education, Recreation, and Dance, 56,* pp. 30–34.

Anthrop, J., & Allison, M. T. (1983). Role conflict and the high school female athlete. *Research Quarterly for Exercise and Sport, 54,* 104–111.

Bakan, D. (1966). *The duality of human existence: An essay on psychology and religion.* Chicago: Rand McNally.

Bandura, A. (1977). *Social learning theory.* Englewood Cliffs, NJ: Prentice-Hall.

Bem, S. L. (1974). The measurement of psychological androgyny. *Journal of Consulting and Clinical Psychology, 42,* 155–162.

Bielby, W. T., & Baron, J. N. (1984). A woman's place is with other women: Sex segregation in organizations. In B. Reskin (Ed.), *Sex segregation in the workplace: Trends, explanations, remedies* (pp. 27–55). Washington, DC: National Academic Press.

Boutilier, M. A., & SanGiovanni, L. (1983). *The sporting woman.* Champaign, IL: Human Kinetics.

Brigham, J. C. (1971). Ethnic stereotypes. *Psychological Bulletin, 76,* 15–38.

Brodie, H. K. H. (1989, March 14). Society fails to support sports-related careers for women. *Charlotte Observer,* p. 21A.

Broverman, I. K., Vogel, S. R., Broverman, D. M., Clarkson, F. E., & Rosenkrantz, P. S. (1972). Sex-role stereotypes: A current appraisal. *Journal of Social Issues, 28,* 59–78.

Brown, S. M. (1979). Male versus female leaders: A comparison of empirical studies. *Sex Roles, 5,* 595–611.

Butt, D. S. (1987). *The psychology of sport: The behavior, motivation, personality, and performance of athletes.* New York: Van Nostrand Reinhold.

Butt, D. S., & Schroeder, M. C. (1980). Sex role adaptation, socialization, and sport participation in women. *International Journal of Sport Psychology, 11,* 91–99.

Cacioppo, J. T., Petty, R. E., & Sidera, J. A. (1982). The effects of a salient self-schema on the evaluation of proattitudinal editorials: Top-down versus bottom-up message processing. *Journal of Experimental Social Psychology, 18,* 324–338.

Cann, A. (1986, April). *Evaluative biases in sex stereotypes.* Paper presented at the meeting of the Southeastern Psychological Association, Orlando, FL.

Cann, A., & Garnett, A. K. (1984). Sex stereotype impacts on competence ratings by children. *Sex Roles, 11,* 333–343.

Cann, A., & Haight, J. M. (1983). Children's perceptions of relative competence in sex-typed occupations. *Sex Roles, 9,* 767–773.

Cann, A., & Newbern, S. R. (1984). Sex stereotype effects in children's picture recognition. *Child Development, 55,* 1085–1090.

Cann, A., & Palmer, S. (1986). Children's assumptions about the generalizability of sex-typed abilities. *Sex Roles, 15,* 551–558.

Clifton, A. K., McGrath, D., & Wick, B. (1976). Stereotypes of woman: A single category? *Sex Roles, 2,* 135–148.

Cohen, C. E. (1981). Person categories and social perception: Testing some boundaries of the processing effects of prior knowledge. *Journal of Personality and Social Psychology, 40,* 441–452.

Connor, J. M., Serbin, L. A., & Ender, R. A. (1978). Responses of boys and girls to aggressive, assertive, and passive behaviors of male and female characters. *Journal of Genetic Psychology, 133,* 59–69.

Darley, J. M., & Fazio, R. H. (1980). Expectancy confirmation processes arising in the social interaction sequence. *American Psychologist, 35,* 867–881.

DeBacy, D. L., Spaeth, R., & Busch, R. (1970). What do men really think about athletic competition for women? *Journal of Health, Physical Education, and Recreation, 41,* 28–29.

Desertrain, G. S., & Weiss, M. R. (1988). Being female and athletic: A cause for conflict? *Sex Roles, 18,* 567–582.

Duquin, M. E. (1978). The androgynous advantage. In C. A. Oglesby, (Ed.), *Women and sport: From myth to reality* (pp. 89–106). Philadelphia: Lea & Febiger.

Eagly, A. H., & Steffen, V. J. (1984). Gender stereotypes stem from the distribution of women and men into social roles. *Journal of Personality and Social Psychology, 46,* 735–754.

Eitzen, D. S., & Sage, G. H. (1978). *Sociology of American sport.* Dubuque, IA: W. C. Brown.

Fagot, B. I. (1974). Sex differences in toddlers' behavior and parental reaction. *Developmental Psychology, 10,* 554–558.

Felshin, J. (1974). The social view. In E. W. Gerber, J. Felshin, P. Berlin, & W. Wyrick (Eds.), *The American woman in sport* (pp. 179–279). Reading, MA: Addison-Wesley.

Fiske, S. T., & Taylor, S. H. (1984). *Social cognition.* Reading, MA: Addison-Wesley.

Gerber, E. W. (1974). Chronicle of participation. In E. W. Gerber, J. Felshin, P. Berlin, & W. Wyrick (Eds.), *The American woman in sport* (pp. 3–176). Reading, MA: Addison-Wesley.

Gettys, L. D., & Cann, A. (1981). Children's perceptions of occupational sex stereotypes. *Sex Roles, 7,* 301–308.

Gilbert, L. A. (1985). *Men in dual-career families: Current realities and future prospects.* Hillsdale, NJ: Erlbaum.

Goldman, J. D. G., & Goldman, R. J. (1983). Children's perceptions of parents and their roles: A cross-national study in Australia, England, North America, and Sweden. *Sex Roles, 9,* 791–812.

Greendorfer, S. L. (1977). Role of socializing agents in female sports involvement. *Research Quarterly, 48,* 304–310.

Greendorfer, S. L. (1979). Childhood sport socialization influences of male and female track athletes. *Arena Review, 3,* 39–53.

Greendorfer, S. L. (1983). Shaping the female athlete: The impact of the family. In M. A Boutilier & L. SanGiovanni (Eds.), *The sporting woman* (pp. 135–149). Champaign, IL: Human Kinetics.

Greendorfer, S. L. (1987). Gender bias in theoretical perspectives: The case of female socialization into sport. *Psychology of Women Quarterly, 11,* 327–340.

Greendorfer, S. L., & Ewing, M. E. (1981). Race and gender differences in children's socialization into sport. *Research Quarterly for Exercise and Sport, 52,* 301–310.

Greendorfer, S. L., & Lewko, J. H. (1978). Role of family members in sport socialization of children. *Research Quarterly, 49,* 146–152.

Griffin, P. S. (1973). What's a nice girl like you doing in a profession like this? *Quest, 19,* 96–101.

Hamilton, D. L. (Ed.). (1981). *Cognitive processes in stereotyping and intergroup behavior.* Hillsdale, NJ: Erlbaum.

Harris, D. V. (1975). Research studies on the female athlete: Psychosocial considerations. *Journal of Physical Education and Recreation, 46,* 32–36.

Harris, D. V. (1980). Femininity and athleticism: Conflict or consonance? In D. F. Sabo & R. Runfola (Eds.), *Jock: Sports and male identity* (pp. 222–239). Englewood Cliffs, NJ: Prentice-Hall.

Hyde, J. S., & Linn, M. C. (Eds.). (1986). *The psychology of gender: Advances through meta-analysis.* Baltimore: Johns Hopkins University Press.

Klatzky, R. L., Martin, G. L., & Kane, R. A. (1982). Influence of social-category activation on processing of visual information. *Social Cognition, 1,* 95–109.

Kuiper, N. A., & Rogers, T. B. (1979). Encoding of personal information: Self-other differences. *Journal of Personality and Social Psychology, 37,* 499–514.

Leahy, R. L., & Shirk, S. R. (1984). The development of classificatory skills and sex-trait stereotypes in children. *Sex Roles, 10,* 281–292.

Lewko, J. H., & Ewing, M. E. (1980). Sex differences and parental influences in sport involvement of children. *Journal of Sport Psychology, 2,* 62–68.

Liben, L. S., & Signorella, M. L. (1980). Gender-related schemata and constructive memory in children. *Child Development, 51,* 11–18.

Lott, B. (1978). Behavioral concordance with sex role ideology related to play areas, creativity, and parental sex-typing of children. *Journal of Personality and Social Psychology, 36,* 1087–1100.

Loy, J. W., McPherson, B. D., & Kenyon, G. (1978). *Sport and social systems.* Reading, MA: Addison-Wesley.

Maccoby, E. E., & Jacklin, C. N. (1974). *The psychology of sex differences.* Stanford, CA: Stanford University Press.

Malumphy, T. M. (1971). Athletics and competition for girls and women. In D. V. Harris (Ed.), *DGWS research reports: Women in sports* (pp. 15–20). Washington, DC: American Association for Health, Physical Education, and Recreation.

Mangan, J. A., & Park, R. J. (Eds.). (1987). *From "fair sex" to feminism: Sport and the socialization of women in the industrial and post-industrial eras.* London: Frank Case.

Markus, H. (1977). Self-schemata and processing of information about the self. *Journal of Personality and Social Psychology, 35,* 63–78.

Martin, C. L., & Halverson, C. F., Jr. (1983). The effects of sex-typing schemas on young children's memory. *Child Development, 54,* 563–574.

Matteo, S. (1988). The effect of gender-schematic processing on decisions about sex-inappropriate sport behavior. *Sex Roles, 18,* 41–58.

McCauley, C., Stitt, C. L., & Segal, M. (1980). Stereotyping: From prejudice to prediction. *Psychological Bulletin, 87,* 195–208.

McHugh, H. C., Duquin, M. E., & Frieze, I. H. (1978). Beliefs about success and failure: Attribution and the female athlete. In C. A. Oglesby (Ed.), *Women and sport: From myth to reality* (pp. 173–191). Philadelphia: Lea & Febiger.

McPherson, B. D. (1978). The child in competitive sport: Influence of the social milieu. In R. A. Magill, M. J. Ash, & F. L. Smoll (Eds.), *Children in sport: A contemporary anthology* (pp. 219–249). Champaign, IL: Human Kinetics.

Mrozek, D. J. (1987). The "Amazon" and the American "Lady": Sexual fears of women as athletes. In J. A. Mangan & R. J. Park (Eds.), *From "fair sex" to feminism: Sport and the socialization of women in the industrial and post-industrial eras* (pp. 282–298). London: Frank Cass.

Myers, A. M., & Lipps, H. M. (1978). Participation in competitive amateur sports as a function of psychological androgyny. *Sex Roles, 4,* 571–588.

Nixon, H. L., Maresca, P. J., & Silverman, M. A. (1979). Sex differences in college students' acceptance of females in sport. *Adolescence, 56,* 755–764.

O'Neill, W. (1971). *The woman movement.* Chicago: Quadrangle.

O'Sullivan, C. S., & Durso, F. T. (1984). Effects of schema-incongruent information on memory for stereotypical attributes. *Journal of Personality and Social Psychology, 47,* 55–70.

Park, R. J. (1987). Sport, gender and society in a transatlantic Victorian perspective. In J. A. Mangan & R. J. Park (Eds.), *From "fair sex" to feminism: Sport and the socialization of women in the industrial and post-industrial eras* (pp. 58–93). London: Frank Cass.

Robinson, C. C., & Morris, J. T. (1986). The gender-stereotyped nature of Christmas toys received by 36-, 48-, and 60-month old children: A comparison between nonrequested vs. requested toys. *Sex Roles, 15,* 21–32.

Rogers, T. B. (1981). A model of the self as an aspect of human information processing. In N. Cantor & J. Kihlstrom (Eds.), *Personality, cognition, and social interaction* (pp. 193–214). Hillsdale, NJ: Erlbaum.

Rohrbaugh, J. B. (1979, August). Femininity on the line. *Psychology Today,* pp. 30–42.

Rothbart, M., Evans, M., & Fulero, S. (1979). Recall for confirming events: Memory processes and the maintenance of social stereotyping. *Journal of Experimental Social Psychology, 15,* 343–355.

Rubin, J. Z., Provenzano, F. J., & Luria, Z. (1974). The eye of the beholder: Parents' views on sex of newborns. *American Journal of Orthopsychiatry, 44,* 512–519.

Sage, G. H., & Loudermilk, S. (1979). The female athlete and role conflict. *Research Quarterly, 50,* 88–96.

Salisbury, J., & Passer, M. W. (1982). Gender-role attitudes and participation in competitive activities varying stereotypic femininity. *Personality and Social Psychology Bulletin, 8,* 486–493.

Sandidge, S., & Friedland, S. J. (1975). Sex-role-taking and aggressive behavior in children. *Journal of Genetic Psychology, 126,* 227–231.

Selby, R., & Lewko, J. H. (1976). Children's attitudes toward females in sports: Their relationship with sex, grade, and sports participation. *Research Quarterly, 47,* 453–463.

Snyder, E. E., & Spreitzer, E. (1973). Family influence and involvement in sports. *Research Quarterly, 44,* 249–255.

Snyder, E. E., & Spreitzer, E. (1976). Correlates of sports participation among adolescent girls. *Research Quarterly, 47,* 804–809.

Snyder, E. E., & Spreitzer, E. (1978). Socialization comparisons of adolescent female athletes and musicians. *Research Quarterly, 49,* 342–350.

Snyder, E. E., & Spreitzer, E. (1983). *Social aspects of sports* (2nd ed.). Englewood Cliffs, NJ: Prentice-Hall.

Snyder, M., & Uranowitz, S. W. (1978). Some cognitive consequences of person perception. *Journal of Personality and Social Psychology, 36,* 941–950.

Spence, J. T., & Helmreich, R. L. (1978). *Masculinity and femininity: Their psychological dimensions, correlates, and antecedents.* Austin: University of Texas Press.

Stein, P. J., & Hoffman, S. (1978). Sports and male role strain. *Journal of Social Issues, 34,* 136–150.

Struna, N. L. (1987). "Good wives" and "gardeners," "spinners" and "fearless riders": Middle- and upper-rank women in the early American sporting culture. In J. A. Mangan & R. J. Park (Eds.), *From "fair sex" to feminism: Sport and the socialization of women in the industrial and postindustrial eras* (pp. 235–255). London: Frank Cass.

Taylor, S. E., Fiske, S. T., Etcoff, N. L., & Ruderman, A. J. (1978). Categorical bases of person memory and stereotyping. *Journal of Personality and Social Psychology, 36,* 778–793.

Tutko, T., Ogilvie, B., & Lyon, L. (1969). *The Athletic Motivational Inventory.* San Jose, CA: Institute for the Study of Athletic Motivation.

Werner, P. D., & LaRussa, G. W. (1985). Persistence and change in sex-role stereotypes. *Sex Roles, 12,* 1089–1100.

Williams, J. E., & Best, D. L. (1982). *Measuring sex stereotypes: A thirty nation study.* Beverly Hills, CA: Sage.

Wilson Report. (1988). *Moms, dads, daughters, and sports.* River Grove, IL: Wilson Sporting Goods.

11

ATTRACTION AND PHYSIQUE: GOING FOR THE RIGHT BODY

Louis Diamant and Gary Thomas Long

University of North Carolina at Charlotte

Michael L. Masterson

Charlotte, North Carolina

A few semesters ago my young workout partner and I were leaving the university weight room. He turned one way and I the other. Some junior high school girls who were attending summer cheerleading camp looked at him as he walked away. "A ten," said one. "Uh-uh," said another, "the butt is a seven." Should I say that their sophistication about such matters was surprising? They had so finely drawn their criteria of muscle and definition that I found it incredible. A few exercise narcissists (positive narcissists, of course) might be into that sort of discrimination—but these children? Who could have predicted it?

Although some studies of physique and attraction exist in the psychology literature, nothing in it could have prepared us to postulate the responses that I observed. A new day is dawning and an attempt to rise to it was made in the investigation described in this chapter. It is our opportunity, within the framework of the hard-body sell, to see how much and how hard people perceive as good.

THE RIGHT BODY

It is hardly news when one reports that the muscled, athletic physique is in vogue; at least media advertising would so assert. Rippled bodies sell us exercise. At this writing, *Sports Illustrated,* hyping a set of bodybuilding videotapes complete with a pair of dumbbells, also announces that you now can "choose

your own body." Workout machines, health club memberships, workout cloth-
ing, diet food, food supplements, and even soft drinks offer the same. A two-
page advertising spread in the *New York Times Magazine* displays photographs
of nine men and women with a variety of muscular developments to tempt the
reader's choice. The text begins, "The fact is you can choose your own body.
The proper diet, the right amount of exercise and you can pretty much have any
body you desire." The advertisement is for a brand of mineral water. But denial
is virtually impossible; there is a thrust to physical and muscular development
that has come so far from the Charles Atlas bodybuilding ads in pulp magazines
that it is in another dimension and the target group is no longer the reader of
comic books and ten-cent pulp magazines. An assumption is made and documented that attractiveness comes from tough exercise and the right products and
that even the beer gut is "ripped" (muscularly defined). The exercise equipment, diet supplement, and bodybuilding gymnasiums are a billion-dollar industry. Health and strength were reasons given by all the male bodybuilders we
recently surveyed for a future project, but most also said they worked out to be
attractive to members of the opposite sex. Of course the purveyors of workout
products are aware of the attractiveness factor, and that mesopmorphy, the most
muscular of Sheldon's (1942) body designates, was preferred by college students (Robbins, 1983). So it may well be the masculinity and femininity factors, and not the struggle for muscular definition, that are the focus of much of
today's workout mentality.

A literature search did not help in our dilemma. What is really the right
body—not in terms of ectomorphy, endormorphy, or mesomorphy (in our quest
for determination we are indebted to Michael Robbins [1983] for offering us his
extensive review of the literature on body build and behavior)—but in the currently popularized approach to visible muscular definition? Although there are a
few research studies on bodybuilders and their personalities, there are, we
think, no scientifically acquired data on why they do it (our future project) and
no quantified studies, despite the exercisers' desire to be attractive, on how
much muscle is thought to be attractive (liked best and thought best) by same-
sex and opposite-sex choosers.

For the present investigation we pulled from the file drawer a collection of
data from the spring semester of 1988 that we hadn't thought to use for this
book because the topic was mistakenly thought to be covered by a social psychologist who had compiled an enviable record in researching attraction and
attractiveness. The goal of the present study was to quantify observations (or
hunches) concerned with the "true" preferences of men and women in terms of
body build. What is truly thought to be the body beautiful at a time when we are
huckstered daily to trim down and muscle up and when at the pressure of a
finger on the remote control a dozen men or women appear on cable television
posturing, posing, and modeling with the hope of becoming Mr. or Ms. Olympia.

METHOD

Subjects

The participants in this study were students in two upper-level courses in psychology. The designation "upper-level" refers to the year in school of the students and does not indicate that they are psychology majors or advanced students in psychology. There were 50 male and 39 female subjects. The mean age was 21.9 years, which in effect gave them young adult status.

Instruments and Procedure

In order to assess the "like most" and "best" body selections in terms of tone, cut, and muscular structure and to eliminate judgment on the basis of the skinny, fat, and medium spectrum, the bodies in a selection of photographs on which respondents were asked to express preference were without weight "problems," that is, were neither skinny nor obese. The essential difference between the models was to be their degree of muscular definition and development. Photographs were examined from several magazine sources including *Muscle and Fitness, Playboy, Play Girl,* and even some merchandising catalogs. A panel of six serious bodybuilders made unanimous choices of pictures classified in the following categories (for both men and women); (a) low-defined = swim suit and underwear models, (b) well-defined = athletic or regional body build contestants, and (c) super-defined = the Mr. or Ms. Olympia stratification.

The faces were cut from the photographs and then the photographs were xeroxed to equal darkness to avoid any racial inferences. Later three gymnasium managers agreed with the classifications. From this process one 8.5 × 11-inch sheet with three men's photographs—low-defined, well-defined, and super-defined—was produced and another sheet with three women's photographs with the same classifications was produced. The positions of the photographs on the sheet were varied to avoid an order effect. The two sheets were placed in a manila envelope along with seven copies of the Catell 16 Personality Factor (16PF) Test Profile sheets (Catell, 1962). Biographical information sheets requesting the subjects' age and sex were included along with several other measures not used for this study.

Each participant was instructed in writing to examine the photographs and for the same-sexed photographs to choose (a) "Which body is most like mine?"; (b) "Which is the best body?"; and (c) "Which body I like most?". The subjects answered questions b and c for the opposite-sex bodies as well.

Subjects were also instructed in writing to complete one of the 16PF profile sheets for each of the six photographs of models, indicating the degree to which they felt the model would have each of the 16 personality characteristics. Each subject also completed a 16PF profile sheet describing him- or herself. Instructions were as follows: "For example, if you think you are shy, you would mark 1, 2, 3, or 4. If you think you are about average you would score 5 or 6. If you think you are quite the opposite of shy, that is, more venturesome, you would score 8, 9, or 10. Please do all of them." The instructions for the photographs were very similar to this. All of the materials were group administered and completed in less than an hour by the subjects.

RESULTS AND DISCUSSION

Because of the multitude of measurements, and the many comparisons/contrasts that are made in the following analyses, certain specific terminology is used. The models in the photographs are referred to as men and women. The subjects are referred to as males and females. Also, the results are grouped so as to attend to the following questions.

1. What were the male's perceptions of and preferences for the three levels of muscular definition in the men and women in terms of . . .

   Body like own,
   Best body,
   Body liked most,
   Opposite-sex best body,
   Opposite-sex body liked most.

2. Likewise, what were the female's perceptions of and preferences for the men and women with the different levels of muscular development?
3. What level of intelligence did the males attribute to these men and women of different physiques?
4. When the females looked at the photographs, how did they perceive the level of intelligence in these men and women of different degrees of muscular definition?
5. What statistically significant differences in perceptions of intelligence attributed to the more or less muscularly defined men and women showed up between the male and the female subjects?
6. What were the statistical relations between a subject's perceptions and a subject's preferences? For example, when subjects chose the body most like their own, did their choice correlate with their choice of the best body or body liked most?

Questions 1 and 2

What were the male and female subjects' judgments of best body and body most like their own and preference for body most liked? Among the males, 84% judged the body with *low* muscular definition as most like theirs. Only 16% saw their bodies as most similar to the well-defined bodies. One male rated his body as superdefined. A similar distribution of judgments emerged from the females: 74% saw the low-defined body as most like their own, and 26% indicated that they had a well-defined level of muscular development.

When asked to rate what they considered the best body of the men, 46% of the males saw the low-defined body as best, 22% said the well-defined body, and 32% said that the superdefined level of muscular development was the best body. There was no meaningful difference between that which men thought best and liked most in male bodies with 50% liking low-defined, 26% liking well-defined, and 24% the superdefined. The females heavily favored the well-defined woman's body as best: 30 of 39 subjects chose this, whereas 20% judged the low-defined woman's body as best, and 1 female judged the superdefined woman as best. That 77% of the females selected the well-defined body as the best body of the three women fits with the current notion that the well-defined body represents health, fitness, and athleticism. Although the superdefined body may readily be seen as that of a fit and strong person, it probably strays too far from current notions of female body structure and feminine attractiveness.

Sixty-seven percent of the female subjects favored the well-defined woman, while the low level of muscular definition was preferred (liked) by 31% of females. Only one female subject preferred the superdefined woman. Twenty-four percent thought the superdefined man's body best, 50% thought the low-defined body best, and 26% judged the well-defined physique to be best.

A hypothesis might be formulated that females in this study could have been expressing dissatisfaction with their own muscular development, because they both judged the well-defined body as best and preferred the well-defined body most. There is an obvious divergence between what men and women think of the classic bathing beauty. The males' view of what a man's body ought to resemble (best body) was quite discrepant from our female participants' views of the same. Amazing, but perhaps not so, was the degree of difference between what was preferred by females and what body type they considered most like their own.

Males and females showed a pattern of agreement in judging the best body for a woman, but they disagreed on what is the best body for a man. Fifty-eight percent of the males selected the well-defined woman's body as best (77% of females judged the well-defined body as best for a woman), 12% of the males selected the superdefined body as best (2% of the females chose this body as best), and 30% of the males (20% of the females) judged the low-defined woman's body as best. As to the disagreement on what is the best body for a man, only 10% of the females selected the low-defined body as best for a man, and the other 90% of females said they thought either the well-defined body (54%) or the superdefined body (36%) was the best of the men's bodies. This finding is in contrast with the results obtained from males.

In addition to the females' judgments that the best body for men is well- or superdefined, 67% of the females preferred (opposite-sex body liked most) the superdefined body in men, 28% of the females liked most the well-developed body, and only 5% said they liked the low-defined man's body.

When males indicated the level of muscular definition in women that they preferred, 56% of them liked best the well-defined body, and 42% liked best the low-defined body. Only one male liked best the superdefined woman's body.

Question 3

What level of intelligence did males attribute to these men and women of different physiques? In judging the intelligence of the well-defined man on the 16PF, the male subjects gave it an average rating of 3.24, while they rated themselves 6.74 on average. The difference between the mean rating was 3.50, a significant difference, $t(49) = 3.33, p < .01$. The attribution of differences in intelligence between the ratings of the superdefined body and the well-defined body was not significant (mean difference $= 0.50$). The test of difference between the well-defined body and the low-defined (the body often selected as the body most like their own by the males) indicated that the male subjects thought the man with the low-defined body more intelligent than the well-defined man, $t(49) = 4.49, p < .001$. The ordinary man (low-defined) was rated as significantly more intelligent than the superdefined Mr. Olympia type, $t(49) = 2.77$, $p < .01$. The males in this study judged themselves to be significantly more intelligent than the Mr. Olympia contestant, $t(49) = 3.81, p < .001$. And they saw the underwear model (low-defined body) as somewhat less intelligent than themselves, $t(49) = 2.00, p < .05$.

Given the analysis above, we now have an idea of how the males saw themselves relative to the three men in the photographs with regard to judged intelligence. The rank order of intelligence attributed to the men and the women in the photographs along with the degree of intelligence that males attributed to themselves is shown in Table 1. Below is further commentary on the statistically significant contrasts that surfaced among the ratings of intelligence by males.

When the male participants made judgments as to who had higher intelligence, the well-defined man or the well-defined woman, they saw the well-

TABLE 1 Rank order of IQ ratings by subjects

Body rated	Mean IQ
Male subjects	
Self	6.74
Low-defined man	5.94
Low-defined woman	5.38
Well-defined woman	4.96
Superdefined man	3.74
Superdefined woman	3.58
Well-defined man	3.24
Female subjects	
Self	6.87
Low-defined man	5.97
Well-defined woman	5.03
Low-defined woman	4.64
Well-defined man	4.23
Superdefined woman	3.69
Superdefined man	3.33

defined woman as more intelligent, $t(49) = 2.33, p < .05$. The low-defined woman was rated as being significantly more intelligent than the well-defined male bodybuilder, $t(49) = 3.94, p < .001$. The males in this study saw the woman who was developed to Ms. Olympia condition (superdefined musculature) as no more or less intelligent than a man in that category; both, however, were thought to be less intelligent than the low-muscled man and low-muscled woman. The woman who was not muscularly defined (low defined) was thought to be significantly more intelligent than a man at the Mr. Olympia level, $t(49) = 2.64, p < .02$. The male subjects had a tendency to see a low-developed man as more intelligent than a muscularly well-defined woman, $t(49) = 1.98, p < .10$. They judged a low-defined man to be significantly more intelligent than a superdefined muscular woman, $t(49) = 4.43, p < .001$. They rated the low-defined man and the low-defined woman as having the highest intelligence of all the models, and saw no differences in their intelligence levels. When it came to judging the intelligence of the well-defined and the superdefined women, the male subjects appeared to think the superdefined woman was more intelligent than the well-defined athletic woman, $t(49) = 3.45, p < .01$. The males did not think the low-defined woman's body housed more intelligence than the well-defined athletic woman; that is, differences in judgments were not significant.

The males in this study were apparently of the opinion that they were more intelligent than the well-defined woman. The comparison between the well-defined woman and themselves gave this portrayal, $t(49) = 3.61, p < .001$.

Males indicated that they saw the low-defined woman model as more intelligent than the superdefined woman, $t(49) = 1.80, p < .02$. They rated the superdefined Ms. Olympia-level model as being significantly less intelligent than themselves, $t(49) = 3.88, p < .001$. And they saw themselves as somewhat more intelligent than the low-defined woman model; however, this was only a trend, $t(49) = 1.36, p < .10$.

Question 4

What level of intelligence did females attribute to these men and women of different physiques? The females judged themselves to be more intelligent than the low-defined woman (whose body they also judged to be most like their own), $t(38) = 2.32, p < .05$. When comparing themselves with the superdefined woman, the females rated themselves as very much higher (mean difference = 3.18 scale points) in intelligence, $t(38) = 4.12, p < .001$. The females, who it may be recalled largely perceived themselves as muscularly undefined, rated themselves as more intelligent than the well-defined woman, $t(38) = 3.63, p < .001$. The well-defined woman as judged by the females rated a higher intelligence level than a Ms. Olympia contestant, $t(38) = 3.34, p < .01$. As one might expect, from tradition, the females rated themselves to be more intelligent than the well-defined man, $t(38) = 4.54, p < .001$. Although females judged the superdefined man's body as the one they liked best, they judged that model to be much less intelligent than themselves (3.50 rating points on the 16PF profile sheet).

The rank order of intelligence attributed by the females to the men and the women in the photographs along with the degree of intelligence that females attributed to themselves are shown in Table 1. Below is further commentary on the statistically significant contrasts that surfaced among the ratings of intelligence by female subjects.

Females judged the man with the well-defined physique to be more intelligent than the superdefined man. Females, judging intelligence by physique, rated the low-defined man higher in intelligence than the well-defined man, $t(38) = 3.00, p < .01$. The male subjects made the comparison with similar results.

When comparing the photographs of the low-defined woman and the low-defined man, the females rated the man higher in intelligence, $t(38) = 3.69, p < .001$. The low-defined man was thought to be quite a bit higher in intelligence than the superdefined woman (mean difference = 2.28), $t(38) = 4.77, p < .001$. The females judged the low-defined woman's body (the one the females most often chose as most like their own) to be more intelligent than the man with the body that they most often liked (preferred), that is, the superdefined man, $t(38) = 2.79, p < .01$. Females rated the well-defined woman higher in intelligence than they rated the superdefined man, $t(38) = 2.10, p <$ .05. As did the males, the females thought that the low-defined man would be more intelligent than the superdefined man, $t(38) = 2.78, p < .01$.

Question 5

What were the differences in the way males and females rated intelligence of the six models? One difference that emerged between males and females as to their attribution of intelligence to the six models was in the case of the well-defined man's body. The mean rating by the females (4.23) of the well-defined man's body was significantly higher, $t(87) = 7.93, p < .001$, than the mean rating by the males (3.24).

Question 6

What relations were there between subjects' perceptions and their preferences? These associations were determined using the Chi-square statistic. Among the males, there was an association between which body was thought most like their own and which body was chosen as the best body; that is, the body chosen as best body by males correlated with the body type they specified as theirs, $\chi^2(2, N = 50) = 4.07, p < .05$. Half of the male subjects thought the body they liked and the body that they judged best was a developed body (well- or superdefined) indicating (a) a wish for change, possibly, or perhaps (b) a transition toward a preference for physical fitness and development, $\chi^2(4, N = 50) = 35.56, p < .001$. Males generally liked most the woman's body that they thought was the best, except for the superdefined body, which was thought best more often than was liked most, $\chi^2(4, N = 50) = 24.62, p < .001$.

In examining the relation between the body the males chose as most liked and the body they chose as most like their own, we observed a significant association, $\chi^2(4, N = 50) = 9.54, p < .05$. When the males judged the men's bodies they showed a preference for the normally (low) defined body type. They had a tendency to continue this preference with their judgment of women's bodies, preferring the low-defined woman over the well-defined and the superdefined women, $\chi^2(2, N = 50) = 4.58, p < .10$. Males thought that the best man's body was the low-defined body by 2 to 1 over either the well- or superdefined. When asked to judge the best of the women's bodies there was about a 2 to 1 ratio favoring the well-defined woman over the low-defined woman. Further, there was a 5 to 1 ratio favoring the well-defined woman over the superdefined woman, $\chi^2(4, N = 50), = 7.97, p < .10$.

A test of the strength of association between the males' judgment of which body was like their own and their judgment of the best opposite-sex body indicated that when males saw themselves as most like the low-defined man, they chose as best opposite-sex body the low- or well-defined woman, $\chi^2(4, N = 50) = 8.53, p < .10$. The males who chose the low-defined man's body as most like themselves also showed a preference for low-defined and moderately (well-) defined bodies in women. The inference to be drawn is that the judgment of low muscular development in themselves is extended to their body preference in women, $\chi^2(4, N = 50) = 50.70, p < .001$. Among the males their choice of best body for a man appears to have been associated with the body type they most liked in women, $\chi^2(2, N = 50) = 10.95, p < .02$.

Among the females, little discrepancy was observed between bodies thought to be best and those liked most. Females who preferred (liked most) the well-defined woman's body also thought it was the best body, $\chi^2(4, N = 39) = 22.78, p < .001$. In the female responses no positive association was found between the body they liked most and the body they owned (judged most like theirs), in contrast to the male group. In fact, an inverse relation was reflected in the results, $\chi^2(2, N = 39) = 3.28, p < .20$.

The females were somewhat consistent in what they liked in both sexes—they preferred well-defined and highly (super) defined muscular bodies in men, and well-defined bodies in women. The attraction to the superdefined body in men, however, did not extend to the preference for this level of definition in women.

The females' selection of best body for a woman was associated with their judgment of the best body for a man, $\chi^2(4, N = 39) = 9.70, p < .05$. The females' choice of the low-defined body as most like theirs appeared to have no association with their choice of best bodies in the opposite sex (again, in contrast to the association found among the males). The possibility of an association between what females saw as the best body for a man and the type of man's body they liked the most was examined. The result showed an association in the positive direction, $\chi^2(4, N = 39) = 14.04, p < .01$. There appeared to be an association between the females' self-appraisal and their choice of the most liked body of men. Specifically, females who saw themselves as having low muscle definition were those who most often selected the superdefined man as the one they most liked. Those who saw themselves as well-defined women liked equally the well- and superdefined man, $\chi^2(2, N = 39) = 7.90, p < .02$.

SUMMARY AND CONCLUSIONS

It behooves us to question whether Edgar Rice Burrough's hero and protagonist would have lasted his decades on the silver screen had he been fully clothed, intellectual, and not quite so sturdy. When one Hollywood Tarzan aged and became flabby, another appeared, sometimes more muscled than his predecessor. The first Tarzans preceded a procession of world-class bodybuilders as movie heroes, reflecting the change in time and notions of bodybuilding until a true star,

Arnold Schwarzenegger, was born. But Schwarzenegger was born in and of a different world than Elmo Lincoln (yes, there was one before Weismuller). He comes from a world that spawned the new Senator Strom Thurmond, who at age 87 announced his intention to seek reelection and accompanied the announcement with another that he lives the fit life, exercising and "lifting weights." Lifting weights—what would Albert Einstein have thought about such a senator? (Einstein is reported to have said that the immature exercised.) (We know what Robert Harlow [1951] thought as he confirmed more psychoanalytically attributed concepts that weight lifters and bodybuilders were struggling with a shaky masculine identity.) All of the authors of this chapter use Nautilus machines and free weights and even the psychoanalytic one of us thinks that the negative perception of bodybuilding and weight lifting has a strong conceptual flaw, unless of course you agree with Freud that all men and women have ongoing concerns with homosexuality. The research on bodybuilding and personality is quite a thin soup, but one morsel (Fuchs & Zaichowsky, 1983) plucked from it reports that weight lifters and bodybuilders are made of sterner (or at least cooler) stuff and present superior profiles on the Profiles of Mood Scales (McNair, Lorr, & Droppleman, 1971). This profile—"the iceberg profile"—was observed to be highly positive in winning athletes by Morgan (1980).

But having gotten that out of the way—the personalities of bodybuilders— we return to the functional dimensions of the present study: the attractiveness of men and women bodybuilders' physiques to the same- and opposite-sex observers and the way this related to the body subjects saw as most like their own. Further, the dimension of personality in the present study dealt with perceptions of intelligence that were attached to muscles and the way they related to the respondents' view of their own intelligence and body build. The results and analysis do not require much embellishment. Generally the females in this study found men who were the most muscular to be their premier choice for best and liked most. Our males, in turn, preferred the swimsuit model as their best and most liked woman's body. Males, to our surprise, chose the least defined man's body (underwear model) as the best, most liked, and most like themselves. Females thought themselves most like the swimsuit model, liked the athletic woman's body the most, and eschewed the Ms. Olympia competitor.

The trail we decided to examine for its perceived relation to muscles was intelligence (or lack of it), which of all the perceived traits seems attached to muscles, strength, and athletes. Long (Chapter 12) makes this connection with the "dumb jock" phenomenon. Ryckman, Robbins, Kaczor, and Gold (1989) have noted it too: "The dumb jock stereotype appears more applicable to male mesomorphs" (p. 250). Male mesomorphs were also seen by their undergraduate raters as more unintelligent than the endomorphs. None of the stimulus persons in our current study could be classified as ectomorphs or endomorphs— not fats, no thins, but rather increases in muscular definition. Muscles (strength) seem to carry the stereotype of lower intelligence. In the case of our male subjects, we could speculate a male envy of the magnificently muscled man, or employing the "just world" theory (Lerner, 1980), we might speculate a compensatory attitude; i.e., no man can have all that power—a superior mind and body. In a recent Schwarznegger film *Twins,* his superior intelligence comes from the bizarre pooling of genes from a collection of fathers who contributed both intellect and muscle; because the magnificent twin is the product of amazing scientific manipulation he is acceptable as fiction. Men simply do not think Mr. Olympia is admirable physically or intellectually. It is possible that our male subjects were not so venturesome or were somewhat more vulnerable, which made them see a lack of physical or intellectual desirability in muscled women, thus preserving a traditional view of the female physique. Women also saw muscled models as less intelligent than themselves and models who looked most like themselves, but this had no bearing on their positive view of the well-defined (but not superdefined) woman, or on their liking most and rating best the well-defined and superdefined male models. The females in this study showed a strong prefernce for supermuscled men and if they have themselves absorbed the "dumb jock" myth, it did not seem to have had a negative effect on attraction. Jane always seemed happy with Tarzan even before he broadened his vocabulary and displayed his true upper-class intellect.

REFERENCES

Catell, R. B., Eber, E. H., & Tatsuoka, M. M. (1970). *Handbook for the Sixteen Personality Factor Questionnaire (16PF).* Champaign, IL: Institute for Personality and Ability Testing.

Fuchs, C. Z., & Zaichowsky, L. D. (1983). Psychological characteristics of male and female body builders: The iceberg profile. *Journal of Sport Behavior, 6*(3), 136–145.

Harlow, R. G. (1951). Masculine inadequacy and compensatory development of physique. *Journal of Personality, 19,* 312–323.

Lerner, M. J. (1980. *The belief in a just world: A fundamental delusion.* New York: Plenum Books.

McNair, D. M., Lorr, M., & Droppleman, L. F. (1971). *Profile of Mood States Manual.* San Diego, CA: Educational and Industrial Testing Service.

Morgan, W. P. (1980, July). Test of champions: The iceberg profile. *Psychology Today,* pp. 92–99.

Robbins, M. A. (1983). *Body build and behavior: A review and critical evaluation of the literature.* Unpublished manuscript, University of Maine, Orono.

Ryckman, R. M., Robbins, M. A., Kaczor, L. M., & Gold, J. A. (1989). Male and female raters' stereotyping of male and female physiques. *Personality and Social Psychology Bulletin, 15,* 244–251.

Sheldon, W. H. (1942). *The varieties of temperament: A psychology of constitu-*

12

SOCIAL PERCEPTIONS OF SPORTS FIGURES: DUMB JOCKS, FLAWED HEROES, AND SUPERSTARS

Gary Thomas Long

University of North Carolina at Charlotte

Chances are that everyone that you know has a rich array of sports images. Even people who are not sports fans have their perceptions of the figures who play as well as those who watch sports. These perceptions constitute a major portion of the average American's view of the world. The images that are common to large portions of our culture can be informative about attitudes and values that are held but not directly expressed.

The nature of the social perceptions of sports figures and fans may be deduced from the images that are projected by the mass media, such as national and local newspapers, national magazines, television, movies, books, and even cartoon characters and children's toys. The importance in our society of the images of sports figures is evidenced by the long-time popularity of the media and media events that portray these images.

In midafternoon on May 17, 1939, the first telecast of a sporting event in the United States was broadcast. Only a few dozen people were able to watch the game between Columbia University and Princeton for fourth place in the Ivy League baseball standings. The single iconoscope television camera used had such a narrow view that it couldn't show the batter and the pitcher in the same picture. Bill Stern's play-by-play was crucial for following the game because the camera had to chase the ball around the field showing a rather limited background (Cantwell, 1973). The next three decades saw a dramatic change in the role of television in presenting sports. In 1969 men first walked on the moon, and it was shown on television. In that same year more people watched the Super Bowl than watched the moon walk (more than 60 million; "Super

Bowl '69," 1969). In 1989 probably more than 100,000,000 people worldwide watched the Super Bowl, and in 1990 30 seconds of commercial time on the Super Bowl broadcast cost $700,000. This increase of the popularity of sports on television illustrates the widespread exposure to sports figures in our society.

The images of those who play the games are everywhere, from Nike billboards, to cereal boxes, to thousands of magazine advertisments and radio and television commercials. Without even counting the thousands of movies and books that portray real and fictional sports personalities, I'm sure we are all convinced that the images of sports figures are myriad and pervasive in our society. In this chapter I explore some of the implications of this state of affairs. From the perspective of a social psychologist and a consumer of many of the sports offerings in our society, I analyze some of the common images of sports figures and sports fans and share some observations and conjectures about the significance of the nature of the attitudes about sports. I use some of the theories and concepts that social psychologists have proposed to explain how people tend to form images of other people to explain how sports fans perceive the players.

Social images may be referred to as *schemata* or as *stereotypes* (Atkinson, Atkinson, Smith, & Bem, 1990). These images make up a person's implicit personality theory. This is the person's own view of what characteristics of people are often found together. The image of a professional boxer calls to mind a set of physical and psychological characteristics. Individuals have their own images of a professional boxer that probably include attributions of aggressiveness and toughness and even judgments about likely intelligence, social skills, and social class background. Although each person has his or her own set of attributions that go with the image, there are some images about which there is widespread, though not universal agreement. These are ways of dealing with the world more efficiently. They cannot, of course, always include the correct attribution of characteristics to individuals, because boxers, as well as every other category of people, are not all alike. Commonly held perceptions are not always accurate, but their validity is not the reason they are interesting. How people see the world tells us more about the people who see things that way than it tells us about the world. The attributions associated with the images of sports figures tell us about how people view the world and not what the sports figures are actually like. Because there is some influence of reality and experience on the way people view the world, the images are not entirely fictional either. They may include attractions that are often, but not always, true.

THE DUMB JOCK

Although there may be hundreds of definable images for sports figures, probably the most pervasive and general one is the "dumb jock." The dumb jock is usually male, physically large and strong, and slow thinking, with few intellectual interests beyond academic eligibility when that is an issue. There is of course some variability in the dumb jock image with respect to his other characteristics. He is sometimes gentle and sweet off his playing field, as is Dr. Death in the Home Box Office television series "First and Ten," and sometimes he is consistently aggressive and loutish, as portrayed by the same actor in his role of Ogre in the movie "Revenge of the Nerds." His sport is most often football and his position is usually one of the "brawn over brain" areas, such as the offensive or defensive line or linebacker.

William Beezley (1985), in an amusing chapter called "Counterimages of the Student Athlete in Football Folklore" in *American Sport Culture: The Humanistic Dimensions,* quotes a story about Knute Rockne that illustrates the stereotypic relation between athletic skill and intelligence. It was said that Knute took his players to a wooded field to separate them into the positions they would play for his Notre Dame football team. Lining the players up on one side of the field, he instructed them to run across the field. The players who dodged the trees became backs and those who ran directly into the trees became linemen.

The dumb jock could play many sports, but he is most likely to be linked with sports that require the greatest physical strength, size, and aggressiveness. Football, boxing, wrestling, weight lifting, and ice hockey are well suited for the dumb jock, but he may also be frequently found in basketball and baseball. He is rarely seen playing competitive golf, swimming, or at the tennis court because these sports are seen as employing less size and strength as major contributors to success. In fact there are data cited in Chapter 11 that show that the more muscular the individual's body the less intelligent the individual is perceived to be. This relation holds for men and women perceivers and for men's and women's bodies.

Why is this dumb jock image so pervasive in our fiction and drama? The image is so often presented and so convincingly portrayed that it is tempting to say that it is based on fact and that is why it is so common. Well, here is one image that has been examined for validity. We have an opportunity to assess the accuracy of the dumb jock image by looking at data on the relation between athletic participation and indices of intelligence.

When examining the dumb jock image for its basis and validity it is interesting to note that the cousin of Charles Darwin, Sir Francis Galton (1822–1911) did not subscribe to the dumb jock view of the relation between strength and intelligence. Galton was a pioneer in the conceptualization and quantification of mental ability. Galton felt that innate mental capacity could be indicated by measures of muscular power, body proportions, reaction time, sensory acuity, and even head size (Myers, 1986). His expectations were that our "dumb jock" would more likely be a genius than a dummy. Galton's work, as it turned out, showed that neither brilliance nor stupidity was identified by measuring these physical attributes.

James Michener (1977), in his entertaining but unscholarly style, referred to "studies" that show that athletes are superior in intelligence to the non-athlete. According to him, there are "substantial studies" indicating that athletes tend to be "somewhat more intelligent than the general run of the school, college or adult population" (p. 301). These studies were not specified, however, so we don't know what types of athletes were included, but Michener's interpretation was a general one: Athletes as a group are smarter than average. If this is correct, it indicates at least that there are not enough dumb jocks in the group of athletes to pull down the group performance to average.

The question is not whether or not any dumb jocks exist, for they surely do. They exist as surely as computer nerds exist. The question is, Do they exist in the numbers and to the degree that would justify the widespread use of the stereotype of dumb jock? I found no studies explicitly dealing with the dumb jock image, but there are several studies of the relation between athletic participation and academic performance. Coakley (1986), in his treatment of the issues surrounding sports in society, reviewed the studies on athletes and academics in high school and in college. His review indicated that high school athletes generally have better grades than nonathletes. In looking at attitudes toward academic achievement, Coakley explained higher grades and higher academic goals among athletes in high school as resulting from the fact that interscholastic sports "attract students with self-confidence, above-average academic abilities, and favorable attitudes toward school" (p. 256). He denied that participation in athletics *causes* these desirable qualities in high school students, but that is not the point in question here. Rather, we are trying to determine what evidence there is that athletes have lower intelligence. Even though the evidence deals with our question only indirectly, there seems to be no support for the "dumb jock" image in high school.

Coakley (1986) cited mixed results from studies of college athletes' scholastic performance. Some studies showed athletes to have better performance whereas others show them to be worse. It may be the college setting that gives rise to most of the examples of the dumb jock image. High schools for the most part do not select students. Virtually the entire population attends high school. This means that all types are represented. If physical and mental abilities and characteristics are largely independent of each other, that is, uncorrelated, then high school would have equal numbers of smart jocks, dumb jocks, smart weaklings, and dumb weaklings. (These are rather crude descriptive terms, but I hope they make the point more easily understood.) Colleges do select students for academic and athletic skills. Colleges are likely to accept all academically qualified students as well as some whose academic qualifications are weaker if they have other skills valuable to the school, such as athletic skills. In college, the whole population of the smart and dumb and the athletic and the nonathletic is no longer present. These two variables, simplified to two levels of each variable for illustrative purposes, create four groups of people in the population: (a) the athletic and smart, (b) the athletic and dumb, (c) the nonathletic and smart, and (d) the nonathletic and dumb. The nonathletic and dumb group are eliminated from the college population. The only dumb ones there are likely to be jocks, thus fostering the dumb jock image. The dumb weaklings were not admitted, so they are nowhere to be seen on the college campus. The college ranks produce many of the fiction writers as well as reporters of interpreted fact who produce the images of our society. It seems plausible that the college experiences of these image makers have given rise to the dumb jock image as it is known today.

A social psychological theory that explains some of the aspects of person perception provides a plausible explanation for the vast appeal of the dumb jock image to the general population. Once provided by the image makers, the dumb jock image satisfies in people some needs that are proposed by the "just world" theory (Lerner, 1980). This theory states that people are motivated by a need to believe that the world is a place where justice prevails. People need to see the world as a place where people get what they deserve and deserve what they get. This implies a need to see the things that others get, both good and bad things, as a fair deal compared with the things we ourselves get. Whenever anyone else gets something good, that person must be seen as either having some superior qualities to deserve the good outcome or also getting something bad to even out the deal. This need to see justice and fairness in the world makes it more desirable to see people as being given an equal amount of talents or abilities as an innate endowment. There is then a general appeal to see compensation in nature. With every strength comes a compensating weakness. The dumb jock has been endowed with superior strength but has inferior intellect to make his deal with nature as fair as ours. The just world theory implies that there is an appeal to perceiving the world as a place where these kinds of fair deals happen. Because this view gives a sense of orderliness and security that people like, people have a tendency to distort things a bit to see them this way when they can.

Given the findings about athletes in high school being generally better in academics than nonathletes, the dumb jock image may be a distortion of reality fostered by this need to see the world as fair. The average person may feel the jock has been given greater strength, and to make up for this overendowment in one area he is given less intellectual ability.

THE FLAWED HERO

The image of the superior athlete who is lacking in some other area can be found in other configurations. It seems to me that the flawed hero is a phenomenon of social perception similar to the dumb jock image. There are numerous fictional examples and some well-known real life stories of the athlete who excels in his sport but falls short in some other area that is not necessarily intelligence. The flaw is often one related to the character of the individual. Perhaps he drinks, gambles, gets into bar fights, or has unfortunate personal relationships with the wrong sort of opposite sex, too many of the opposite sex, or even the same sex. Some have referred to Mike Tyson, Pete Rose, Jim Thorpe, Babe Ruth, Steve Garvey, Billie Jean King, and Billie Martin as examples of having one or more of the flaws, although they were all highly successful in their sport and their performances apparently were not affected by the flaws.

There are also dozens of professional athletes whose careers have been terminated by drug use either by affecting their performance or by league action being taken when the drug was illegal and its use became known. The excitement and enthusiasm shown by many media personnel and fans when one of these young millionaires of professional sports, such as Chris Washburn, is suspended for drug use is consistent with the idea that people often want to see those who were overrewarded in some way (e.g., being given millions of dollars for being tall and agile with a ball) suffer. In a just world, this suffering makes up for the unjust overreward.

THE SUPERSTAR

The need to see the world as just doesn't always require that we see outstanding athletes as having compensating weaknesses. Another way of seeing justice in, for example, Joe Montana's earning $3 million a year is to see him as having many truly superior qualities in addition to athletic skills. It is not enough to see the superstar as a truly superior athlete. To justify the superstar's success he must also be seen as having other outstanding qualities such as high moral character and a great personality. He should be a model for children and adults in every way. The true superstar may also be a super family man, community leader, and all around super person. If the male superstar is not married, he must then be a super bachelor like Joe Namath at his peak. Dr. J was a superstar, as was O. J. Simpson. Now Wayne Gretzky, Joe Montana, and Michael Jordan are real life superstars who are admired greatly for their personal qualities in addition to their athletic performance.

Viewing the superstar as having this wide array of admirable characteristics allows the fan to idolize him with less tension than would otherwise result from seeing him or her as unfairly overrewarded. This general admiration for the sports superstar makes it possible for many stars to make more money outside their game than in it. The superstar image can be sold to advertisers for millions of dollars. The products promoted often have no connection to the star's sport. Joe Namath has sold pantyhose. Joe DiMaggio sells Mr. Coffee. Chris Evert sells soft drinks. Arnold Palmer sells motor oil. Football players sell beer and automobiles. Baseball players sell razor blades, shaving cream, and underwear. It is certainly no surprise when athletes sell sports equipment or fitness-related products, but surely the average fan knows as much about shaving as John McEnroe does.

There is an explanatory concept in social psychology that deals with the apparently illogical tendency to value the opinions of sports heroes on matters on which they have no expertise. This tendency, which does not only apply to sports figures, is called the "halo effect" (Sears, Peplau, Freedman, & Taylor, 1988). When someone judges another person to be good or superior in one way there is a tendency to see them as good in many other ways as well. This is a positive halo effect. The principle underlying this tendency is said to be one of consistency. This consistency is said to simplify our very complex world for the perceiver. It is much easier to deal with the world if the good are all good and the bad are all bad. Of course, if people were asked if they thought this way they would recognize the oversimplification and deny it. This perceptual process takes place without our awareness and when we're not being particularly thoughtful.

Very few fans carefully think through the logic of choosing their heroes or their favorite teams. The images we create or adopt from others satisfy needs we have of which we are not aware. We need heroes who are models of skill, strength, courage, character, and all the other things we admire. When Michael Jordan is idolized to the extent that he is, he must be more than a great or even the greatest basketball player of his time. He must be of admirable character, modest but confident; he must like children; he must not lie, cheat, or take drugs. He, as an example, must be consistently good, and very good at that, to justify the great rewards he receives without threatening our need to see the world as just.

The huge salaries received by today's sports heroes can be a threat to the fans' belief in a just world unless the hero is seen as truly superior in many ways. Mature sports fans, those over thirty years old, have seen their sports heroes go from being nicely rewarded in the 1960s to the mind-boggling multi-million-dollar contracts of the nineties.

A comparison of the 1962 NBA first draft choice Bill McGill with the 1989 first choice Danny Ferry illustrates the change in the financial rewards that are available for our sports heroes. In the 1962–1963 college basketball season the leading scorer in the nation was Bill McGill of the University of Utah, with a 38.8 points per game average (Nixon, 1984). McGill was the first draft pick of the NBA. He was given a signing bonus of $5,000 and signed a 2-year contract with the Chicago Zephyrs for $17,000 per year. This was the highest salary he ever made in professional basketball, although he played in the NBA and the ABA until 1970.

To give some comparison to the nonsports world of the time, I graduated from Wake Forest College (now University) in 1962 with a bachelor's degree and went to work for E. I. DuPont de NeMours & Company, Inc., as a buyer of construction materials for $7,200 per year. This was a pretty good salary for a college graduate at the time. So McGill was making about $2\frac{1}{3}$ as much as a good college graduate's salary. That's not bad, but given the length of the average NBA career and the rarity of his skill it's not so much either.

In 1989 Danny Ferry of Duke University was the NBA's first draft pick. He signed a contract to play in Italy for $1,000,000 a year plus a car, house, maids, and food. A good salary for a college graduate in 1989 was about $20,000. This means our basketball hero of today is earning more than 50 times the salary of the average college graduate, considerably up from the $2\frac{1}{3}$ factor of the early 1960s. This state of affairs can have an impact on how sports fans view their heroes. Although it is very difficult to measure such things, it may be said that fans are now less tolerant of flaws in the hero. The hero can quickly and easily lose the hero status to become the goat.

In their first season the NBA expansion team, the Charlotte Hornets, won only about one of every four games, but they were the darlings of the city. Their leading scorer and highest paid player, Kelly Tripuka, was a local hero even though he had played for Notre Dame in college. Charlotte, North Carolina, is Atlantic Coast Conference college basketball territory and Notre Dame is a team that local fans love to hate. In spite of this, Kelly was cheered and admired. Season tickets to Hornets games were almost impossible to get and the Charlotte team led the entire NBA in attendance for the 1988–1989 season. In the early stages of the 1989–1990 NBA season the Hornets were slightly less successful in the win–loss column and Kelly was in a noticeable shooting slump. You could almost see the goat's horns growing on the one-time hero of the Hornets. The fans at the home games of the Hornets began to boo Kelly regularly until he was so disturbed that he made a tearful postgame speech to the fans. He told them that the home he had found, where he had wanted to finish his career, was becoming very unpleasant for him and his family.

Would the fans have turned on him so quickly if he were not a "million-dollar" man? Maybe they would have still been unhappy with his performance, but I think that the attack on Tripuka would not have been so harsh if he were not so highly paid. One of his teammates, Robert Reid, remarked to this effect in a television interview. He said the highest paid players on a team have to expect to take the heat from the fans when the team is not doing so well, even though it is not their fault.

It seems plausible that the high rewards that professional athletes are receiving today will make fans demand more from them. It is also likely that fans will be less tolerant of slumps in performance. Such predictions can be derived from the just world theory. High rewards, according to the just world theory, must be justified by superior performance. Extremely high rewards must be justified by superior performance and superior personal qualities. If those receiving the million-dollar contracts don't live up to these requirements, they threaten our need to believe the world is just and we want to see them punished and their rewards lowered. Fans will quickly boo and demand that the top-paid athletes who fall into a slump be traded or benched.

The contrast of fan behavior in college sports with that of fans of professional sports may further illustrate this point. In my 35 years of following college sports, mainly basketball and football, an occasion of the college fans booing their own team's players has been extremely rare. It may have happened somewhere, but in comparison I have to recall only as far back as the 1989–1990 professional football season and the Philadelphia Eagles and the 1989–1990 NBA season and the aforementioned Charlotte Hornets to cite occasions of home fans of professional sports booing their own players.

Sometimes college coaches are the target of abuse from fans of their own team, but this very rarely happens to a college player. This situation is again consistent with the just world model. College coaches can now approach the million-dollar contracts of the professional players, and when they do they are held to the high standard of the superstar professional athlete. If they don't justify their high rewards through their superior performance they are quickly out of favor.

Even further, for the very well-rewarded coaches, they must not only win but should also have entertaining personalities and high morals. There is a lot of fan talk in the local bars that says Dick Crum was fired as football coach at the University of North Carolina at Chapel Hill because he was "dull." His television personality was widely described as bland. He was reportedly paid approximately $800,000 for the remainder of his contract and his win–loss record was much better than the coaches before and after him, so it gives some credibility to the notion that his "lack of personality" was an important factor in his dismissal. There is no direct evidence of this, but it serves as an illustration of how high rewards lead to very high expectations as predicted by the just world model.

CONCLUSION

Some of the most widely held stereotypes of sports figures have been explored and some theoretical concepts of social psychology have been applied to explain the thought processes of the perceivers. At this point the reader's own storehouse of anecdotes concerning superstars, flawed heroes, and just world examples may be bursting for expression. Students often cite examples of the flawed hero by saying, "but he [or she] is queer [or stupid or crooked]" while the superstars are seen as "walk on the water" types with no moral or personality flaws and clearly superior performance in their sport. If the super athlete develops the slightest flaw he will be quickly rejected and despised. He must be considered despicable to be paid all that money and perform so poorly, because this situation antagonizes our strong need to believe the world is just. Our needs sometimes lead us to perceptual distortions. Attribution theory contributes to our understanding of how spectators' perceptions of athletes may be affected by attributional biases (Kelley & Michela, 1980) like the need to believe in a just world. I hope this application of social psychological theory has provided some insights into the dynamics of the public's perception of some of the people who play our games.

REFERENCES

Atkinson, R. L., Atkinson, R. C., Smith, E. E., & Bem, D. J. (1990). *Intro-duction to psychology.* New York: Harcourt Brace Jovanovich.

Beezley, W. H. (1985). Counterimages of the student athlete in football folk-lore. In W. Umphlett (Ed.), *American sport culture: The humanistic dimen-sions* (pp. 212–225). Cranbury, NJ: Associated University Press.

Cantwell, R. (1973). Sport was box office poison. In J. Talamini & C. Page (Eds.), *Sport and society: An anthology.* Boston: Little, Brown.

Coakley, J. J. (1986). *Sport in society: Issues and controversies.* St. Louis: Times Mirror/Mosby College Publications.

Kelley, H. H., & Michela, J. L. (1980). Attribution theory and research. *An-nual Review of Psychology, 31,* 457–501.

Lerner, M. J. (1980). *The belief in a just world: A fundamental delusion.* New York: Plenum Books.

Michener, J. A. (1977). *Sports in America.* New York: Fawcett Crest.

Myers, D. G. (1986). *Psychology.* New York: Worth.

Nixon, H. L. (1984). *Sport and the American dream.* New York: Leisure Press.

Sears, D. O., Peplau, L. A., Freedman, J. L., & Taylor, S. E. (1988). *Social psychology.* Englewood Cliffs, NJ: Prentice-Hall.

13

RUNNING—A PSYCHOSOCIAL PHENOMENON

Michael L. Sachs

Temple University

Running. Just look outside and you will see runners of all different sizes, shapes, and abilities. Running is more than just an activity—it is a phenomenon.

There have been runners in all societies for thousands of years. However, a popular focus on running has been evident only for several decades, propelled initially by Dr. Kenneth Cooper's (1968) book *Aerobics*. Frank Shorter's victory in the Olympic marathon in Munich in 1972 spurred running to dizzying heights of popularity in the rest of the 1970s and into the 1980s. Although some who started running have dropped out or shifted to other activities (e.g., cycling, or combining sports, such as triathloning), many continue to participate. A recent article (Henderson, 1989) cited a figure of 5,500,000 Americans running at least three times per week throughout 1988. Although this number represents only 2% of the U.S. population, there are many millions more who run (or jog or walk) less often but still participate. Delhagen (1990) reported that an often cited figure of the number of runners in the United States is 25,000,000, which represents 10% of the U.S. population. Importantly, the earlier figure of 5,500,000 represents a 10% increase from 1987. The count of people who ran at least one race in 1988 also increased, indicating a healthy status for running.

Running is the only sport/recreational activity specifically addressed in this book. The reasons for this are twofold. First, it is the physical activity of choice for many individuals in search of health and physical fitness. Second, it is the physical activity of choice for researchers interested in these individuals. There are many hundreds of studies that have examined runners from psychological, physiological, sociological, philosophical, and historical perspectives (Sachs, 1987).

Why have so many individuals selected running as the physical activity of choice? Running is a natural activity, one in which we have engaged (to greater or lesser degrees) since childhood. Our bodies have evolved over time to walk and run efficiently. Running is relatively inexpensive—a t-shirt, shorts, pair of socks, and good running shoes need cost no more than $60 or so (although one can certainly find more expensive attire, and some running shoes cost around $200). Running can be done at any time of the day, throughout the year, with few constraints on location (one doesn't need a pool, a court, a golf course, etc.), and no need for others with whom to participate. Running provides an excellent activity for charting progress—increasing in time and distance run as the days/weeks/months pass. In addition, although there are many facets of physical fitness (e.g., cardiovascular fitness, strength, muscular endurance, and flexibility), running addresses the area in which most individuals are interested—cardiovascular fitness.

Although I may appear, to some degree, to be extolling the virtues of running to the point of preaching the gospel of running, this is not the case. The psychological benefits I discuss in this chapter may be obtained through a variety of physical activities. Indeed, many other aerobic activities, such as walking, swimming, cycling, aerobic dance, and cross-country skiing, are just as, if not more, effective as running for particular individuals. For many persons, activities that may not be aerobic in orientation, such as tennis, racquetball, or weight lifting, may have similar salutary effects. Running may simply represent the most efficient activity to achieve the psychological and physiological benefits desired.

However, running is not for everyone! Some individuals find running boring, painful (because of injuries or biomechanical imbalances), inconvenient, etc. For these individuals other physical activities may be preferable. The activity selected must be the choice of the individual! If the motivation to begin participating in physical activity is present the environment must be structured so that adherence (sticking with it) is likely. The first step in this process is to select an activity that the individual enjoys. Few individuals stick with exercise if they are not deriving something positive and enjoyable from the activity.

MOTIVATION: STARTING OUT

For many individuals, the activity of choice is running. Why do people start running in the first place? For many, it is a desire to "get in shape." This means increasing one's level of cardiovascular fitness. There is often a desire to lose weight and look and feel better. A few individuals may have heard about the psychological benefits of running and want to achieve these positive effects.

There may also be external motivating factors, such as a friend, colleague, or relative who starts to run and encourages the person to participate. There may even be a bet in place to achieve a certain time/distance. One pizza store franchise owner was supposedly promised a luxury automobile if he would run and complete a marathon. He did and he got his car.

These factors are present in the initial stages of participation. As the runner sticks with the activity the same motivating factors remain but the relative importance of the factors changes. After a number of months (it depends on the individual), the primary factors often become the psychological ones—the reductions in stress and anxiety, and the increases in creativity and feelings of well-being. Being in shape, looking better, and losing weight all remain reasons to run, but these become somewhat secondary in importance (Carmack & Martens, 1979; Morgan & Goldston, 1987; Sachs & Buffone, 1984).

HOOKED ON EXERCISE: ADDICTION TO RUNNING

The concept of addiction to running appears regularly in newspapers and magazines. This concept was first popularized by Glasser (1976) in his book *Positive Addiction*. Glasser suggested that although most addictions are harmful to an individual both physically and psychologically, addiction to some activities, such as meditation and running, might actually be positive. He saw these activities as enhancing, rather than decreasing, the physical and psychological strength of the person. Kostrubala (1976), in his book *The Joy of Running*, suggested a similar notion.

Sachs and Pargman (1984) defined addiction to running as "psychological and/or physiological addiction to a regular regimen of running, characterized by withdrawal symptoms after 24–36 hours without the activity" (p. 233). This definition emphasized a relationship to running that may affect the physical and the psychological realms of the person. The person in this state needs to run when he or she had planned to run; taking a day off is okay if the person had planned a day off. Indeed, many runners run only 5 or 6 days a week and feel quite comfortable on their rest days. However, if the runner cannot run on a day when he or she had planned to run, withdrawal symptoms may manifest themselves. The symptoms may include anxiety, restlessness, guilt, irritability, tension, bloatedness, muscle twitching, and discomfort. Glasser (1976) noted reports of apathy, sluggishness, weight loss due to lack of appetite, sleeplessness, headaches, and stomach aches. The withdrawal symptoms cited by runners are varied, and encompass both psychological and physiological reactions. However, it should be noted that the level of experience of the symptoms is generally "only" mild to moderate. Runners are not twitching in corners, in agony

from feelings of guilt or anxiety, but the symptoms are still felt and are quite
real for the runner.

The notion of an addiction to running suggests that some runners are
"hooked on running," needing a daily dose of running to maintain physical and
psychological health. They develop a compulsion, a need to run that outweighs
other considerations in their lives. Family, friends, and work, for example,
assume secondary importance to the *need* to run. The element of choice disappears. The need to run controls the individual, and such thought and energy
may be directed toward the next run. Morgan (1979a, 1979b) suggested that the
concept of a positive addiction left something to be desired and discussed negative addiction. He cited numerous examples of runners who run despite circumstances (particularly injuries) that suggest a cutting back or time off from running. Many of us know of one or more individuals whose life appears to
revolve around running and whose existence seems to be defined by the concept
of being a "runner." These individuals may be thought of as negatively addicted, as persons whose lives are such that running controls them rather than
they control their running.

Although most individuals would not want to admit being addicted to anything, the notion of addiction to running has become so popularized and wa-
tered down that many runners agree that they are indeed addicted to running.
However, most individuals are actually indicating that running has become a
healthy habit, as Peele (1981) discussed at length. Running can move on a
continuum from healthy habit through dependence and compulsion to addiction. Most runners remain on the healthy habit side of the continuum,
with running having an important place in their lives but one considered
alongside other responsibilities of family, work, friends, etc. As an individual's
relationship with running moves toward the addiction side of the continuum, he
or she starts to lose control and the need to run becomes more and more
encompassing.

Only a small percentage of runners reach the stage where they lose control
of their running and running controls them. This is the stage that Peele would
call addiction and Morgan would term negative addiction. These runners may
be as difficult to treat as persons addicted to other experiences or substances.
Other physical activities may not suffice if the person cannot run because of
injury. Appointments will be missed and important social engagements skipped
if the need to run becomes overpowering. Efforts at developing programs to
help negatively addicted runners are underway. Those by Morrow (1988) and
Chan (personal communication, October 9, 1989) are most noteworthy. A recent (Benyo, 1990) trade book on exercise addiction entitled *The Exercise Fix*
includes a chapter called "How to Recover from Aerobic Exercise Addiction."

We can take comfort in the realization that most runners view running as a
healthy habit (even if many call it an addiction). It is an activity that is healthy
when participation is within reasonable limits, taking into consideration other

aspects of life. A few individuals carry their relationship with running to the addiction end of the continuum, but they are a distinct minority.

THE MIND OF THE RUNNER

What do runners think about when they run? Runners use one of two cognitive strategies: association or dissociation. Association may be defined as focusing on bodily sensations, in particular breathing, posture, and muscular feedback (i.e., heaviness in calves and thighs, abdominal sensations). Runners stay aware of physical factors when they associate. This strategy can aid runners in maximizing performance while minimizing physical pain or discomfort. Runners will use association to reach that fine line between maximum performance and overextension, but this ability depends on skill in reading one's bodily sensations and knowing what the sensations are at 100% effort (maximum performance) as opposed to 101% (overextension).

Dissociation is being used when the runner "purposely cuts himself off from the sensory feedback he normally receives from the body" (Morgan, 1978, p. 39). When runners dissociate they think about anything else but how they feel. There are three categories of dissociation that can be identified: diversions (meditating, fantasizing), problem solving, and spontaneity ("it just happens") (Lorentzen & Sime, 1979). Diversions may encompass specific tasks, such as writing letters, playing music, building a house, counting the number of blue cars, focusing on the side of the road, etc. The fantasy component can be brought in with a particular fantasy that an individual may have (e.g., finishing the marathon in under 2 hr, or winning the Olympic 10,000-m race in world record time). Problem solving usually refers to dealing with a problem at work or home and letting the rhythm of the run and potential increases in creativity that some find from running facilitate creative solutions or clarity of thinking in dealing with the problem. Spontaneity may be characterized as free flow of thoughts, drifting, aimless thinking, free floating, letting the mind wander, letting the mind freewheel, absence of set thought patterns, and random thoughts.

Runners shift frequently between association and dissociation. Competitive runners may associate more in races to maximize performance, but will use both strategies extensively in training. It is difficult to maintain a constant associative strategy for extended periods of time unless an individual has trained him- or herself to do so. This measure of concentration, or attention span, is a psychological skill that can be developed with practice (Lynch, 1987; Martens, 1987). Most runners find, however, that they will associate more at the beginning of a run, to facilitate getting into a rhythm, and at the end of the a run, to facilitate finishing strongly/comfortably. During the middle portion of the run (which could be the largest component, because the beginning and end

could each be only a mile or less out of a run of 6 miles or more, for example)
runners will tend to dissociate the majority of the time, with occasional associative checks to make sure the body is feeling comfortable and performing at the
level desired for that training session/competition.

THE RUNNER'S HIGH

*Unlike a lot of runners, this one chooses to run at noon, when the sun over
the shimmering blue Pacific burns hottest. The first half hour, as he trots through
the seaside parks of La Jolla, is pure agony, "exaggerated body pain and philosophical crisis." But he knows there's relief; "Thirty minutes out and something
lifts. The fatigue goes away and feelings of power begin. I think I'll run 25 miles
today. I'll double the size of the research grant request. I'll have that talk with the
dean and tolerate no equivocating." Then, another switch, from fourth gear into
overdrive. "Sometime into the second hour comes the spooky time. Colors are
bright and beautiful, water sparkles, clouds breathe, and my body, swimming,
detaches from the earth. A loving contentment invades the basement of my mind,
and thoughts bubble up without trails. I find the place I need to live if I'm going to
live." (Black, 1979, p. 79)*

This dramatic description of experience of the runner's high comes from
the noted psychopharmacologist Arnold Mandell. However, many less famous
runners have had similarly exhilarating experiences.

The popular literature seems to suggest that many runners experience the
runner's high. Indeed, Lilliefors (1978) found that 78% of a select group of
runners reported experiencing a sense of euphoria during their runs. Forty-nine
percent of the runners noted that the euphoria was occasionally spiritual in
nature. Sachs (1984) found similar results, with 77% of the runners in his study
having experienced the runner's high.

There are many terms used to describe the experience of the runner's high,
including euphoria, strength, speed, power, gracefulness, spirituality, sudden
realization of one's potential, glimpsing perfection, moving without effort, and
"spinning out" (Sachs, 1984). One definition of the runner's high that has been
suggested is "a euphoric sensation experienced during running, usually unexpected, in which the runner feels a heightened sense of well-being, enhanced
appreciation of nature, and transcendence of barriers of time and space"
(Sachs, 1984, p. 274).

It is clear from talking with runners that there is a continuum of experiences that runners categorize as "the runner's high." For some runners this
experience is basically a glorified sense of well-being. For other runners this
experience is a peak experience, as in this report by a national-caliber runner:

A highly unique transcended state wherein the other senses (sight, sound, and smell) took on peculiar degrees of sensual acuity. He described his visual experience as being somewhat similar to that which a blind man might go through shortly after having an operation which provided him with the miracle of sight, that is, a very sudden and astounding experience. (W. E. Sime, personal communication, 1983)

These peak experiences occur relatively infrequently. Maslow (1962, 1964, 1968) described peak experiences as encompassing characteristics such as the following: greater integration than at other times; more ability to fuse with the world; feeling oneself at the peak of one's powers; using capabilities to their fullest; effortlessness and ease of functioning; being a center of activities and perceptions; being more creative; and being more spontaneous, expressive, and natural. Some of these terms are certainly similar to the ones noted earlier as characteristic of the runner's high, but others represent a higher level of attainment. A possible continuum would feature a general sense of well-being on one end and peak experiences on the other.

Reports from runners (Sachs, 1984) indicate that this kind of characterization may be meaningful. Of the 60 runners in Sachs's study, 46 (77%) said they had experienced the runner's high. Thirty-seven percent said they had experienced the runner's high during an average of 29.4% of their runs. The remaining nine runners had only experienced the runner's high an average of 3.5 times. One might suggest that the "percentage" runners were more toward the general sense of well-being end of the continuum, given the comparative frequency of occurrence of the runner's high for them, whereas the "number of times" runners were more toward the peak experience end of the continuum, given the comparatively rare occurrence of the runner's high for them.

The runner's high is definitely a personal experience, resisting categorizations that apply to all who experience this altered state of consciousness. For example, while many runners said they experience the runner's high only while running slowly and comfortably, others noted experiencing it "only during and after hard runs." However, there are some characteristics of the runner's high that the majority of runners noted. First, it is an experience that cannot be predicted—the runner can usually not say before a run begins that he or she will experience the runner's high during this run. Second, cool, calm weather with low humidity and few distractions are conducive to experiencing the runner's high (i.e., running in midtown Manhattan in 95° temperature and 99% humidity is not likely to result in experiencing the runner's high).

Third, the runner must be able to run comfortably for a relatively long distance (6 miles or more, at least 20–30 min of running). Almost all experiences of the runner's high describe it coming into play after 30 min or more of running. Fourth, a comfortable pace is conducive to experiencing the runner's high. If an individual is straining to complete a particular distance, and/or running at a pace considerably faster than his or her norm, it is unlikely that the individual will experience the runner's high.

Approximately half of the runners talked about experiencing different levels of the runner's high, which would be in agreement with the idea of the continuum presented above. Although the concept of a general sense of well-being is less exciting than the idea of a peak experience, or what one runner called a "super high," it is important to note that this experience is a particularly positive one for the runner. As such, it may have important implications for motivation and continued participation in running.

RUNNING AS THERAPY

The concept of using exercise in general, and running in particular, as therapy has been examined extensively in the literature (Morgan & Goldston, 1987; Sachs & Buffone, 1984). Although the Greek ideal of *mens sana in corpore sano*—a healthy mind in a healthy body—has been with us for thousands of years, it is only recently that the use of exercise as a therapeutic approach to caring for depression and anxiety has been suggested (Eischens, Greist, & McInvaille, 1978; Glasser, 1976; Greist & Greist, 1979; Greist & Jefferson, 1984; Greist, Jefferson, & Marks, 1986; Harper, 1979; Johnsgård, 1989; Kostrubala, 1976).

The use of running as therapy has been recommended primarily as an adjunct to cognitive approaches. Although running has occasionally been used as the sole psychotherapeutic tool, it is generally aligned with other approaches in a more holistic approach. This suggests that both cognitive ("talking therapies") and behavioral ("running therapy") approaches can be used in working with clients with presenting problems such as anxiety and depression.

More than a decade of research and hundreds of studies have been conducted in this area, from Greist's significant initial work (Greist et al., 1978) to more recent studies (e.g., Martinsen, Strand, Paulsson, & Kaggestad, 1989). Results have tended to be mixed, although there is much evidence to support the use of running in ameliorating anxiety and depression. The main problems have come in the quality of the research; that is, the many methodological problems encountered make it difficult to attribute improvement in psychological states to running itself. Other considerations, such as characteristics of the participants; characteristics of the exercise instructors; and frequency, intensity, and duration of the exercise program may result in different findings that do not reflect the impact of exercise per se on the individual's psychological state.

Several of the findings of a group of experts in the field who participated in a state-of-the-art workshop in April 1984 sponsored by the Office of Prevention of the National Institute of Mental Health are as relevant now as they were then:

> *Physical fitness is positively associated with mental health and well being. . . . Exercise is associated with the reduction of stress emotions such as state anxiety. . . . Anxiety and depression are common symptoms of failure to cope with mental stress, and exercise has been associated with a decreased level of mild to moderate depression and anxiety. . . . Longterm exercise is usually associated with reductions in traits such as neuroticism and anxiety. (Morgan & Goldston, 1987, p. 156)*

The key word in these findings is *associated*. It would be nice to be able to say that a cause-and-effect relation exists—that the use of exercise (cause) results in reduced anxiety and depression (effect). However, the best we can confidently offer at present is that exercise is associated with reductions in these areas, although recent work suggests that we may be closer to being able to offer cause–effect rationales than we have been in the past (North, McCullagh, & Tran, 1990). Future work will most likely clarify this association versus cause–effect issue, as well as extend knowledge toward physiological/blood chemistry perspectives (e.g., Dienstbier, 1989).

RUNNING IN THE 1990s AND BEYOND

The practitioner—the runner—will find the future beckoning with more and better races, both shorter (e.g., 5 km and 5 miles) and longer (ultramarathons), from which to choose. Shoes will improve with advances in technology, progressing from the current ones with computer chips to ones that you can program to go out for a run while you stay in bed, getting your exercise and more sleep at the same time (well, maybe not that advanced!). Certainly, no indications of a downturn in interest in running are apparent and, if anything, numbers of runners should gradually increase.

Researchers in the field will find more work on the psychological/physiological links that result from running regularly, as well as work on getting people starting to run in the first place and keeping them at it (Dishman, 1988). There is still significant work waiting to be accomplished on running and psychology, and the future looks exciting.

REFERENCES

Benyo, R. (1990). *The exercise fix*. Champaign, IL: Leisure Press.

Black, J. (1979). The brain according to Mandell. *The Runner, 1*(7), 78–80, 82, 84, 87.

Carmack, M. A., & Martens, R. (1979). Measuring commitment to running: A survey of runners' attitudes and mental states. *Journal of Sport Psychology, 1*, 25–42.

Cooper, K. (1968). *Aerobics.* New York: Bantam Books.

Delhagen, K. (Ed.). (1990). Health watch: Exercise and fiscal fitness. *Runner's World, 25*(1), 14.

Dienstbier, R. A. (1989). Arousal and physiological toughness: Implications for mental and physical health. *Psychological Review, 96,* 84–100.

Dishman, R. K. (Ed.). (1988). *Exercise adherence: Its impact on public health.* Champaign, IL: Human Kinetics.

Eischens, R., Greist, J., & McInvaille, T. (1978). *Run to reality.* Madison, WI: Madison Running Press.

Glasser, W. (1976). *Positive addiction.* New York: Harper & Row.

Greist, J. H., & Greist, T. H. (1979). *Antidepressant treatment: The essentials.* Baltimore, MD: Williams & Wilkins.

Greist, J. H., & Jefferson, J. W. (1984). *Depression and its treatment.* Washington, DC: American Psychiatric Press.

Greist, J. H., Jefferson, J. W., & Marks, I. M. (1986). *Anxiety and its treatment: Help is available.* Washington, DC: American Psychiatric Press.

Greist, J. H., Klein, M. H., Eischens, R. R., Faris, J., Gurman, A. S., & Morgan, W. P. (1978). Running through your mind. *Journal of Psychosomatic Research, 22,* 259–294.

Harper, F. D. (1979). *Jogotherapy: Jogging as a therapeutic strategy.* Alexandria, VA: Douglass.

Henderson, J. (1989). Joe Henderson's journal. *Runner's World, 24*(12), 14.

Johnsgård, K. W. (1989). *The exercise prescription for depression and anxiety.* New York: Plenum.

Kostrubala, T. (1976). *The joy of running.* Philadelphia: J. B. Lippincott.

Lilliefors, J. (1978). *The running mind.* Mountain View, CA: World Publications.

Lorentzen, D., & Sime, W. E. (1979). *Association/dissociation and motivation in marathon runners.* Unpublished manuscript, University of Nebraska, Lincoln, NE.

Lynch, J. (1987). *The total runner: A complete mind-body guide to optimal performance.* Englewood Cliffs, NJ: Prentice-Hall.

Martens, R. (1987). *Coaches guide to sport psychology.* Champaign, IL: Human Kinetics.

Martinsen, E. W., Strand, J., Paulsson, G., & Kaggestad, J. (1989). Physical fitness level in patients with anxiety depressive disorders. *International Journal of Sports Medicine, 10,* 58–61.

Maslow, A. H. (1962). Lessons from the peak experience. *Journal of Humanistic Psychology, 2,* 9–18.

Maslow, A. H. (1964). *Religions, values, and peak-experiences.* New York: Viking.

Maslow, A. H. (1968). *Toward a psychology of being.* Princeton, NJ: D. Van Nostrand.

Morgan, W. P. (1978, November). The mind of the marathoner. *Psychology Today, 11,* pp. 38–40, 43, 45–46, 49.

Morgan, W. P. (1979a). Anxiety reduction following acute physical activity. *Psychiatric Annals, 9*(3), 36–45.

Morgan, W. P. (1979b). Negative addiction in runners. *The Physician and Sportsmedicine, 7*(2), 56–63, 67–70.

Morgan, W. P., & Goldston, S. E. (Eds.). (1987). *Exercise and mental health.* Washington, DC: Hemisphere.

Morrow, J. (1988, October). *A cognitive–behavioral intervention for reducing exercise addiction.* Paper presented at the annual meeting of the Association for the Advancement of Applied Sport Psychology, Nashua, NH.

North, T. C., McCullagh, P., & Tran. Z. V. (1990). Effect of exercise on depression. *Exercise and Sport Sciences Reviews, 18,* 379–415.

Peele, S. (1981). *How much is too much: Healthy habits or destructive addictions?* Englewood Cliffs, NJ: Prentice-Hall.

Sachs, M. L. (1984). The runner's high. In M. L. Sachs & G. W. Buffone (Eds.), *Running as therapy: An integrated approach* (pp. 273–287). Lincoln, NE: University of Nebraska Press.

Sachs, M. L. (1987). Bibliography: A retrieval system for exercise and mental health. In W. P. Morgan & S. E. Goldston (Eds.), *Exercise and mental health* (pp. 161–191). Washington, DC: Hemisphere.

Sachs, M. L., & Buffone, G. W. (Eds.). (1984). *Running as therapy: An integrated approach.* Lincoln, NE: University of Nebraska Press.

Sachs, M. L., & Pargman, D. (1984). Running addiction. In M. L. Sachs & G. W. Buffone (Eds.), *Running as therapy: An integrated approach* (pp. 231–252). Lincoln, NE: University of Nebraska Press.

14

THE AFRICAN–AMERICAN ATHLETE: A PSYCHOLOGICAL PERSPECTIVE

Les Brinson
Elwood L. Robinson

North Carolina Central University

The predominant participation of African-Americans in athletics is controversial and is difficult to explain on either a "common sense" basis or with traditional behavioral science theories. The success of the African-American athlete in America is well documented (Ashe, 1988; Hoose, 1989; Kane, 1971; Russell & Branch, 1979). Despite this success, racial biases and stereotypes, genetic theories, motivation, and psychological dimensions continue to influence their participating practices in sports.

Sports has long been considered the great equalizer, the opportunity for athletes and spectators of all races to come together for a common cause. But since the first Kentucky Derby, run in 1875 with 15 jockeys, 14 of whom were black, the thousands of games that blacks and whites have played in public together have not served to bring us appreciably closer.

It is not our intention to here document the role of psychological processes in athletic performance or comment on the frequent use of psychological concepts for explaining poorly understood phenomena in sports. Several volumes have already been devoted to these topics (i.e., Christina & Landers, 1976; Cratty, 1989; Harris, 1973; Michener, 1976; Morgan, 1970). Moreover, we do not feel that these processes are appreciably different in the African-American athlete. Instead we informally reflect on some motivational, psychological, physical, and racial barriers that have affected the participation of African-Americans in sports today. Because of space limitations, we do not delve into an extensive history of blacks in sports (see Ashe, 1988); nor do we belabor the controversy regarding the physical difference in the races accounting for the success of black athletes.

HISTORICAL PERSPECTIVE

Athletic participation has been an important part of the African-American's heritage. Africans enjoyed contests and most of them were connected in some way with religious ceremonies, fertility rites, rites of passage, and the entertainment of visitors (Ashe, 1988). Sporting events had significance that went beyond mere enjoyment. They taught young people general fitness, economic survival, civic and cooperative values, and military skills that served the dual purposes of health and survival.

The African-American personality, some believe, cannot be understood outside the boundaries of rhythm, dance, and sports. African people throughout the world have a view that is conceived as a universal oneness (Akbar, 1976). The coming together and sharing with each other in a harmonious manner reaffirms the rhythmic flow between self and others. Dancing is highly symbolic and significant when viewed within this context. The rhythmic nature of music, which shatters the illusion of insulation and fuses the listeners into a shared oneness, becomes an affirmation of unity between the people, especially when physical or psychological threat is imminent. Therefore, it seems that sports may represent a twofold process for African-Americans: first, a symbolic expression of personality development and, second, a mechanism for their basic survival.

The spiritualistic songs of the early black church, the protests of black people during the 1960s, the rhythmic "steps" of black fraternities and sororities, and the gathering of blacks for songs and speeches following crises throughout history all punctuate a reflexive proclivity for sports or sportslike involvement of African-Americans when dignity, pride, or security are at risk. Perhaps the old pejorative of "natural rhythm" among African-Americans and the mockery that has been made of black ritual song and dance represent a tragic lack of understanding of the psychological coping strengths and the symbolic meaning and utility of these forces in the lives of African-Americans.

There is a historical economic antecedent to the participation of blacks in sports. In early Africa and in America, black-controlled athletic contests were accompanied by rhythmic dance and song. In early Africa, such performances were intended to please the gods. Medicine men sometimes divined special omens from the outcomes of athletic games and ordered appropriate dances to suit the occasion. Combining the athletic with the social remained a peculiar facet of African-American life through the 20th century. It is noteworthy that during the early 1920s the financial success of many black-run basketball, football, and track contests depended on whether a dance was held for the spectators immediately afterward (Ashe, 1988).

These personality dynamics, cultural norms, and sports skills are deeply rooted in the history of African-Americans. Once in America, these natural skills along with the love of sports combined with a new structured and organized sports system to form a perfect marriage. This combination has resulted in the production of some of the greatest and most spectacular athletes the world has ever seen.

RACISM IN SPORTS

The fundamental proposition that has historically affected African-Americans in America has been cultural domination with its double-edged sword of racism and economic exploitation. Consequently, racism and exploitation are at the source of any understanding of African-Americans and their participation in sports in America.

African-Americans make up 77% of all NBA players and 62% of all NFL starters (Hoose, 1989). Some of these athletes earn millions of dollars. On the surface, sports would seem to be a model of racial progress. However, although appearances may have changed four decades after Jackie Robinson's Major League debut, racial prejudice remains as deeply rooted in American sports as it is in American society in general.

Hoose (1989) raised some interesting issues regarding racial stereotypes at work in sports. He contended that there are two major principles regarding African-Americans in sports today:

1. The nearer a position is to where the ball usually is, the less likely that a black will occupy it.
2. The more responsibility or control involved in a position, the less likely that a black will play it.

A statistical analysis of football, basketball, and baseball positions seems to add support to Hoose's thesis. African-Americans are more likely to be defensive backs, wide receivers, and outfielders. They are least likely to be quarterbacks, pitchers, or catchers. Black baseball players are today nine times as likely to be outfielders as pitchers; four of five blacks who play defensive positions are either outfielders or first basemen. Only about 40% of all white players play these positions (Hoose, 1989). The expects in sports state that African-Americans are most often in these positions because these are the speed positions, and managers want to use the speed element that has often been associated with blacks. However, this practice often wastes leadership ability and intelligence by not giving African-Americans the opportunity to compete for other positions.

In 1968, CBS telecast a special program on the black athlete. In 1971, *Sports Illustrated*'s lead story was devoted to the issue of why blacks had come to dominate certain sports, namely, football, basketball, baseball, boxing, and track and field. In 1987 two prominent sports personalities, Al Campanis and Jimmy "the Greek" Snyder, lost their jobs because of statements they made about black athletes and blacks in sports. In addition, in 1989 NBC revitalized *Sports Illustrated*'s 1971 thesis on the black athlete and broadcast a 60-min special that attempted to address reasons for their apparent success in the major sports in the world. As the commentary continues, the theories regarding the African-American's perceived dominance in certain sports remain unsubstantiated.

The genetic explanation for African-American superiority has varied greatly in the past 400 years. The myth of the black "natural" athlete has remained constant throughout this century. All too often, African-Americans have had their success explained in terms of their African ancestry, selective breeding, huge thighs, content of their blood, and even their eye color (Hoose, 1989). Seldom is their success credited to their mental talents or intelligence.

Allport (1954) wrote that a stereotype is "an exaggerated belief associated with a category. Its function is to justify, or rationalize, our conduct in relation to that category" (p. 241). The conduct that has been associated in relation to the category "black athletes" has been to demean them by rendering them subhuman; they don't succeed by virtue of human attributes, such as thought, planning, or control. They just react and respond to their "God-given" talents.

Forces that complicate matters further are the psychopathological effects in institutional and personal racism that lead to a host of insecurity, adjustment, or general self-affirmation problems (Brinson, 1987). To cope with these forces, African-American athletes have often developed coping strategies that are self-destructive or lead to negative outcomes. The double conscious of W. E. B. DuBois, the sense of always feeling the stress of living two lives—an American and an African-American, has been a way of coping with societal pressures. Also the plight of the African-American athlete in America is well documented in the biography of one of America's greatest black athletes, Paul Robeson. These extreme coping measures are adjustment responses to the frustrations of racism.

Adler's personality theory offers some insights into the African-American's personality and his or her response to racism. Institutional racism places its victims in a no-win, defenseless, or existentially inferior status (Adler, 1907). The Adlerian notion of "compensation" in which individuals respond to racism by becoming completely submerged in a task to the exclusion of any critical thinking, self-monitoring, or self-planning seems to address what has happened to some African-American athletes. As evidence of this blind, consuming loyalty, a recent study commissioned by the National Collegiate Athletic Association (NCAA) of intercollegiate student athletics showed that the most respected or dominant person in their lives is their coach (National Collegiate Athletic Association, 1988). In this context, poor academic records, particularly of African-Americans (which created the bases for NCAA rules 42 and 48), drug abuse, and abusive and general conduct disorders in general may be understood and treated. In addition, the dynamics associated with the participation and dominance of African-Americans in sports can be understood in this context.

One of the most important statistics in the history of black participation in American sports is the conspicuous absence of black owners. It seems odd that, given the enormous salaries of some black athletes and the enormous amount of money that many blacks have obtained in the United States, their participation in the sports ownership industry is almost nonexistent. Today, even with professional franchises selling for $60 and $70 million a piece, capital is no longer the main obstacle for blacks who wish to acquire teams.

Recently, Brewington (1989) reported that a group of black investors made history by purchasing the NBA's Denver Nuggets. This marks the first minority-owned major sports franchise. One hundred twenty years after the Cincinnati Red Stockings first took the field, blacks are just beginning to develop an initial financial stake in the destiny of an integrated sports team.

In 1989, after A. Bartlett Giamatti had been chosen to succeed Peter Uberroth as baseball's commissioner, a group of National League owners named Bill White, a black man, to replace Giamatti as president of the National League. Only time will tell whether White's historic appointment will defuse or reinforce efforts to increase blacks' representation among baseball's owners, boardrooms, and front offices.

THE NEGRO BASEBALL LEAGUE

From 1889 until 1946, black men were barred from organized baseball by a "gentleman's agreement." For nearly half a century some of the nation's greatest baseball players performed in the obscurity of the Negro League. Even today, many of them have not been recognized for their outstanding accomplishments. The Negro League has been viewed as a "second class" experience for black players by white America. It has not been legitimized by the Major League's Hall of Fame. Only a handful of players (Satchel Paige, Josh Gibson, Buck Leonard, Oscar Charleston, Cool Papa Bell, Judy "Sweet Juice" Johnson, John Henry Lloyd, Martin Dihigo, Ray Dandrige, Rube Foster, and Monte Irvin) have been inducted into the Cooperstown Hall of Fame based on their performance in the Negro League (*Baseball Encyclopedia*, 1988). Their names are listed with asterisks. Even Monte Irvin, who hit .293 in eight major league seasons, has an asterisk beside his name.

To suggest that those players represent the only noteworthy talent from the Negro League is clearly not adequate. We now are realizing that the Hall of Fame has merely recognized the legends and there are still players who should be seriously considered for induction.

After the Civil War, integrated baseball teams were formed in the north, and there were a number of talented black players on them. Chu (1982) indicated that the first black to play professional baseball was John (Bud) Fowler who played for New Castle, Pennsylvania, in 1872. He was followed by Moses Fleetwood who played for the Toledo (Ohio) Mudhens in 1883. Like those who followed them, it was necessary for them to be outstanding athletes, and more talented than their white peers. Further, they had to be psychologically equipped to cope with the twin evils of insult and physical danger in the practice of their crafts. When Toledo was scheduled to play in Richmond, Virginia, during this period, the team sent the following message to the Toledo manager:

> *We the undersigned do hereby warn you not to put up Walker, the negro catcher, the evenings that you play in Richmond, as we could mention the names of 75 determined men who have sworn to mob Walker if he comes on the ground in a suit. We hope you will listen to our words of warning, so that there will be no trouble; but if you do not there certainly will be. We only write this to prevent much bloodshed, as you alone can prevent. (Peterson, 1970, p. 23)*

Peterson provided additional insights into the difficulties faced by black players with another statement of a white player in 1888:

> *While I myself am prejudiced against playing on a team with a colored player, I still could not help pitying some of the poor black fellows that played in the International League. Fowler used to play second base with the lower part of his legs encased in wooden guards. He knew that about every player that came down to second base on a steal had it in for him and would, if possible, throw the spikes into him. . . . About half the pitchers try their best to hit these colored players when at the bat. (Petersen, 1970, p. 41)*

Despite all these barriers the seemingly indomitable spirit and strength of character of the African-American athlete prevailed. The struggle came to a climax when Jackie Robinson, a 27-year-old rookie in 1946, began to play Major League baseball. He and his wife became one of the most publicized black couples in the country for a time. In spite of his talents and publicity, Jackie Robinson, along with countless other black professional baseball players, still had a very difficult time gaining acceptance in baseball.

MOTIVATION

Despite the recent emphasis on the physical attributes of African-American athletes, their success has not been entirely due to physical characteristics. African-
American athletes, who today make up a large percentage of the major sports
labor forces, have begun to make some inroads into the country club sports.
However, their success has been continuously credited to their superior physique,
African ancestry, and natural talents, rather than their mental capacities or their
motivation.

Bill Russell, arguably the greatest player to play professional basketball,
had strong reactions toward the 1971 *Sports Illustrated* story that suggested that
the superiority of blacks in certain sports was due to genetic and racial factors.
Russell stated,

> *I worked at basketball eight hours a day for twenty years—straining, learn-
> ing, sweating, studying—but* Sports Illustrated *didn't mention such factors as
> reasons for blacks' success in sports. Or all the forces that turned my ambition to
> basketball instead of, say banking. No, I was good at basketball because of my
> bone structure. All of which shows you how far out in the twilight zone your
> thinking can drift if it comes from a weird starting point. All the racial upheaval of
> the 1960's had taught* Sports Illustrated *that it's okay to be a racist as long as you
> try to sound like a doctor. (Russell & Branch, 1979, p. 199)*

Motivation begins with self-confidence and self-efficacy. Young athletes of
all races who feel good about themselves and exhibit high levels of confidence
are more likely to enter into a competitive sports situation than children lacking
in self-confidence or self-efficacy.

How is self-efficacy developed? Bandura (1977) proposed a model of self-
efficacy that states that self-efficacy is enhanced by successful performance,
vicarious experience, verbal persuasion, and emotional arousal. The most important of these four is successful performance. According to Bandura, successful performance raises expectations for future success; failure lowers these
expectations. Once strong feelings of self-efficacy develop through repeated
successes, occasional failures will be of small consequence. Feelings of self-
efficacy lead to improved performance, while a lack of these feelings results in
slackening of performance.

The most critical aspect of Bandura's theory for African-Americans is its
focus on repeated successes through participatory modeling. In participatory
modeling, the person first observes a model perform a task. Then, the person is
given the opportunity to replicate what he or she has seen. Moreover, it's equally
important that the observed model be a member of the same ethnic group. The
tacit message to African-Americans or other ethnic groups is that this sport wel-
comes and rewards their participation. Psychological barriers are removed when

blacks see other blacks participating in certain sports. Therefore, the reason that there are only a few black swimmers, golfers, and tennis players is not because they lack the athletic ability but rather because blacks have had limited access to black models and limited opportunities to participate in these sports.

African-Americans have seen other blacks excel in basketball, football, boxing, and track and field for many years. They watch these models and then through participatory modeling (often 8–12 hr a day) gain strong feelings of self-efficacy. The feelings, according to Bandura, lead to improved performance, thereby increasing the opportunity to excel. Considerable support for Bandura's model exists in sports-related research (Feltz, Landers, & Raeder, 1979; Feltz & Mugno, 1983; Gould & Weiss, 1981).

A different type of motivation is also important for African-Americans. Sports have been viewed as an avenue to a much better life. Today, thousands of young African-Americans seek the fulfillment of their dreams through sports. For some it is a dream that has taken on pathological obsession. For many, sports is perceived as the only road to prestige and wealth. Few other roads have been open to young blacks. Sports in recent years have given blacks some special opportunities. While they may be discouraged from pursuing some careers, African-Americans can point to a number of examples of success in sports.

Although the chances of a career in sports are remote, the African-American athlete continues to persevere and harbor expectations of success. Kennedy (1988) compared black and white collegiate male basketball players on their expectations to play professionally subsequent to their college careers. Kennedy controlled for size of the university and history of the school in producing professional athletes. He found that only 50% of whites expected to play sports professionally whereas 97% of the blacks had such expectations.

Because the rewards in athletics are substantial, motivation is stronger. The African-American athlete has something tangible to aspire to when he picks up a baseball, football, or basketball. He has the examples of a Bo Jackson, Doug Williams, or Michael Jordan to inspire him.

INTELLIGENCE AND SPORTS

In Western culture, intelligence is viewed as a reflection of linguistic and logical–mathematical competencies. The ability to plan, orchestrate, and execute are essential components. In addition to the emphasis on linguistic facility, Wechsler (1958), whose early works in intelligence set the standard for current definitions and conceptualizations, curiously incorporated "performance" as a coequal aspect of intelligence. We agree with Wechsler that athletic performance should be conceptualized as a form of intelligence.

There is an apparent truism in sports: When a sports position is perceived as requiring intelligence, responsibility, or control, that position is least likely to be occupied by an African-American. The quarterback is considered to be the most intelligent football player. In the four decades that blacks have played in the NFL, only nine players have thrown more than 25 passes, one of them a halfback (Walter Payton) (Hoose, 1989). This small number certainly doesn't reflect their ability to play the position. It is estimated that between 75 and 100 African-Americans have played quarterback in the Canadian Football League. In the 1988–1989 football season, there were six black quarterbacks on eight Canadian team rosters, while in the United States there were only five black quarterbacks scattered among the NFL's 28 teams.

Athletes are often the most recognizable figures in the world. They inspire idolatry which often borders on deification, with many youths desiring to follow their successful paths. These youths are typically attracted to their athletic ability and not their intelligence. One adjective that is not used to describe either the athletes personally or their performance, particularly for African-Americans, is *intelligent*. Are Magic Johnson, Bo Jackson, Michael Jordan, Carl Lewis, or Mike Tyson geniuses? Gardner (1983) would like for us to begin to conceptualize their talents as intelligence. His theory posits the existence of several relatively autonomous intellectual competencies, or multiple intelligences. He has identified six competencies, but more may be discovered. They are linguistic intelligence (e.g., syntactic and pragmatic capacities involved in the use of language and communication), logical–mathematical intelligence (e.g., logical thinking and numerical ability), musical intelligence (e.g., rhythmic and pitch abilities involved in composing, singing, and playing music), spatial intelligence (e.g., perceiving the visual world, transposing and modifying one's initial perception, and recreating aspects of one's visual experience), personal intelligence (e.g., knowledge of self and others, including the ability to discern other individuals' moods, temperaments, motivation, and intentions), and bodily–kinesthetic intelligence (e.g., dancing, acting, athletics, and inventing). These competencies may be viewed as building blocks out of which thought and action develop. They constitute the basis of human symbol-using capacities and interact to produce a diverse mixture of human talents that may be deployed for societal ends.

We must not assume that what is valued by our culture is all there is to intelligence. The athletes mentioned above should be, according to Gardner, considered to possess a special kind of intelligence based on their athleticism. Perhaps, then, the incredible abilities of a Michael Jordan are in reality an exhibition of his "intelligence," which may be similar to that of a Mozart or Einstein. This or any concept of intelligence is related to context and culture.

CONCLUSION

The issues discussed in this chapter are both complex and controversial. We are concerned that whenever a group of people, such as African-Americans, is given such wide attention and scrutiny, there is a danger of losing the individuality of each person in that group. Such labeling leads to stereotyping, which in its extreme form is the root of prejudice.

African-American athletes have been successful in some American sports. Despite their accomplishments, racial ambiguities remain in American sports. These attitudes and their vicissitudes have directly affected the participation of African-Americans in all aspects of sports. Full participation in American sports, by all Americans, can only occur when we remove racial barriers.

REFERENCES

Adler, A. (1907). Organic inferiority and its compensation. In M. L. Ansbacher & R. R. Ansbacher (Eds.), *The individual psychology of Alfred Adler* (p. 241). New York: Harper & Row.

Akbar, N. (1976). The rhythm of black personality. *Southern Exposure, 3,* 14–19.

Allport, G. W. (1954). *The nature of prejudice.* Reading, MA: Addison-Wesley.

Ashe, A. R. (1988). *A hard road to glory: A history of the African-American athlete.* New York: Warner Books.

Bandura, A. (1977). Self-efficacy: Toward a unifying theory of behavioral change. *Psychological Review, 84,* 191–215.

Baseball encyclopedia. (1988). New York: Macmillan.

Brewington, J. A. (1989, June 17). Denver Nuggets to become first minority-owned sports franchise. *USA Today,* p. 1C.

Brinson, L. C. (1988, May 2). NCCU prof: Racism helps create symptoms of "learned helplessness." *Durham Sun,* p. 1.

Christina, R. W., & Landers, D. M. (Eds.). (1976). *Psychology of motor behavior and sports* (2 volumes). Champaign, IL: Human Kinetics.

Chu, D. (1982). *Dimensions of sport studies.* New York: John Wiley & Sons.

Cratty, B. J. (1989). *Psychology in contemporary sport.* Englewood Cliffs, NJ: Prentice-Hall.

Feltz, D. L., Landers, D. M., & Raeder, U. (1979). Enhancing self-efficacy in high avoidance motor task: A comparison of modeling techniques. *Journal of Sport Psychology, 1,* 112–124.

Feltz, D. L., & Mugno, D. A. (1983). A replication of the path analysis of the causal elements in Bandura's theory of self-efficacy and the influence of autonomic perception. *Journal of Sport Psychology, 5,* 263–277.

Gardner, H. (1983). *Frames of the mind: The theory of multiple intelligences.* New York: Basic Books.

Gould, D., & Weiss, M. (1981). The effects of model similarity and model task on self-efficacy and muscular endurance. *Journal of Sport Psychology, 3,* 17–29.

Harris, D. V. (1973). *Involvement in sports: A somatopsychic rationale for physical activity.* Philadelphia: Lea & Febiger.

Hoose, P. M. (1989). *Necessities: Racial barriers in American sports.* New York: Random House.

Kane, M. (1971, January). An assessment of "black is best." *Sports Illustrated,* pp. 72–83.

Kennedy, S. (1988, August). *Addressing academic and career planning of collegiate athletes.* Presented at the annual meting of the American Psychological Association, Atlanta, Georgia.

Michener, J. A. (1976). *Sports in America.* New York: Random House.

Morgan, W. P. (Ed.). (1970). *Contemporary readings in sports psychology.* Springfield, IL: Charles C Thomas.

National Collegiate Athletic Association. (1988). *Summary of results from the 1987–1988 national study of intercollegiate athletes.* Washington, DC: American Institute for Research.

Russell, B., & Branch, T. (1979). *Second wind: Memoirs of an opinionated man.* New York: Ballantine Books.

Wechsler, D. (1958). *The measurement and appraisal of adult intelligence.* Baltimore: Williams & Wilkins.

15

MENTAL RETARDATION AND RECREATIONAL FITNESS PROGRAMS

Albert A. Maisto
Janet R. Stephens

University of North Carolina at Charlotte

American society places a great deal of importance on recreation and leisure activities. Hundreds of millions of dollars are spent every year on sports, games, hobbies, and toys. If asked, most children would cite an athlete or some famous person connected with sports and leisure activities as their hero or heroine. Both adults and children alike excitedly anticipate time off from work or school so that they can engage in favored leisure activities. The role of recreation in the lives of Americans is already very powerful and still seems to be expanding.

Recreation opportunities for a large segment of our population, specifically mentally retarded individuals, are very limited, however, and do not appear to be expanding and developing as rapidly as those for the general population. Cheseldine and Jeffree (1981) and McConkey, Walsh, and Mulcahy (1981) interviewed families and caretakers of mentally retarded persons and found that most of the leisure activities that they engaged in were passive and solitary in nature. McConkey et al. (1981) found that one-half the sample population did not participate in any activity outside the home, two-thirds did not take part in any community activity, and four-fifths had no nonhandicapped friends. Other research (Wilkinson, 1982) revealed that leisure services for mentally retarded individuals are almost nonexistent in many communities and that the services that are available are segregated and limited. Though research indicates mentally retarded persons have few leisure and recreation opportunities, it also suggests they may need them as much as, if not more than, their non-mentally-handicapped peers.

Stein and Sessoms (1977) suggested that appropriate recreation experiences can have a positive influence on a mentally retarded person's physical, emotional, intellectual, and social development. Although there is not an abundance of research to support this argument, several studies have been conducted in support of this contention.

Loovis (1978) reviewed a variety of studies that have consistently shown that the motor proficiency of mentally retarded persons can be improved as a result of participation in planned physical education. Oliver (1958) was the first to study the effect of systematic physical education programs on the motor performance of mentally retarded persons. Oliver found significant improvements in athletic achievement, physical fitness, and strength.

Anderson, Grossman, and Finch (1983), in a review of different techniques that measured the effects of recreation on social skills development in the mentally retarded individuals, divided the research into four categories. Behavior modification was the first technique they discussed. Using tangible and social reinforcers, Hopkins (1968) reported an increase in smiling among mentally retarded subjects. In another study candy was used as an effective reinforcement to teach two severely mentally retarded children to pass a ball back and forth (Whitman, Mercurio, & Caponigri, 1970). A behavior modification program designed by Knapczyk and Yoppi (1975) taught cooperative and competitive play with a token system; however, they reported a lack of carryover when the token system was discontinued.

Arranging tasks so as to require cooperation was the second technique into which Anderson et al. grouped studies on social skills. This technique was illustrated by Mithaug and Wolfe (1976), who designed puzzle tasks that required that mentally retarded subjects communicate in order to complete them. They found that level of social interaction and verbalization increased with task interdependence.

The third technique discussed by Anderson et al. involved modeling. O'Conner (1969, 1972) and Keller and Carlson (1974) found that their most isolated subjects changed socially very little after watching filmed models of normal children, but less isolated children increased positive social interaction. By pairing high and low interactive children and using shaping procedures and immediate reinforcement of modeling behavior, Morris and Dolker (1974) produced a high frequency of cooperative play.

The fourth technique of Anderson et al. was the control of environmental factors. Quilitch and Risley (1973) found that various toys were different in the amount of social play they evoked.

The importance of exercise in maintaining good physical and mental health is well documented. Regular exercise is valuable in controlling obesity and in decreasing heart, lung, and circulatory system diseases. Exercise helps some sleep better, helps some feel more alert and energetic, and helps others relax. It may help relieve emotional stress, anger, tension, and even depression. A regular program might help build muscles that would improve self-help abilities in some mentally retarded persons. Recreation and exercise build confidence in some people and simply relieve boredom for others. The benefits of exercise apply to the mentally retarded persons as much as to the nonretarded persons, in some cases more. For example, the need to reduce excess weight and maintain cardiac efficiency is particularly important to individuals with Down's syndrome, a disorder that not only involves intellectual impairment, but is often associated with obesity and a propensity toward cardiac complications (Robinson & Robinson, 1976).

Stein (1977a) stated that the aims of recreation and adapted physical education for handicapped individuals are no different than for nonhandicapped individuals: personal fulfillment, health and fitness, relaxation, behavior change, social adjustment, aesthetic appreciation, maximization of independence, and fun and pleasure.

Although it seems logical and clear that mentally retarded persons would benefit from recreation opportunities, such opportunities are not available for them. Cheseldine and Jeffree (1981) surveyed the families of 214 mentally retarded individuals and reported that mentally retarded persons' choices of activities are severely limited by lack of provision, lack of community acceptance, lack of skills, and restrictions by cautious caretakers.

Wilkinson (1982) interviewed institutional recreation personnel and concluded that those involved with integrated play (i.e., programs that included handicapped and nonhandicapped persons) cited attitudes as the major barrier to successful integration. Those not involved with integrated play cited design, cost, safety, lack of responsibility, staff shortages, and education as the major barriers. In many programs mentally retarded individuals were found to be allowed, but not encouraged, to participate. Sometimes integration was permitted only if the retarded person already possessed all the necessary skills to participate. As a result of these many barriers, most mentally retarded persons participate very rarely in recreation activities, and when they do it is often in limited and segregated programs.

Project LIFE (Leisure Is For Everyone) (1987) has cited programmatic and physical barriers to integration. Programmatic barriers are present when the individual lacks the specific skills or capabilities that have been identified as necessary for inclusion in an activity. Physical barriers include environmental and administrative limitations. Examples of physical barriers are human resource, transportation, fee, architectural, training, communication, and legal liability limitations.

Clearly, there are many potential difficulties with providing mentally retarded persons with appropriate and desirable recreation opportunities. However difficult it may be, it is necessary because it is required by law. Federal special education legislation Public Law 94-142 includes recreation as a related service area. Section 504 of the Rehabilitation Act of 1973 states that all agencies receiving federal funds must ensure that facilities and programs are accessible to persons with handicaps. Antidiscrimination acts in many states guarantee the rights of all people to enter and receive services from nonfederal agencies, businesses, and commercial establishments (Project LIFE, 1987). Not only does the law require that the recreation needs of mentally retarded persons be met, it is their right as human beings.

Having established that recreation opportunities for mentally retarded persons are less than adequate, the question is how to enable retarded persons to exercise their right to appropriate recreation. One model is Special Olympics. Special Olympics is an annual international program of physical fitness, recreation, and sports for the handicapped persons of all ages that provides competition at all ability levels (Maxwell, 1984). According to Orelove, Wehman, and Wood (1982), the original goal of Special Olympics was to increase public awareness of the need for sports programs for handicapped persons and to actually create such programs. Positive aspects of Special Olympics include (a) the increased opportunity for success, because participants compete with others roughly on their own level; (b) the reinforcement of social contact by a nonthreatening atmosphere; (c) the teaching of motor abilities, specific athletic skills, social skills (e.g., taking turns and cheering on others), and language skills (following directions) by training for the event; (d) the promotion of parental and volunteer involvement; and (e) the generation of community awareness and support (Orelove et al., 1982). Orelove et al. also cited several limitations of the current Special Olympics model: (a) It evokes sympathy and pity and carries a generally negative stigma; (b) it segregates handicapped persons, thus emphasizing deviance; (c) it does not provide an opportunity for normalization with nonhandicapped peers; (d) its one-day focus is impractical given the need for ongoing community recreation activities; (e) the extended amount of time spent in training for Special Olympics is not a good use of educational time; and (f) because it has become highly competitive at some levels, the primary purpose of participation may have been lost. Orelove et al. recommended that handicapped peers be gradually and systematically added so as to normalized Special Olympics. Project LIFE (1987) remarked that handicapped persons deserve to be just as unspecial as anyone else. More recently, Hourcade (1989) also praised the past accomplishments of Special Olympics, but suggested it is time to move to a more integrated model of recreational opportunity.

Though Special Olympics is one source of recreation for the mentally retarded population, it alone is insufficient. Appropriate and accessible community programs are needed. Stein (1974) argued that the focus of recreation personnel needs to switch from finding ways to incorporate all individuals with certain characteristics into a given program to identifying personal, social, emotional, physical, and related traits of individuals that will make it more likely for each to succeed under certain circumstances with specific methods.

McConkey et al. (1981) advocated that leisure skills be taught to the mentally retarded in a systematic and structured way. Nietupski, Ayres, and Hamre-Nietupski's (1983) comprehensive review of recreation/leisure skills training studies conducted with mentally retarded subjects examined such systematic and structured training techniques. In their review, Nietupski et al. arranged studies into four convenient groupings: antecedent environmental factors, behavior modification, task analysis, and maintenance and generalization. Findings from studies investigating antecedent environmental factors indicated that provision of play materials increases toy contact in comparison with austere conditions. However, the level of contact attained merely with the provision of toys is very low. Additional instructional procedures are clearly required for retarded persons to achieve independent leisure skills.

As for what types of materials appeared to elicit the natural expression of play skills, studies are contradictory and unclear and Nietupski et al. (1983) hypothesized that material preferences are highly individualized. Studies employing behavior modification have found modeling, verbal directions, and manual guidance to be effective in leisure skills training used as antecedents or corrective consequences. Social, edible, and tangible reinforcers have been found to be effective in aiding skill acquisition, as has overcorrection of mistakes. Also, the direction-following and verbal communication skills that have been taught through leisure skills training suggest that play might serve as a teaching medium for other skills. Task analysis has also been found to be effective. Task analysis involves first specifying precise behavioral sequences required for the appropriate use of recreation materials. Then, response requirements made of the subject are gradually increased along the behavioral sequence until all the steps are acquired. Using task analysis and training, retarded subjects have been taught to roll a ball, ride a tricycle, slide on a sliding board, play frisbee, operate a tape recorder, jump on a trampoline, play table games, use the telephone, and exercise. To maximize maintenance and generalization, after the skill is taught subjects should be trained across more than one exemplar on the most diverse materials available, approximating as closely as possible the actual environmental context (Nietupski et al., 1983).

Project LIFE (1987) is an excellent resource guide for analyzing recreation activities as well as individual skills. Project LIFE advocates that first the particular recreation activity under consideration is analyzed to determine what kinds and levels of skills are required. Then the specific individual being considered for participation is looked at to determine if he or she possesses the required skills or can acquire them, or whether the activity can be modified to accommodate that individual. However, Project LIFE advocates adapting the activity only when it is necessary and only as much as necessary. Only adaptations that are specific to the lacking skills should be implemented.

Project LIFE (1987) discussed three types of adaptations: (a) obtaining, creating, or modifying equipment or adding an assistive device that allows a person to accomplish a skill or compensate for a lack of ability; (b) using a substitute or alternative method for the individual to perform the skill, such as by providing additional cues or assistance by a leader, coach, instructor, partner, or volunteer; and (c) changing the rules or procedures to allow an alternative skill to the absent one for all participants or to eliminate the necessity of that skill for participation.

There is no prescribed list of activities for mentally retarded persons. They can for the most part participate in any activities that nonhandicapped persons do. (For specific suggestions of recreation activities, see Southern Regional Education Board, 1984; Wehman, 1979; Wuerch & Voeltz, 1982.) Project LIFE (1987) made the following suggestions about aiding recreation participation by mentally retarded individuals:

- get to know the individual as a person;
- do not underestimate the person's abilities and interests;
- break down directions into simple steps that can be learned sequentially;
- repeat directions as needed;
- demonstrate when possible;
- use a hands-on teaching approach and visual aids;
- be patient;
- provide positive feedback and be specific with suggestions for improvement;
- do not give praise when it is not deserved;
- provide a variety of activities—active and passive as well as easy and challenging;
- be creative, adaptive, and resourceful;
- respect the person's dignity at all times.

In addition to specific suggestions for working with mentally retarded persons in a recreation setting, Project LIFE (1987) has also provided suggestions for overcoming some of the other barriers to successful recreation experiences for the mentally retarded population. Human resource problems can be resolved by hiring additional personnel, obtaining appropriate training for existing personnel, obtaining additional funding or donations, and using volunteers. Physical access problems should be approached by following policies for barrier removal, asking service organizations for assistance, providing direct assistance to the individuals, being creative, and fixing it yourself. By reducing fees, checking about special funds, and recruiting sponsors and donations, fee problems can be eliminated. If communication is the barrier to participation, hire or recruit someone who can communicate with the individual in his or her medium, such as someone who uses sign language or understands a communication board system. In order to eradicate transportation barriers, community resources should be tapped. The possibilities of public transportation, volunteer drivers, car pools, and sponsors should be considered. If legal liability is a concern, remember that Section 504 of

the Rehabilitation Act guarantees the rights of mentally retarded persons to participate. The three basic duty criteria for a reasonable professional are (a) providing
adequate supervision, (b) exercising good judgment, and (c) providing proper
instruction (Project LIFE, 1987).

Other authors have proposed that the responsibility for the provision of appropriate recreation opportunities lies more with the whole community (e.g.,
Wilkinson, 1982). Spinak (1975) envisioned recreation in the community as consisting of stepping stones: recreation in the institutional setting; recreation programs for disabled individuals; recreation programs with disabled persons; and
finally normalized, integrated programs. Spinak maintained that because not all
individuals will be able to fit into normal programs the need for special services
will diminish but not disappear. Howe-Murphy (1979) proposed that individual
ability should be maximized and the physical, social, and cultural barriers should
be minimized by changing recreation attitudes and skills and by promoting community education, awareness, and attitudinal acceptance. Hutchinson and Lord
(1979) proposed a more detailed model of integration. First, emphasis should be
placed on building confidence and self-esteem while improving physical and social skills in mentally retarded persons. Then, education about mental retardation
and recreation should be aimed at the disabled individuals, their families, recreation staff, and the general public as a whole. Along with these two processes, the
participation of support and advocacy services should be engaged. Through careful programming, a developmental continuum of services beginning with segregation and leading to integration should be implemented.

In summary, the legal right of mentally retarded persons to have access to
equal recreation opportunity is provided for under various federal statutes. Depriving mentally retarded individuals of this right is more than illegal, however. It
should be considered an affront of their dignity and freedom to enjoy life as
individuals. The existing literature outlines a variety of procedures and techniques
that can enhance participation and implementation of recreation programs for
mentally retarded individuals. In addition, empirical investigations unequivocally
support the value of recreation in enhancing the development and quality of life of
mentally retarded persons. Finally, although many existing programs, such as the
Special Olympics, have played an important role in raising public awareness and
providing recreation opportunity, we should strive to create new programs that
serve to integrate rather than segregate this segment of our population.

REFERENCES

Anderson, S. C., Grossman, L. M., & Finch, H. A. (1983). Effects of a
    recreation program on the social interaction of mentally retarded adults.
    Journal of Leisure Research, 15(2), 100–107.
Cheseldine, S. E., & Jeffree, D. M. (1981). Mentally handicapped adolescents:

Their use of leisure. *Journal of Mental Deficiency Research, 25*(49), 49–59.

Hopkins, B. L. (1968). Effects of candy and social reinforcement, instruction and reinforcement schedule learning on the modification and maintenance of smiling. *Behavior Modification, 1,* 121–129.

Hourcade, J. J. (1989). Special Olympics: A review and critical analysis. *Therapeutic Recreation Journal, XXIII,* 58–65.

Howe-Murphy, R. (1979). A conceptual basis for mainstreaming recreation and leisure services. *Therapeutic Recreation Journal, 13*(4), 11–18.

Hutchinson, P., & Lord, J. C. (1979). *Recreation integration.* Ottawa: Leisurability Publications.

Keller, M. F., & Carlson, P. M. (1974). The use of symbolic modeling to promote social skills in pre-school children with low levels of social responsiveness. *Child Development, 45,* 912–919.

Knapczyk, D., & Yoppi, J. (1975). Development of cooperative and competitive play responses in developmentally disabled children. *American Journal of Mental Deficiency, 80,* 245–255.

Loovis, E. M. (1978, November/December). Effect of participation in sport/physical education on the development of the exceptional child. *American Corrective Therapy Journal,* pp. 167–179.

Maxwell, B. M. (1984). The nursing role in the Special Olympic program. *Journal of School Health, 54*(3), 131–133.

McConkey, R., Walsh, J., & Mulcahy, M. (1981). The recreational pursuits of mentally handicapped adults. *International Journal of Rehabilitation Research, 4,* 493–499.

Mithaug, D., & Wolfe, M. S. (1976). Employing task arrangements and verbal contingencies to promote verbalizations between retarded children. *Journal of Applied Behavior Analysis, 9*(3), 301–314.

Morris, R., & Dolker, M. (1974). Developing cooperative play in socially withdrawn retarded children. *Mental Retardation, 12,* 24–27.

Nietupski, J., Ayres, B., & Hamre-Nietupski, S. (1983). A review of recreation/leisure skills research with moderately, severely, and profoundly mentally handicapped individuals. *Australia and New Zealand Journal of Developmental Disabilities, 9*(4), 161–176.

O'Conner, R. D. (1969). Modification of social withdrawal through symbolic modeling. *Journal of Applied Behavior Analysis, 15*(2), 15–22.

O'Conner, R. D. (1972). The relative efficacy of modeling, shaping, and the combined procedures for the modification of social withdrawal. *Journal of Abnormal Psychology, 79,* 327–334.

Oliver, J. N. (1958). The effect of physical conditioning exercises and activities on the mental characteristics of educationally subnormal boys. *British Journal of Educational Psychology, 28,* 155–165.

Orelove, F. P., Wehman, P., & Wood, J. (1982). An evaluative review of

Special Olympics: Implications for community integration. *Education and Training of the Mentally Retarded, 17*(4), 325–329.

Project LIFE. (1987). *Project LIFE: Leisure is for everyone* (technical report). Chapel Hill, NC: University of North Carolina at Chapel Hill.

Quilitch, H., & Risley, T. (1973). The effects of play materials on social play. *Journal of Applied Behavior Analysis, 6*(4), 573–578.

Robinson, N. M., & Robinson, H. B. (1976). *The mentally retarded child* (2nd ed.). New York: McGraw-Hill.

Southern Regional Education Board. (1984). *Recreation for the mentally retarded.* Atlanta: Author.

Spinak, J. (1975). Normalization and recreation for the disabled. *Leisurability, 2*(2), 31–35.

Stein, J. U. (1974, March/April). What research and experience tell us about physical activity, perceptual-motor, and recreation programs for children with language disorders. *American Corrective Therapy Journal,* pp. 35–41.

Stein, J. U. (1977a). Physical education, recreation, and sports for special populations. *Education and Training of the Mentally Retarded, 12*(1), 4–13.

Stein, J. U. (1977b, Jan/Feb). Recreation and leisure for special populations. *American Corrective Therapy Journal,* pp. 10–19.

Stein, T. A., & Sessoms, H. D. (1977). *Recreation and special populations* (2nd ed.). Boston: Holbrook Press.

Wehman, P. (Ed.). (1979). *Recreation programming for developmentally disabled persons.* Baltimore: University Park Press.

Whitman, T., Mercurio, J., & Caponigri, V. (1970). Development of social responses in two severely retarded children. *Journal of Applied Behavior Analysis, 3*(2), 133–138.

Wilkinson, P. F. (1982). Providing integrated play environments for disabled children: A design or attitude problem? In *Environmental Design Research Association* (Proceedings of the 13th international conference, pp. 329–338). College Park, MD: Environmental Design Research Association.

Wuerch, B. B., & Voeltz, L. M. (1982). *Longitudinal leisure skills for severely handicapped learners.* Baltimore: Paul H. Brookes.

Index